Thriving

Thriving

The Complete Mind-Body Guide
for Optimal Health and Fitness
for Men

Dr. Robert S. Ivker
and Edward Zorensky

Crown Publishers, Inc.
New York

To Harriet—my best friend, lover, playmate, healer, teacher, and wife of twenty-nine years—without whom there would be no thriving.   RSI

To self-healing, and to those whose love and wisdom have helped instill in me a sense of spirit, clarity, and wholeness. Especially, to Nancy, Kate, and Ben.   EZ

Published by Crown Publishers, Inc., 201 East 50th Street, New York, New York 10022. Member of the Crown Publishing Group.

Random House, Inc. New York, Toronto, London, Sydney, Auckland

http://www.randomhouse.com/

CROWN is a trademark of Crown Publishers, Inc.

Printed in the United States of America

Design by Lynne Amft

Library of Congress Cataloging-in-Publication Data is available upon request.

ISBN 0-517-70460-9

10   9   8   7   6   5   4   3   2   1

First Edition

Contents

Acknowledgments

I am most grateful to my father, Morris Ivker, for providing me with such a solid foundation upon which to thrive. During the first twenty-five years of my life, he was a bastion of caring and security. Until he developed Parkinson's disease at age fifty-seven, he was one very contented guy. At the top of his game professionally, he had achieved all of his life's goals. For me, he was a model of a truly successful man and a wonderful father, husband, brother, and uncle as well. The Yiddish word *mensch* best describes him: a man whose heart is always in the right place. The values he taught me comprise the bulk of the fabric with which this book was woven. He's been my greatest teacher—through both his healthy and even his unhealthy years. His passion for medicine inspired me to become a physician.

Since 1972, I've helplessly watched his disease gradually erode both his physical and mental capabilities while robbing him of every last vestige of self-esteem and any enjoyment in life. His painstakingly slow dying process has allowed me to experience every stage of grieving—from denial and anger to sorrow and acceptance. And lately I've recognized that these years of tears and my growing appreciation for his gentle and compassionate spirit have empowered me to reach a level of emotional and spiritual health that I may never have attained otherwise, certainly not this quickly. In my at-tempts to mitigate his Parkinson's and ease his suffering, I've healed my own *dis-ease* and transformed myself into a healer. Thanks, Dad. I do love my new job, but I would have preferred a less painful training program.

My father died on February 7, 1997. Even with all of the grieving practice I'd had, there was still a feeling of deep loss. But within hours of his passing, I began to sense his presence more closely than I had in many years. I felt his spiritual aliveness so clearly. On the first Sabbath following his death, I did the "Forgiveness Meditation" (page 178). It was the most healing meditation I've ever done, and when I finished, I felt such a deep connection with him. Dad, I'm still hungry for more of your wisdom. It's been so long. But now there are no barriers—I'll be listening closely and holding you forever in my heart. Thanks for everything. You've done a superb job.

Coincidence has been defined as "God's way of remaining anonymous." So it is not surprising to me that Ed Zorensky became my coauthor. His father-in-law, Morty Goldman, is a man who has had a profound impact on both Ed and myself. Morty owned Camp Takajo, a boy's camp in Maine that I attended as a camper for six summers beginning at the age of nine. Morty has taught both Ed and me more about thriving and integrity than perhaps any other man besides my father. Morty had a way of leading, not only boys, but everyone he encountered to their own greatest gift and allowed them to build a sense of confidence they could carry through a lifetime.

We are also very grateful to my agent, Gail Ross, and her assistant, Howard Yoon. With their guidance, we created a book proposal that helped launch this project and that successfully directed us through the remainder of the writing.

Another man who has contributed immeasurable to *Thriving* is our editor, Peter Ginna. With his light but incisive touch, and a wisdom that belies his years, Peter has helped to refine and complete this book in a way that speaks directly to men of all ages. Thank you, Peter, for a job well done!

I am especially proud of the truly unique holistic reference in Part II. It would not have been possible without the expertise, effort, and teamwork of a group of healers with whom I've worked closely over many years. My association with this group has been both a pleasure and an honor. They include: Bob Anderson (chapters 11, 13, and 14), Arrone Appel (chapters 6 and 9), Gabriel Cousens (chapters 11 and 12), Tim Engles (chapter 3), Mark Hoch (chapter 11), Harriet Ivker (chapter 12), Jonas Linkner (chapters 9, 13, and 14), Myron McClellan (chapters 4, 5, and 6), Joel Miller (chapter 12), John Mizenko (chapter 15), Steve Morris (chapter 9), Todd Nelson (chapter 15), Scott Shannon (chapter 12), and David Vaughn (chapter 3).

Ed and I also enjoyed the many benefits of having "in-house" editors—our wives, Nancy and Harriet. The book is replete with their contributions, and that feminine touch helped us to maintain a balanced presentation. During the last several months of the writing and editing, Harriet assumed almost all of my other professional responsibilities. "Thanks" is far too great an understatement to express my gratitude for her efforts.

Preface

Be the Exception to the Rule:
Getting Beyond *Dis-ease* to Thriving

For twelve years I suffered with sinusitis, and like a lot of guys with a chronic disease, I learned to "live with it." But then it began to impact my whole body, my mind, my work, my marriage, and even my friendships. I finally told myself, "Physician, heal thyself." Even though colleagues told me there was no cure, I figured there had to be a better way. I eventually quit my family practice and embarked on a life-changing journey that allowed me to experience the condition of optimal health I call "thriving." Along the way, I put all of my awareness into finding new ways of addressing, understanding, and communicating with my *dis-ease*. It took me five years to complete the first stage of this transformation. I healed my sinusitis and wrote a best-selling book called *Sinus Survival,* telling others how to do the same.

Some of my most important teachers in this process had been the forty-something men I had been treating in my family practice for a multitude of stress-related ailments. What most of these men had in common was a cataclysmic change occurring in their lives, not unlike what I had experienced. Being intimately involved in the midlife crisis of so many men left me feeling shaken and somewhat helpless. What could I do for them?

I figured it was one thing for a doctor to heal himself—that was my job—but how many other men, especially non-doctors, would think to heal themselves as I had done? There were no books specifically for men, putting them in touch with their gut healing instincts and how to use them. Not yet.

As I deepened my commitment to the subject of men's health, I was struck by the frightening statistics on how unhealthy American men really were. I was moved to tears when I allowed myself to feel the emotional pain of the men closest to me—my father and brother—and the overwhelming realization that in addition to the patients I'd worked with, there were millions of other men who silently shared their suffering. It seemed reasonable to me that perhaps I could do something similar to *Sinus Survival* in presenting my journey as a man healing himself through the midlife transition. The message I most wanted to convey was—*it works!* At age fifty, I'm more fit physically, mentally, and spiritually than I've ever been.

My new book for men would help ease the burden and greatly improve the quality of life for many more men than I was able to reach in my holistic medical practice. It would present helpful information that was accessible to men of all ages—midlifers as well as younger boomers, generation X–ers, and older men, too.

While I was hiking one day, the title of the

book came to me, and that was the spark that ignited my commitment to launch *Thriving*. After five months of writing the book proposal, consisting primarily of chapter 1, I presented it to my literary agent, Gail Ross. Her assessment: "You're a great doctor and a good writer, but if this book is to fulfill its potential you need a great writer to work with you."

Guys are funny the way they keep things to themselves. One day, a friend told me he'd had epilepsy for most of his life. He said that for over thirty years his mind had often been foggy from dilantin and phenobarbitol. At two in the morning he would sometimes awaken with a *grand mal* seizure that would put him in an even deeper fog for days afterward. He started having these seizures when he was a toddler, and they persisted until he was in his early thirties. I asked him how he got rid of them. "Starting at age twenty-three, I changed my life from the ground up," he said. "I changed the way I breathed and how I exercised. I took vitamins. I changed my diet and the drugs I put into my body, and how I slept and what I thought about. And after a while they stopped."

It has been the standard medical line to say that a disease like epilepsy sometimes goes away by itself. It's the conventional medical line for many common chronic diseases. But chronic disease doesn't just go away by itself. It usually takes an actively positive change in the body, mind, and spirit to end a disease process that has gone on for years. The more conscious that change, the faster and more dramatic those results will be. My

friend not only healed himself, but today, at age forty-eight, he is in better shape than ever. He teaches karate and holds a fourth degree black belt. He's a Ph.D., a former English teacher, and an accomplished writer, and he happens to be the coauthor of this book. Like me, Ed was the exception to the rule. He had done on his own with epilepsy what I had accomplished with sinusitis. He had changed his life and put himself on the path to thriving.

If the two of us could heal ourselves, we figured that we could take my idea for a book on thriving, combined with my holistic medical expertise and our collective experience with self-healing, and sit down to write a book that would inspire and show men how to do the same without taking five or fifteen years to accomplish it. We put our heads and hearts together and came up with this book as a way of teaching other men how to be "exceptions to the rule." What we learned about curing and healing our lives turned into a "no-nonsense" approach for getting beyond disease, beyond feeling just "okay," to achieving that optimal state of health called thriving.

The intuitions we men have about how we can heal ourselves can be extraordinarily powerful. And yet how often do we suppress those gut feelings by going along with the herd and taking direction only from a "qualified" medical authority? Believe it or not, we are probably—each one of us—our own best authority for understanding what's wrong with us and making it right. We truly know our own bodies better than anyone else, and those bodies have the capacity to heal themselves of almost any disease. How we go about creating that optimal state of health on every level of awareness is another story. It happens to be the story of this book.

To start thriving, men need to rethink some commonly held assumptions about what feels good, because when it comes to health, men have typically settled for less. From boyhood on, we were conditioned to believe that feeling good was equated with success: an abundance of money, power, and sex. We learned to equate these goals with happiness and even health. But as you begin your own process of healing, you will soon realize that the most critical ingredients in the recipe for optimal health and happiness are passion, creativity, and intimacy.

If you are like most men, you probably grew up on a steady diet of competition. As boys we were taught that the bulk of life's rewards derive from winning—*being the best* in whatever field we've chosen to excel. What about just *being*? What does it mean to live as *a whole human being*? How well do we know ourselves beyond our talents and capabilities as a performer or competitor, as someone with feelings, attitudes, relationships, and a spirit that makes each one of us a unique individual? This book describes the methods to consciously create that state of balance and grace we call thriving. *It is the experience of peak moments on a regular basis—daily, hourly, and potentially moment by moment.*

No man is able to reach this condition of health and harmony alone. We need lots of help, and ironically most of us live with at least one terrific teacher. The problem is that we've become such competitive creatures—so defensive and self-absorbed—that we often have trouble *listening to the life-enhancing messages* our wives, partners, and children have been giving us for years. We can't hear our own inner messages, and we've lost touch with that sense of intuition and rightness we trusted as boys. *Thriving* is about recovering those instincts.

No matter what condition you're in, *Thriving* shows you how to do better: how to avoid quitting on yourself, how to read those painful messages your body and mind are constantly sending, how to change attitudes and belief systems, how to get in touch with and direct those deeper resources that we all carry around inside and that have extraordinary healing powers. By the end of the book, you'll be writing your own plan for a new, sensible way of living, and you'll do it in a way that lets you keep your balance, your sense of humor, and your job, if you want it. *Thriving* teaches you to combine the acute focus and high energy awareness of "peak" experiences with the practical and powerful healing therapies of medicine's newest specialty: holistic medicine. The thriving program will enable you to enjoy the process of re-creating your life. This process of learning to thrive will become a life-changing adventure.

In our work together over the last two-and-a-half years, *Thriving* has been a true collaboration. Ed and I have plumbed the depths of our own life experiences with self-healing and thriving. In sharing a broad range of personal and professional insights—from medicine, to teaching, to martial arts—we have brought our own experience to bear on the best medical, physical, mental, and spiritual authorities we could find to provide a program for men that not only makes sense and is easy to learn, but is one that works.

Thriving is laid out in two parts. Part I maps your journey of self-discovery. It shows you how to build a sense of thriving in body, mind, and spirit by getting in touch with a basic intuitive power that you knew as a kid. Part I also outlines the bulk of the holistic treatment plan for the diseases of Part II.

The material in Part II was prepared by a group of leading holistic medical authorities to provide a comprehensive guide for treating the most common chronic diseases afflicting men today. Never before compiled in such detail, the information in this invaluable reference includes explanations of symptoms and conventional treatment. In addition, the holistic medical treatments—including vitamins, herbs, exercise, diet, and the identification of underlying emotional causes—have already proven to be consistently effective in clinical practice.

Why settle for just feeling okay? Put yourself in charge of your most important possession—your health. *Thriving* is about loving your life and living it as a peak experience. We hope you gain as much from reading this book as we have from writing it.

Rob Ivker and Ed Zorensky

Part One

Training to Thrive

The Basics of Thriving

Our deepest fear is not that we are inadequate.
Our deepest fear is that we are powerful
*   beyond measure.*
It is our Light, not our Darkness, that most
*   frightens us.*
We ask ourselves, who am I to be brilliant,
*   gorgeous, talented, fabulous?*
Actually, who are you NOT to be?
You are a child of God. Your playing small
*   does not serve the World.*
There is nothing enlightened about shrinking
*   so that other people won't feel insecure*
*   around you.*
We were born to make manifest the glory of
*   God that is within us.*
It is not just in some of us; it is in everyone.
And as we let our own Light shine, we
*   unconsciously give other people permission*
*   to do the same.*
As we are liberated from our own fear, our
*   presence automatically liberates others.*

Nelson Mandela, 1994 inaugural
speech, quoting Marianne Williamson's
book *Return to Love*

How This Book Will Change Your Life

Guys are supposed to be tough. Ever since we were kids, we were taught to gloss over pain and to "hang in there." Most of us have been gritting our teeth for so long we don't even know what "feeling good" is anymore. Medical health is defined as the absence of illness. But there is a big difference between what your doctor calls "healthy" and the way you can and should be feeling. Optimal, or holistic, health is a state of well-being that encompasses *body, mind,* and *spirit.* The best way to describe optimal health is one word: *thriving.* Learning to thrive will make you feel better and function with more energy and clarity than you ever knew before. To reach this state of thriving, there are no shortcuts, pills, or magic potions. It requires passing through four basic stages: a *commitment* to change, a willingness to explore both physical and emotional *pain,* a desire to connect with the *power* that comes from working through these reactions, and an openness to the *harmony* with which you let your life unfold in dynamic new directions.

It took me fifteen years as a practicing family physician to discover this dimension of well-being—thriving—which is far beyond the absence of illness. As a holistic physician, it has taken me another ten years to explore a multitude of alternative and complementary therapies for effectively treating and preventing chronic disease. These methods have become the basis for a new approach to creating optimal health that can help men of all ages change their lives and thrive.

This book is both a guide and reference. Part I will show you a systematic method for developing a greater awareness of body, mind, and spirit. You will not only learn to see yourself and your world differently, you will quickly see positive changes in the way you feel. Your body will look and feel stronger and younger. Your mind will be calmer and more creative. You will become more in touch with your spirit and feel more alive than ever before. In Part II you will learn to use a comprehensive index to the holistic medical treatment of the most common chronic men's diseases. These holistic treatment plans will help you to diagnose and heal your specific chronic health problem, if you have one.

If you are resistant to letting go of your current habits, beliefs, and limited understanding of life's potential, then this book is *not* for you. *Thriving requires a willingness to change.* I discovered this for myself after having suffered for ten years with America's most common chronic disease—sinusitis. Most doctors will tell you that a chronic condition is one that you will have to learn to live with—one that is essentially incurable. (Common chronic diseases include arthritis, high blood pressure, and heart disease.) Doc-

tors will also tell you that you are healthy as long as you're not sick or in pain. How many times have you gone to the doctor, had a thorough physical exam, been told you are healthy, and yet you still feel lousy?

In my own case, I started on this quest for greater health when I refused to accept the dismal prognosis of chronic sinusitis, even though I had been plagued with congestion, headaches, and diminished energy for years and they showed no signs of going away. Ear, nose, and throat specialists told me that even though surgery could provide temporary relief, they couldn't guarantee a cure. Here I was, a doctor on the receiving end of the same message that I had delivered to countless patients. But when it happened to me, I realized how depressing this feeling truly was. The poetic justice of my situation underscored the limitations of conventional medicine. I had always been frustrated with merely treating symptoms while telling patients, "We don't really understand the cause of your ailment or why you got sick." By focusing on the diagnosis and treatment of disease, medical school never taught us to answer that question. With those patients suffering chronic illness, I always cringed at the sense of hopelessness that I was instilling in them, but my hands were tied by the limitations of my training. Now I resolved to do something about it.

As a family doctor, merely treating the symptoms of chronic disease went against every ideal and aspiration I had as a healer. I was now determined not only to cure my own sinus disease, but to change my whole approach to health and healing. I realized that when it comes to health, both doctors and patients have been conditioned to settle for less. We've been told that if we are not sick, we are healthy, and most of us—especially men—accept chronic aches and pains as part of the aging process without doing much about it. These chronic conditions not only diminish quality of life, they erode passion and drain creativity without our even knowing it. We become more detached from and even unconscious of how our body and mind really feel.

How aware are you of your true physical, mental, and spiritual condition? You're about to find out! The following *Thriving* Self-Test will give you a true indication of your present state of health. It will also introduce you to some core principles of well-being that we explore in this opening chapter to get you started on a new experience of optimal health and fitness. *Take the Thriving Self-Test now before reading the rest of this book.* You will take it again in two to three months after working on the training program described in Part I. By then, I guarantee you will feel much better and you will be well on your way to thriving.

For now, as you answer the questions on the self-test, be aware of the six main aspects of optimal health. Most of us can probably distinguish between experiences of *body, mind,* or *spirit.* Yet these categories can be further subdivided into six distinct ways that optimal health shows up in your life. These can overlap and strongly affect one another. These aspects are body—***physical*** and ***environmental*** health; mind—***mental*** and ***emotional*** health; and spirit—***spiritual*** and ***social*** health

The *Thriving* Self-Test

Thriving is a state of optimal health that starts with a heightened awareness of the relationship between six fundamental dimensions of health: physical, environmental, mental, emotional, spiritual, and social. This book will give you a greater understanding of their interaction to help you live a longer, healthier, more enjoyable life.

In "re-creating" your life, and learning to *thrive,* you will be able to identify the critical sequence of "four stages" that accompany every conscious act of self-change. They consist of *commitment, pain, power,* and *harmony.* These four stages occur in any creative process, and the degree to which you consciously participate in them—no matter what the undertaking—provides an indication of how healthy you are.

The test that follows measures your current state of *thriving* in each of the six states of health. Choose one of the four responses for each question and place the appropriate score next to the question. Questions in **bold** count **double.** Total the points and see where your score places you on the "Thrivometer." The responses are scored in the following way:

Never = 0 points
Rarely = 1 point
Sometimes = 2 points
Regularly = 3 points

The *Thriving* Self-test

The Body (Physical and Environmental Health)

Commitment	Score
Do you maintain a healthy diet (low fat, low sugar, fresh fruits, grains and vegetables)?	
Is your daily water intake adequate (at least $\frac{1}{2}$ oz/lb body weight: 160 lbs = 80 oz)?	
Do you live and work in a healthy environment with respect to clean air, water, and indoor polution?	
Do you do household chores, such as cooking, cleaning, or food shopping?	
Do you make time to experience both sensual and sexual pleasure?	
Do you schedule regular massage or deep-tissue work?	
Do you engage in regular physical workouts?	
TOTAL	

Pain	Score
Are you free of chronic aches and pains (indigestion, constipation, back pain, bad knees?	
Are you free of chronic diseases (arthritis, high blood pressure, prostate problems)?	
Do you maintain physically challenging goals?	
Are you free of any tobacco, drug, or alcohol dependency?	
Are you within 20% of your ideal weight?	
Are you free from sexual dysfunctions such as impotence and premature ejaculation?	
Do you have an understanding of the relationship between your chronic physical problems and the emotional stresses in your life?	
TOTAL	

Power	Score
Are you physically strong?	
Is your body flexible?	
Do you have an awareness of life-energy or chi within your own body?	
Do you feel physically attractive?	
Do you feel strong sexual energy?	
Do you feel energized or empowered by nature?	
Do you have good endurance and aerobic capacity?	
TOTAL	

Harmony	Score
Are you agile and well-coordinated?	
Are your five senses (seeing, hearing, touch, taste, and smell) acute?	
Do you breathe abdominally?	
Do you regularly awaken in the morning feeling well-rested?	
Do you have daily, effortless bowel movements?	
Do you have a gratifying sexual relationship?	
Are you aware of specific ways in which your home and your environment affect your physical well-being?	
TOTAL	
BODY TOTAL	

The Mind (Mental and Emotional Health)

Commitment	Score
Do you have specific goals in your personal and professional life?	
Do you have the ability to concentrate for extended periods of time?	
Do you make a point of being on time?	
Do you have a sense of humor?	
Is your outlook basically optimistic?	
Are you willing to take risks or make mistakes in order to succeed?	
Does your job use all of your greatest talents?	
TOTAL	

Pain	Score
Are you free from a strong need for control or the need to be right?	
Is your job enjoyable and fulfilling?	
Do you give yourself more supportive messages than critical messages?	
Is your sleep free from disturbing dreams?	
Are you able to adjust beliefs and attitudes as a result of learning from painful experiences?	
Do you allow yourself to feel fear, anger, sadness, and hopelessness instead of repressing those emotions?	
TOTAL	

Power	Score
Are you aware of and able to express anger safely and nonviolently?	
Can you freely express sadness or cry?	
Do you use visualization or mental imagery to help you attain your goals or enhance your performance?	
Can you meet your financial needs and desires?	
Do you explore the symbolism and emotional content of your dreams?	
Do you remember your dreams?	
Do you believe it is possible to change?	
Do you have the ability to express fear?	
TOTAL	

Harmony	Score
Do you enjoy high self-esteem?	
Do you maintain peace of mind and tranquillity?	
Do you make time for activities that constitute the abandon and absorptions of play?	
Do you engage in counseling, meditation, journaling, or some other practice that helps you to understand your feelings?	
Do you take time to "let down" and relax?	
Are you accepting of all your feelings?	
Do you experience feelings of exhilaration?	
TOTAL	
MIND TOTAL	

The Spirit (Spiritual and Social Health)

Commitment	Score
Do you actively commit time to your spiritual life?	
Do you listen to your intuition?	
Do you have an appreciation of nature?	
Do you have a regular place either in the house or in nature set aside for meditation, prayer, or reflection?	
Do you make time to connect with young children, either your own or somebody else's?	
Are creative activities a regular part of your work or leisure?	
Have you demonstrated the willingness to commit to a marriage or comparable long-term relationship?	
TOTAL	

Pain	Score
Do you have one or more close friends to whom you talk openly about your emotions?	
Are you free from anger toward God?	
Do you or did you feel close with your parents?	
Do you feel close with your children?	
Did you grow up with a loving and emotionally supportive father?	
If you have experienced the loss of a loved one, have you fully grieved that loss?	
Do you feel that your experience of emotional pain enabled you to grow spiritually?	
Are you able to let go of your attachment to expected outcomes and to embrace uncertainty?	
TOTAL	

Power	Score
Do you act upon your intuition and take risks?	
Do you have a faith in a God, higher being, or spiritual power?	
Can you routinely let go of self-interest in deciding the best course of action for a given situation?	
Are playfulness and humor important to you in your daily life?	
Do you have the ability to forgive yourself and others?	
Do you regularly experience intimacy, besides sex, in your committed relationship?	
TOTAL	

Harmony	Score
Do you go out of your way or routinely give your time to help others?	
Do you feel a sense of belonging to a group or community?	
Are you regularly grateful for the blessings in your life?	
Do you take regular walks or have daily contact with nature?	
Do you affectionately touch another human being each day?	
Do you observe a day of rest completely away from work, dedicated to nurturing yourself and your family?	
Do you allow yourself to experience unconditional love from yourself and others?	
TOTAL	
SPIRIT TOTAL	
Thriving Total	

Scoring the *Thriving* Self-Test

Condition	Total Points:
Thriving	258–288
I Feel Great	228–257
I'm Okay	198–227
I'm Not Sick	168–197
I'm Getting By	138–167
I'm Hangin' In There	108–137
Survival	Below 108

"Physician, Heal Thyself"

My father, a successful radiologist in Philadelphia, loved his work with a passion. I grew up wanting to be just like him. I marveled at is methodical and precise way of reading X rays by tracing his finger across the film, which enabled him to detect the smallest aberrations in human tissue or bone. Early on in my life, the idea of using acquired knowledge and skills to diagnose illness and to heal others became my passion. By the age of twelve, my goal was to become a family doctor in the Marcus Welby tradition—as a healer, friend, teacher, and counselor. He was a physician who helped his patients to heal their lives as well as their illnesses. All through high school, college, and medical school, I prepared with this one purpose in mind. In the early 1970s I moved to Denver, Colorado, where I completed my residency in family practice—at the time, medicine's newest specialty. Soon afterward, I established what eventually became a highly successful family practice. Although I thought I had attained my lifelong goal, I gradually realized that the family medicine I had diligently been practicing for fifteen years was no longer generating the exhilaration or even the satisfaction that I had enjoyed in my first years of medicine after my residency. The evolution of medical science was responsible for converting the general practitioner, or GP, into the more highly trained board-certified specialist in family medicine. But I felt as if it had transformed me from the healer I had envisioned as a child into a highly skilled repairman, fixing broken or malfunctioning body parts.

It was probably the timing and the cumulative effect of seeing so many patients that finally caused this realization to hit me like a two-by-four between the eyes. It happened, one afternoon, when I walked into the examining room and there sat a forty-five-year-old corporate executive with hypertension (high blood pressure), who had come in for his regular blood-pressure check. For more than a year, I had prescribed the accepted medications and recommended that he modify his diet and lifestyle. Yet his condition had not changed for the better. Although his blood pressure was now within an acceptable range, he was still taking strong drugs, he was still overweight, he was still not exercising, he was still eating poorly, and he had still done nothing to reduce the stress in his life. On top of everything else, the side effects from his blood-pressure medication, as is often the case, had made him impotent. Since it was his third different prescription and he seemed pleased that his blood pressure was under control, we agreed to maintain the treatment plan in spite of his impotence. He shook my hand and agreed to see me in six months. As the door shut behind him, I had the sinking feeling that his health would improve very little by the next time I saw him. In fact, his health was already worse, because he had lost a wonderful dimension of physical intimacy with his wife. He was content to eliminate the symptoms of his condition without ever confronting its causes. He wasn't alone. There were hundreds, perhaps thousands, more just like him in my practice alone, who considered themselves healthy as long as they experienced no symptoms of illness. Furthermore, they believed the responsibility for this condition of health was solely the physician's. Something was drastically wrong.

I had been trained in a highly regarded family practice residency and had built my prac-

tice, to the best of my ability, according to the highest standards of family medicine. Still, I was failing in my commitment as a healer, and I wondered how many other doctors were failing their patients in the same way. For the first time in my professional life, I questioned the value of conventional medicine and its sole focus on disease. What troubled me most was that the best this highly scientific system could offer in treating chronic diseases—such as hypertension, arthritis, or diabetes—was the relief of symptoms. Conventional medicine was great at treating life-threatening illness and was often successful at slowing the progression of chronic disease, but it did little in the way of giving the patient a true sense of health. Another shortcoming was its inability to provide an opportunity for the patient to heal himself. My executive patient no longer had high blood pressure (as long as he took his medication), or the headaches that often accompany it, but he also had no greater understanding or experience of what optimal health actually was . . . nor did I.

I discovered that in spite of what we've been told by Madison Avenue, the surgeon general, the American Medical Association, or the FDA, the truth is that conventional medicine is failing all of us, but men in particular. The United States is the most powerful nation in the world, it enjoys one of the highest standards of living, and it spends more on health care per capita than any other nation; but American men rank only fifteenth in the world in longevity. Despite the advances in medical technology and research, statistics show that

American men have experienced—much more than American women—a steady decline in both physical and emotional health.

- Life expectancy for men is seven years less than that for women: men, seventy-five; women, eighty-two.
- Eighty percent of all suicides are men.
- Prostate cancer afflicts one out of nine men and kills thirty-five thousand each year. The death rate for this most common cancer in men has grown at almost twice the death rate of breast cancer in the last five years.
- In 1993, over one hundred thousand men contracted lung disease and 85 percent of them are expected to die from it. By comparison, fifty thousand men died during the war in Vietnam.
- Eighty percent of serious drug addicts are men.
- Men are three times as likely as women to be alcoholics. Men are seven times as likely as women to be arrested for drunk driving.
- Men are twenty-five times more likely than women to end up in prison.

When I took my first peek behind the "wizard's curtain" and realized the limitations of conventional medicine, I had been practicing medicine for fifteen years. I was forty years old with a wife, two teenage daughters, and a financially secure future. I thought I had everything I ever wanted. Yet I felt emotionally and spiritually bankrupt, and I knew I couldn't keep running on this same treadmill. I didn't want to end up as one of the 25 percent of family doctors who were dead by the age of fifty. So I sold my practice to a local hospital and decided to start over.

I had all the symptoms of a midlife crisis, which I had seen in hundreds of my male patients. For some reason, men in their late thirties and forties run up against an invisible wall that makes them question many of their lifelong assumptions. Why should I have been any different? If I was going to question beliefs and attitudes, I had to start with a definition of optimal health. I first needed to find out what it was, and I couldn't do that until I found out what it felt like. Step one was to cure my own chronic sinusitis. I was about to reinvent myself as a physician and a man. I was going to revisit Hippocrates' command to all doctors: "Physician, heal thyself." But this time I would take it to heart.

The Power of Peak Experience

I started by trying to find out what excited men and made them really feel good about themselves. Whatever it was, I reasoned, it would probably also make them healthier. The more I thought about it, the more I kept coming back to sports. By the mid-eighties, almost every physician's prescription for better health included exercise. I kept thinking about the allure of sports for men. Most men had once passionately played sports in their youth, but, in middle age, they gave their energy to sports in the form of dollars for ticket sales, television, and merchandise. Sports has been one of the first and most enduring activities to make men of my generation feel good about themselves. And thanks to the technology of television, its greatest moments are constantly revived in the collective consciousness of men so they can be shared with sons and daughters.

Most men have a favorite sports highlight. Usually, it is a moment of uncommon beauty, precision, and grace that marks a turning point in the final moment of a World Series, a Super Bowl, or an NBA championship. These moments of peak performance often come up in conversations about "Who was the greatest . . . ?" or "What was the best . . . ?": Bill Mazeroski's bottom-of-the-ninth-inning home run in the seventh game of the 1960 World Series, the U.S. hockey team's victory over the Soviet Union in the finals of the 1980 Olympics, Joe Montana's pass to Dwight Clark with fifty-two seconds left in the 1982 NFC title game. These examples symbolize a pinnacle of achievement in the face of intense demands and astonishing odds. They typify that most male of virtues, the one that Hemingway called "grace under pressure." These images of peak performance go to the very heart of what it means to be male—"to be able to perform."

In our own lives, moments of peak performance don't occur at Yankee Stadium, but their impact remains enormous all the same. We still feel the synchrony, the sudden sense of grace and effortlessness. What man doesn't remember the perfect five-iron, the impossible exam he aced, an "unconscious" bump run down a "black diamond," a transfixing monologue performed in a school play, a great pre-

sentation in front of the boss, or even a night of uncommon erotic bliss? For those few magically creative moments, we transcended our everyday tedium, frustration, and anxiety, and for an instant we glimpsed a different world, a gravityless place where we were in control and we succeeded without effort. Athletes often call this sensation of peak experience "being in the zone." It is a sense of body as mind, a continuous medium through which energy and awareness flow together as one, and action becomes an effortless sequence of intentions. It is a state of optimal health, the ultimate happiness, what Henry James called "the great good place."

Peak experience does not belong to athletes alone. Musicians, artists, and scientists often describe the exhilaration that accompanies their creative work and contributes to a deeper sense of well-being. When men like Pablo Picasso, Vladimir Horowitz, Pablo Casals, Albert Einstein, Linus Pauling, and even George Burns talked about their passion for their work, it was clear that the pure joy these men took in their life's work contributed to their longevity. These exceptional men lived creative lives well into their seventies, eighties, and beyond, and what made them "thrive" was their creative energy, their love of life, and especially *their passion for their life's work.*

Most men identify in their peak experiences many of the same qualities we admire in our sports heroes: unbounded joy, the willingness to take risks and put themselves on the line, and success. But one main difference is that our moments of synchrony usually occur without our expecting them. In the world of elite sports competition, peak performance comes as a result of a systematic program of intensive training. We may have rehearsed a presentation or practiced a backhand, but rarely with the focus and intensity of an elite athlete. They not only train to execute athletic movement with maximum efficiency and full expectation of success, but they also practice relinquishing conscious control to unconscious execution. Most of us rarely anticipate "unconscious" participation or even make the effort to visualize our success that precisely. Whereas the elite athlete expects his training to culminate in a moment of perfection, the rest of us rarely train enough to nurture the expectation of these moments.

As we get older, we can still identify peak experience when we see it on TV. We may even occasionally experience a sense of exhilaration, but these moments seem to happen without our knowing exactly why. Because we diminish our expectation of these moments, they occur less frequently. Some of us seek moments of abandon through alcohol and drugs, but the sensation is never quite the same. With age, we enjoy fewer peak experiences because we stop *training* for them. We no longer maintain the positive emotions that attract them into our lives. We convince ourselves that our capacity for peak moments has dried up like the cartilage in our knees.

It's no wonder that most men by their late thirties have abandoned their pursuit of both health and peak performance. After all, they go hand in hand. Not only have most men forgotten what health feels like, they never

really knew what the word actually meant. The words *health, heal,* and *holy* all derive from the Anglo-Saxon word *haelen*—"to make whole." True health is a state of wholeness. Hence the term *holistic medicine,* which treats the *whole* person—his body, mind, and spirit—unlike conventional medicine, which treats only dysfunctional *parts* of the body. Another way of thinking of this wholeness is the sense of being "centered" or "in harmony"—your body and mind united in a way that allows you to experience the flow of life energy, or spirit, in every dimension of your being. As boys, we got that feeling of wholeness mostly through the release of *play.* In fact, the origin of the word *play* comes from the middle Dutch *pleien,* meaning "to dance, leap for joy, and rejoice." The more fragmented our lives are, the less we allow ourselves to play. If we're lucky, we get to play once a week during a Sunday-afternoon golf game. Maybe we sneak off to the park with the kids for an hour.

In the martial arts—which, like many of the precepts for holistic *(whole-istic)* medicine, developed in the East—body, mind, and spirit are said to act in harmony as prerequisites for every movement. If there is an imbalance, the technique invariably fails: it may look like a punch or a kick, but the technique lacks a certain completeness or energy called *ki* in Japanese or *chi* in Chinese. These cultures believe that this palpable life energy runs like a current through every living thing: plants, animals, and humans. For the Chinese, *chi* animates both body and mind. Although traditional

Chinese medicine is based on *chi* and the balance of *chi* in body and mind, Western medicine does not even recognize the existence of this life energy. Our religions vaguely identify life energy as "spirit," yet few Western men have developed the ability to experience it at will. The power of spirit as life energy is that reality we experience in both mind and body during a peak experience. These moments can include not only highs in athletic performance, but creative highs—completing a watercolor or closing a deal—and the emotional highs of greater intimacy with a spouse or child. *The six aspects of optimal health—physical, environmental, mental, emotional, spiritual, and social— each embody our experience of different states of life energy.* When the experience of these peak moments becomes a habit in our daily lives, they comprise that state of health called *thriving*.

Our longing to return to that childlike sense of joy and fundamental playfulness, in which life energy directs our actions and is the focus of our daily life, is a man's strongest unconscious impulse. Christ attested to the liberating power of the child within the man when he urged, "Except ye be converted, and become as little children, ye shall not enter into the kingdom of heaven." Eighteen hundred years later, the Romantic poet William Wordsworth echoed this sentiment:

> *My heart leaps up when I behold*
> *A rainbow in the sky:*
> *So was it when my life began;*
> *So is it now I am a man;*

> *So be it when I shall grow old*
> *Or let me die!*
> *The Child is father of the Man.*

Thriving is that ever-present spark of childlike exhilaration that we can consciously rekindle into a torchlike flame, if we know how. We can take that spark of exhilaration off the tennis court or mountain peak and bring it into our everyday lives on a regular basis, but it takes practice. We must first prepare the mind to be open to these peak experiences. And once we command the mind, the body will follow.

PNI and a New Approach to Health Care—the Mind-Body Connection

My understanding of the mind's power to direct the body began to develop when I started holistically treating my own sinusitis. The first thing I realized was that I would need to change my belief that it was impossible to cure. Rejecting the "impossible" freed me to imagine my body without the symptoms of sinusitis. I realized that if I was going to get better, I would need to throw out the conventional drug and surgery-oriented therapies and embrace an approach that would work from the inside out, to heal both mind and body. I changed my patterns of diet, exercise, and even breathing. I added nutritional supplements and herbal treatments. It wasn't long before I began to experience greater vitality and endurance than I had known in ten years. What was different? My attitude!

I was discovering that the immune system and physical strength of a man half my age were *not* necessary preconditions for healthy sinuses. I could do it at age forty. By creating the *expectation* of a better state of health, I started to enjoy new moments of peak experience. What's more, even though I knew medically that libido is generally diminished with age, I was finding that my enjoyment of sex was heightened, and that my immune system and physiology had become even stronger. I was discovering in my own physical transformation that *body and mind share a vitally powerful connection.*

In medical school, prospective doctors are taught to diagnose and treat disease. We learn that body and mind are separate and distinct compartments of a human being, with little interaction between the two. Doctors are trained to focus their attention almost exclusively on the body, and we do so in almost military terms. We think of the immune system as a defense force on constant alert to protect the body against invasion by bacteria, viruses, allergens, and cancer cells, but are in a quandary as to how the immune system becomes weakened enough to allow infection, allergy, and cancer to occur. Consequently, conventional medicine plays only a reactive role in treating the body: a specific symptom appears and the doctor prescribes drugs or surgery to vanquish or treat it. In the case of emergency-room trauma or life-threatening infections, this can be truly miraculous; however, it isn't effective over the long haul in treating chronic diseases.

Holistic medicine, on the other hand, seeks to create optimal conditions for good health, by empowering the patient to take responsibility for creating health in body, mind, and spirit. *In addition to focusing on treating symptoms as conventional medicine does, holistic medicine addresses the underlying physical, mental, and spiritual causes of disease.* Because of the expanded focus of holistic medicine, it is often called "alternative." However, this too is, in fact, a misnomer: holistic medicine utilizes both conventional *and* alternative therapies. Therefore, the term *complementary medicine* is far more accurate in describing the cooperative relationship that exists between conventional and holistic medicine. In outlining the holistic treatment of chronic diseases afflicting men, Part II of this book recommends both conventional and alternative therapies working together.

For thousands of years, Eastern medicine has been aware of the need for harmony between mind and body, man and nature, but it wasn't until the late twentieth century that Western medicine started to scientifically confirm the power of the mind-body connection. This new awareness started with studies in the 1950s and 1960s documenting the value of vitamins and good nutrition, which pioneered the preventive medical movement. In the 1970s and 1980s, the discovery of antioxidants' effectiveness against free radicals provided additional scientific support for alternative approaches to conventional medicine. But it wasn't until the 1980s that compelling research provided a revolutionary understanding of the immune system and generated a new field of study called *psychoneuroimmunology (PNI),* based on a multitude of studies in which scientists confirmed the effects of attitudes and feelings on immune function.

One of the most important PNI discoveries revealed the existence of "messenger" molecules called *neuropeptides,* which carry the messages of thoughts, beliefs, attitudes, and feelings through the bloodstream to communicate directly with every cell in the body. The most exciting findings proved that individuals are capable of either weakening or strengthening their immune system by virtue of what they think or feel. Scientists also learned that these messages can originate from any organ in the body, not just the brain. A broken heart or sense of gut-wrenching loss can actually "speak" directly to our immune system. These studies concluded that *the immune system actively functions as a "circulating nervous system" that is exquisitely sensitive to our every thought and feeling.* Evidence suggests that feelings of self-rejection and loss can seriously impair immune function and result in a variety of chronic diseases. Although for thousands of years Chinese medicine has described the relationship between the excess of specific emotions and organ dysfunction, behaviorial medicine and PNI are just beginning to scientifically confirm such a connection.

Scientists have found that feelings of exhilaration or joy actually produce measurable amounts of a neuropeptide identical to interleuken-2—a powerful anticancer drug that normally costs about $40,000 per injection. Feelings of peace and tranquillity have been shown to produce a chemical in the body nearly identical to the drug Valium—a popular tranquilizer. Studies confirmed that regular aerobic exercise releases the euphoria-inducing endorphins that produce "runner's high." This recognition of "the circulating nervous system" is currently producing a paradigmatic shift in medicine's approach to healing, because for the first time doctors possess scientific evidence of an instant and intimate communication between the mind and body. And who could be better qualified to direct that communication than the patient himself?

In dispelling the myth of the separation between mind and body, PNI scientists have helped us to see our physical health as a reflection of our mental, emotional, social, and spiritual well-being. By learning to tap this new awareness, we can put ourselves in the care of a built-in doctor "on call" twenty-four hours a day, who will go to work wiping out diseased cells while providing us with moments of peak experience . . . and he doesn't even bill our insurance! The catch is we have to leave the *right* message on his answering machine: we can't continue to play the same negative, limiting tape that we may have been hearing since childhood. Because the immune system is sensitive to our every thought and feeling, we need to change our unhealthy beliefs and attitudes if we want to thrive.

The body is a wonderfully sophisticated biological mechanism, but it is also very suggestible: it tends to believe everything we tell it and reacts accordingly. States of depression measurably depress the immune system and make us more likely to get sick. Studies have linked a significant sense of loss or grief to a higher incidence of cancer. How conscious, then, are we of our feelings of joy and pain? And how can we create experiences of thriving to retrain and fortify our immune systems on a regular basis?

Marvelous as it is in treating life-threatening emergencies and the symptoms of disease, conventional medicine has severe limitations, most of which are apparent in its treatment of chronic or so-called "incurable" disease. For most men suffering from a chronic illness such as heart disease, diabetes, or prostate cancer, doctors usually impose two basic limiting beliefs. Either the patient is told to learn to live with his condition and accept a diminished quality of life while being treated with medications and/or surgery, or he is given a "death sentence" and told he has a certain number of months to live. In either case, the physician's negative prognosis inevitably elicits in the patient feelings of hopelessness, fear, anger, and grief. If these feelings go unexpressed, they only serve to further depress the immune system and accelerate the disease process. Studies have shown that when cancer patients are told by their doctors they have six months to live, they generally believe the prognosis and adhere to its schedule. For these "compliant" patients who accept the belief of their physician, their deadlines become a self-fulfilling prophecy.

Belief systems can affect us collectively as well, especially the assumptions of popular culture. In a society that worships youth and the romantic sexuality of late adolescence, men are told that we reach our physical prime by age twenty-six and that we're over the hill by age forty. As a result, most middle-aged men shift their priorities from physical well-being to career and financial success. But attainment of these material goals is small consolation for the deterioration of our health. By allowing ourselves to fall victim to the mental pollution of limiting beliefs, we create feelings of deterioration and decline that are predictably borne out in premature aging and chronic illness.

To undo the conditioning of negative beliefs, and to thrive well into our eighties, nineties, and beyond, we must rewrite our belief systems to reflect what we want to achieve, where we want to go, and how we want to be as we age. Afflictions like prostate cancer do not have to be a part of that picture; our capacity to change is more than wishful thinking. PNI research has shown us that it is possible to reverse the old adage "I'll believe it when I see it" to say "I'll see it when I believe it." Early on in treating my own sinusitis, I systematically began to tell myself, "My sinuses are now completely healed," as if it had already occurred. Eighteen months later, using the holistic approach described in Part II, I was free of sinus disease. The power of the mind and the potential of a human being is like a genie sitting in a bottle.

Plugging Into the Energy of Thriving

If you don't feel good about yourself, you're not going to feel good about your work, your marriage, or your relationships. Trying to perform at your best on a low supply of self-esteem is like running a Lexus on a moped battery. Let's say you are frustrated by the mediocre state of health that you have been conditioned to believe an adult male *should* feel. You resolve to do better, just as I did. Your first instinct might be to create a state of health beyond what you have previously experienced. But what exactly is that condition? And how do you create it?

I have already described six dimensions of optimal health: physical, environmental, mental, emotional, spiritual, and social. Think of these states as fields or reservoirs for life energy. If stress constantly drains away life energy, its effects will show up in each of these dimensions. Conversely, a high state of life energy in any one of these dimensions can spill over into the others and nurture us in various ways. As the vital essence that either makes or breaks our state of health, this life energy is more familiar to us than we realize. Portrayed in almost every work of literature, drama, song, and film, its spirit is encapsulated in a four-letter word that is never censored and has proven to be life's most powerful healer. What's more, as an emotion we all have experienced, forever talk about, but rarely *feel* on a consistent basis, this state of being is always guaranteed to make us feel good. The word for it is *love*. Love is simply the purest form of life energy. As life energy manifests in the body, you feel more loving to and nurturing of your body. For optimum mental health, your mind is filled with positive, nurturing, and energizing thoughts, beliefs, and images.

Whether we call it *ki, chi,* the Sanskrit

prana, or the Hebrew *chai,* love as life energy is the basis of treatment for health care's newest specialty—holistic medicine. The greater its degree of unconditionality, the stronger is love's healing potential. Our capacity for experiencing unconditional love will determine the extent to which we thrive. While a conventional doctor focuses solely on treating specific physical symptoms of illness, a holistic physician teaches his patient *to love and nurture his body, mind, and spirit.*

Because most men equate self-love or self-esteem with their ability to perform, the debilitating effects of the deprivation of love in the form of self-criticism can prevent us from performing as well as we would like and hence reduce our self-esteem even further. If it persists over time, this self-criticism can result in chronic *dis-ease.* For most men, when the ability to function on and off the job (to instantly recall details or distant memories, to maintain our physical fitness, or to "perform" sexually) is impaired and we *make mistakes,* then we perceive ourselves as being less worthy or less deserving of love than we once were. *This loss of self-love is experienced as if the flame of life energy itself is being gradually extinguished.* I first witnessed this male pattern of decline as a teenager, when I helplessly watched the physical and mental deterioration of my grandfathers. I continued to observe it in my uncles and older male patients. But most painful of all has been watching the steady deterioration of my father's strong self-esteem and love of life over the past twenty-five years under the heavy weight of Parkinson's disease. The greater his physical limitations and his inability to perform his job, the deeper his depression and the greater his feelings of worthlessness.

As I examined the sources of dis-ease in my own life, I discovered that my perceived inability to *achieve,* and my lack of forgiveness for mistakes, resulted in a subsequent loss of self-esteem. These were important factors in *causing* my chronic sinusitis in the first place. The physical symptoms of dis-ease act like a fun-house mirror that distorts and magnifies the self-inflicted psychic wound. The weapon most men use to drain life energy is the deprivation of love, which we masterfully, and often unconsciously, wield against ourselves and against the ones with whom we are closest. To thrive, we must learn to generate our own sources of self-love instead of relying on others to provide it for us through approval, appreciation, or praise. In subsequent chapters, you will begin to find out how to charge your own batteries, moving beyond performance as the sole measure of your self-esteem, as you discover new sources of empowerment.

The Four Stages of Peak Experience

To tap into new sources of energy, we need to break some old habits. Trying to overcome outmoded attitudes or belief systems from our past, to provide ourselves with optimal health in the present, is like taking the hitch out of your golf swing. It's hard to let go of that ingrained bodily memory long enough to let yourself experience a more efficient swing. You may stumble into that perfect swing once every few holes, but what you really need is a systematic way to dissolve that hitch so you can consciously perform the new swing at will.

The same holds true for trying to break the habit of self-criticism in order to experience self-love and a sense of thriving. For example, in the tranquil setting of a spectacular mountain lake, anyone can have a sense of thriving. Life energy here is plentiful and flows through you like an electric current. Unfortunately, however, most of us don't live our lives in the pristine beauty of woods or mountains, where we can easily trigger this experience spontaneously. In the absence of mountain lakes or any other natural setting, we have to make a more conscious effort to connect with life energy on a regular basis. Like developing a hitchless golf swing, it requires a disciplined and conscious approach to master it. In the following chapters, we will explore more fully four dynamic concepts— *the four stages:* (1) commitment, (2) pain, (3) power, and (4) harmony—that can enable you to experience peak moments on demand rather than by accident.

Full participation in each of these four stages will unite body, mind, and spirit, resulting in a level of awareness so different from our habitual mode of mindfulness, and so far beyond the limits of the ego, that we call it an "altered state of consciousness." Successful athletes and artists have developed idiosyncratic ways of embracing this higher state of awareness at will. Their methods may include relaxation or breathing techniques, as well as private rituals that make them receptive to these periods of "grace," or visualizations that enable them to key their performance to a higher level of awareness. Dr. George Sheehan, a physician who has written extensively on running and athletic performance, describes a similar sequence of awareness that progresses from the body, through the mind, and into the spirit, during a one-hour run:

The first thirty minutes is for my body. During that half hour, I take joy in my physical ability, the endurance and power of my running. I find it a time when I feel myself competent and in control of my body, when I can think about my problems and plan my day-to-day world. In many ways, that thirty minutes is all ego, all the self. It has to do with me, the individual.

What lies beyond this fitness of muscle? I can only answer for myself. The next thirty minutes is for my soul. In it, I come upon the third wind (unlike the second wind, which is physiological). And then I see myself not as an individual but as a part of the universe. In it, I can happen upon anything I ever read or saw or experienced. Every fact and instinct and emotion is unlocked and made available to me through some mysterious operation in my brain.

What most experiences of the "zone" seem to have in common are four consistent stages, or states of being, which build one upon the other, progressing from body, through mind, to spirit, as we bypass the ego and enter a state of expanded awareness. These are the four stages: *commitment, pain, power,* and *harmony.* In Sheehan's description of his one-hour run, his *commitment* put him on the road; his *pain* consisted of the physical feedback experienced in the first half hour; the experience of *power* was his "third wind," and the sense of *harmony* was reflected in his feeling "a part of the universe."

In transforming your own life, you can systematically apply these four stages to the process of *thriving.* You will find that they enable you to rewrite your belief systems and to increase substantially your creative potential. The first of the four stages in this recurring process is *commitment:* the declared intent and marshaling of physical energy in order to change—to set a new goal, to take action. The second stage is *pain*—the body's inevitable physical response to the stimulus of change. On an emotional level, this feedback usually takes the form of fear or anxiety. The key to unlocking painful feelings is to bring ourselves to fully experience them in the present, instead of expending energy trying to avoid or resist them. This is especially difficult for men—to admit that we're afraid and to allow ourselves to feel that fear. The acceptance of these feelings, by fully participating in them as completely as possible, triggers the third stage, *power*—an infusion of life energy that neutralizes their unconscious control over us. With life energy flowing through previously closed channels, we dissolve the ego and experience ourselves in the *here and now.* The resistance of pain gives way to the pleasure of play. This feeling of synchrony leads us to the final stage, a state of *harmony*—the union of body, mind, and spirit. Characterized by a sense of unforgettable grace and beauty, this experience of at-one-ness can occur alone, with others, in a natural setting, or even on a busy city sidewalk.

Once we understand the sequence and resulting synergy of these four stages, we can apply them in our daily lives. This process is particularly important to men, for as we disarm pain and its emotional component, fear, we reduce anxiety and our need for control. Although chapters 2 through 7 of *Thriving* detail how to implement this four-step creative process in your own life, let's look briefly at each of these four stages of peak experience.

Commitment

When the men of the baby-boomer generation (born between 1946 and 1964) were toddlers, our fathers were emerging from nearly twenty years of living in fear. Their lives had been indelibly scarred by the Depression of the 1930s and the Second World War. They were survivors, and what they taught us to value most were survival skills—hard work, toughness, and delayed gratification. Most baby boomers grew up competing for their father's affection. Naturally, we competed with siblings, but even more perhaps we competed with our father's commitment to his job. As boys, the love we craved from our father usually came sparingly and took the form of praise for achievement. It's no wonder that we have been stuck on achieving ever since.

Although style may differ from one genera-

tion to the next, the pursuit of achievement and success still defines the primary commitment for most men today. The majority of men of the baby-boomer generation seem to experience an unusually high level of frustration and unhappiness in their middle years. We call it midlife crisis, but it has less to do with starting to play life's "back nine" than it does with the disparity between our expectations of success and our present state of well-being, which falls somewhere between disappointment and depression. We believed that our commitment to financial security earned through hard work was the way to realize our dreams, only to find that this commitment to wealth often came at the expense of health and the enjoyment of life.

To set aside the survival-based belief system inherited from our fathers, and to recreate ourselves in a *thriving-based* system, first requires committing to a drastically new course of action. To put it in work-related terms, consider *thriving* a full-time job. Like many jobs, you'll have to sign a contract. In this case, the contract is not with an outside party, but with yourself. By committing to an expanded sense of self-awareness, you are contracting to make your commitments more in accordance with your heart than your head. In meeting your own needs, you are learning to exercise intuition *as well as* intellect. Most men pride themselves on a keen mind, but thriving depends more on deep compassion. You needn't formulate a specific plan, but you must be willing to establish specific goals so you can keep yourself on course. Then you will learn to make choices and commitments *based on what truly feels good to you, instead of based on what you have been conditioned to believe feels good.*

To visualize a life of thriving, ask yourself what your ideal life looks and feels like. Where do you want to be five or ten years from now? Maybe your answers include "My chest pain is gone and I jog on a regular basis." "My work is more meaningful and I have my own business." "There is greater intimacy in my marriage." "I have a clearer sense of purpose in my life." These statements of goals and directions are fueled by commitment. Part of this commitment is your willingness to change profoundly, to take risks and to exercise patience. Because this process works at its own pace, there are no deadlines or schedules. Your only requirements are *desire, belief,* and *expectation.* You must *desire* a change in direction and visualize it with clarity. You must *believe* that change is possible, and you must *expect* that your thoughts, beliefs, and actions will direct that change. Remember, we are only limited by the scope of our imagination. In spite of what our parents, education, and society have taught us, the choice is ours. As the second-century philosopher and CEO of the Roman Empire Marcus Aurelius said, "The universe is change; our life is what our thoughts make it." Prepare to surprise yourself.

Pain

As a boy, how many times were you warned not to do something because you would hurt yourself, or how many times were you urged to play in spite of your pain? Most boys are conditioned to either avoid pain or deny it, be it physical or emotional. Rarely are they taught to acknowledge pain and learn from it. One of the most unhealthy beliefs in our society is that pain is simply a negative factor in our lives to be quickly eliminated with painkillers and alcohol.

Although emotional pain is much more pervasive than physical pain, most men are not nearly as conscious of it. The fear of failure, the sadness of loss, the loneliness of isolation, are all common feelings among American men. Yet the majority of us are unable even to identify them, let alone express them. *As science learns more about the mind-body connection, we increasingly understand the body's physical pleasure or pain as an external reflection of our inner condition.* Disease and injuries, as well as record-breaking performances, mirror internal states of mind.

If you suggest to most men over thirty that pain has any redeeming value, they will probably think you are crazy. That's because most men focus on how pain *limits* them instead of on how it can *communicate* with them. Pain can actually provide information and direct us to ways of enlarging the possibilities of a given experience. It's how most of us learn: by trial and error. As an essential part of thriving, *pain is a communicator that tells us how we are doing.* If we think of the nervous system as an electrical circuit, with current freely flowing through its wires, then physical pain is the accumulation of resistance along that circuit. This resistance can stimulate an intense local awareness of any given part of the body, often in ways that preclude awareness of the whole. The greater the resistance, the more localized pain we experience. By contrast, a clear circuit that holds no resistance provides a frictionless medium that we identify with exhilaration. As a guide, pain can provide specific, highly useful information, indicating points of stress, friction, or imbalance. This information is critical for understanding the limits of your physical capabilities. An understanding of the sources of pain can improve efficiency and performance, whether you're playing the violin, lifting weights, or casting a fly rod. Think of pain as the lemon from which we make lemonade.

Much of our emotional pain comes from our perception of having made a mistake. For most men, the ultimate screwup is to have made a mistake in public. Instead of reacting with humiliation, shame, and fear, we can learn to use that pain as feedback to improve our performance. The worst consequence of mistakes is the fear it engenders that even further inhibits performance. Think of any business deal. It involves presentations to a number of different people. If one of those presentations meets with disapproval or disinterest because of something you said, you can't let the pain of that rejection knock you out of the game. Try to understand the feedback. Consider what it was you said that caused the negative reaction, clarify it, and your next presentation will be stronger, bringing you that much closer to achieving your goal.

In the same way we can become used to physical pain, we can habitually carry around emotional pain that triggers an associated physical response. For example, the pounding headache you experience driving home from work might simply reflect the demands and pressures of a particularly trying day. However, as a chronic condition, repeated headaches might serve as a signal that the ongoing stress of your job has contracted the muscles lining your arteries and caused high blood pressure. Medically known as hypertension, high blood pressure is a leading cause of heart disease, which kills more middle-aged American men than any other cause.

By becoming conscious of our pain and tracing it to its source (often located in fear or sadness), we can decide how to manage it or prevent its recurrence. For example, ask yourself, "What made this particular day stressful?" Let's say that you were overloaded with more work than you could handle, or that you felt that a presentation went poorly. We already know that poor performance is extremely painful to most men. As a result, perhaps you even conjured a vivid image of yourself losing your job. Where did that fear of failure come from? Was it a hypersensitive association to a past trauma, or was it a realistic warning? The resistance in our emotional and physical circuits can have many sources, some justified and connected to reality, others not. If we can answer these questions, we can put the stress in perspective and ease up on ourselves by being more compassionate and adjusting our standards to better fit the situation. However, if we mask the pain with alcohol, painkillers, or simple denial, we learn nothing. Instead, we perpetuate the pain and create conditions that further weaken our bodies as well as our performance.

A 1988 *Fortune* magazine survey showed that the most common trait among successful men in business and other fields is the willingness to accept failure and mistakes as part of growth. Our willingness to fully embrace the necessary pain and effort of creative achievement is a vital step toward the condition of thriving. *Risk-taking is the vehicle that carries us to positive change.* Its uncertainty lies in that while we are guaranteed to lose our known reality, we don't know exactly what we will change into. Muhammad Ali, a great risk-taker in his own right, once said, "He who is not courageous enough to take risks will accomplish nothing in life." Boston Celtic great John Havlicek put it this way:

> One of the more interesting compliments I've ever been paid came when somebody said that the best thing about me was that I wasn't afraid to look bad. Some guys are embarrassed when they are knocked down and absolutely mortified when they have a shot blocked. Over the years, I've had hundreds of shots blocked. You've got to go in and take chances.

Michael Jordan, perhaps the greatest player of all time, was willing to take an even greater risk of failure in playing baseball for a year. Jordan understood that the pain of failure is part of athletic excellence. Instead of attempting to learn from physical and emotional pain, most men deny it by seeking relief through addictions: work, alcohol, drugs, sex, and toys.

You need only look as far as print and media advertising to see how American society tacitly endorses all of these escapes. "Workaholism" is by far the most socially reinforced and financially rewarded of our addictions. Masked as a virtue, in many cases it is a denial of emotional pain that inevitably results in dysfunction and dis-ease. Men are typically willing to excuse addictions if they perceive them as necessary to providing success.

Mickey Mantle performed well through both physical and emotional pain within baseball. When Mantle broke in with the Yankees, he was a rare combination of speed and power from both sides of the plate. Although a series of crippling injuries reduced his output, Mantle's physical gifts enabled him to play through pain and kept the Yankee dynasty alive through the middle sixties. Off the field, however, Mantle's private life fell into disarray, and in later years he admitted to having been an alcoholic through the latter part of his baseball career. His decline accelerated when he retired from baseball and the joy of his physical performance was gone. By nature a shy man, Mantle was left unprotected by clubhouse walls or outfield fences. Thrust into a more social world of public relations and promotional appearances, he felt out of place and isolated. He finally sought help for his alcoholism at age sixty-two, entering the Betty Ford Clinic, and he began to talk candidly about confronting his emotional pain. Mantle was just one of many sports heroes who encountered this problem, but one of the few who had the courage to honestly confront it.

This pattern is familiar among professional

athletes: they retire and the pain and stress they routinely endured on the field, but now experience in other arenas, is no longer manageable without the gratification of physical achievement or the joy of victory. In our own lives, we relinquish the playful creativity of boyhood and resign ourselves to the diminished wonder and expectations of that "joyless" stage of life called adulthood. Mantle was an athlete whose life spun out of control once his perceived capacity for achievement abandoned him. This loss resulted in an emotional pain that he masked with alcoholism, which ultimately killed him through the destruction of his liver.

Our own lives are replete with losses—divorce, career change, and business failure. Each, however, can also be seen as a gain, *as long as we are able to acknowledge the pain and learn from it.* If our fear of failure causes us to avoid pain altogether and prevents us from taking risks, we may avoid some of these losses; but we may be equally deprived of victories and peak moments. Our ability to feel pain and to learn from it as a communicator that guides us to our innermost needs is crucial for optimal health. As kids, we were taught "Big boys don't cry." As adults, we must learn that thriving men do.

Power: A Leap of Faith

For our fathers, and subsequently for us, power is the ability to impose our will on our surroundings—*to control.* We also tend to measure power by its material manifestations—power cars, power lunches, power lifters, private jets, seven-figure salaries, and trophy homes. Instead of imposing our ego-centered will on our surroundings, thriving teaches us to access an unlimited source of energy *within* that reflects a larger, universal will. Most men rarely give much thought to the nonmaterial dimensions of power, except when the electricity goes off or the TV reception is poor. Then we call it "power failure." If a man is unable to have an erection, we call him *impotent* or powerless. Men easily identify sexual or material displays of power, but we have a harder time with those invisible expressions of life energy.

Because men typically view power in its visible forms, we don't often allow ourselves to be directed by unseen forces, if we can avoid it. Westerners assume the karate master uses pure muscle to break a stack of boards, when, in fact, the action is *chi* driven. The body acts as a conduit that channels this more subtle energy. This same channeling of *chi* enables the eighty-year-old tai chi master to fling a two-hundred-pound twenty-year-old across the mat. Most of us rarely experience this energy, because it requires our *surrendering* to it instead of *controlling* it—a notion that is highly threatening to most men.

Intuition is the power of accepting or surrendering to the nonrational—to those invisible forces of life energy that constantly envelop and penetrate our lives. Women are characteristically more "intuitive" than men, because men have conditioned themselves to think the vibrations of life energy are too subtle for them to receive. Men assume that these vibrations bypass the empirical, rational thought processes that most of us have been taught to value: if we can't see it, we don't believe it. Because men typically lead with their left brains—the analytical hemisphere—our "sensitivity" tends to show up in the precision of our technology instead of in the accuracy of our intuition. As a result, the sophistication and sensitivity of our tools is much finer than what we have been able to achieve in the refinement of our own sensibilities. We excel at creating webs of *virtual* reality fed by the transmissions of fiber-optic, microwave, laser, and satellite technology, even though all of this virtual reality tends to overcomplicate our lives and burden our minds with information overload. We're so in the habit of taking comfort in our technology and burying our heads in the sand of *virtual* reality, that we can no longer identify the *real* presences of life energy. We've become so consumed with virtual *forms*, we've forgotten the real *content* of our lives.

Men need to realize that the true measure of power lies not in its material expressions, but in expanded awareness, in our ability to access spirit and to allow its regenerative energy to shape our lives. In our day-to-day lives, we recognize the purest communications of the spirit as *passion*—that enthusiasm (from the Greek *en-theos:* "in god") that animates us to achieve at the highest level. Great musicians and artists, whose passion allows them to surrender to their art form, have what we call "inspiration."

Most men are fascinated by the power of spirit embodied in physical achievements,

and time and again its display draws us to the spectacle of sport. *Men love the accomplishments of sport because they offer a clear and quantifiable display of the power of spirit.* Rarely in our own lives do we need to jump the highest, to throw the farthest, to run the fastest, and to score the most points. And yet, if we are guided by our *passions*—instead of being guided by negative belief systems— these passions will, in turn, direct us to accomplishments that push the limits of our imagination. When Joseph Campbell described the heroes of myths "following their bliss," he was talking about men who allowed themselves to be directed by their passions and spirit.

Not until midlife do most men begin to recognize and cultivate an awareness of spirit. We are not alone in requiring maturity before opening ourselves to an experience of spirit: Jewish *Kabbalists* and Hawaiian kahunas alike prohibit initiation into the mysteries of spirit until after age forty. The religions of the world are replete with figures who encountered spirit as part of a midlife crisis: Abraham, Noah, Muhammad, Buddha. For most males, an incipient understanding of the spirit rarely comes before midlife; because only when we have experienced the fluctuations of the ego and desire can we penetrate the illusory nature of the mind and its creations. Just as we cannot cure chronic emotional or physical pain until we trace it to its true source, so the inventions of the ego hold us in their grasp until we realize they are mere illusions. It usually takes until midlife for us to realize the emptiness of this "attach-ment"—that, like the emperor in the fable, the ego is wearing no clothes after all.

Until we balance the needs of the ego with a direct experience of spirit, we cannot thrive. Real power derives from our surrendering to that life energy. But to make that leap of faith, we must first embrace our pain, confront our fear, and bypass the ego. As Lao-tzu said, "And if I cease to desire and remain still, the empire will be at peace of its own accord."

Harmony

You're involved in the action and vaguely aware of it, but your focus is not on the commotion but on the opportunity ahead. I'd liken it to a sense of reverie—not a dreamlike state but the somehow insulated state that a great musician achieves in a great performance. He's aware of where he is and what he's doing, but his mind is on the playing of his instrument with an internal sense of rightness—it is not merely mechanical, it is not only spiritual; it is something of both, on a different plane and a more remote one.

Arnold Palmer, *The Psychic Side of Sports*

At first, thriving, re-creating ourselves along internal guidelines, can feel a little like flying through a cloud. So what keeps us from flying into a mountain? The answer is that internal radar capable of confirming our direc-tion and bearings at any moment. It's called *intuition.* To keep our bearings, we need only use our intuition to harmonize with life energy. It's as simple as learning to shut up and lis-ten . . . to what our minds and bodies are try-ing to tell us.

The displays of balance we witness in great athletes require a flexibility, quickness, and explosiveness that derive from acute proprio-ceptive neuromuscular responsiveness. In simpler terms: the body of a great athlete knows how to listen to itself and respond ac-cordingly. As observers, we assume that by some combination of innate endowment and training, the muscles and nerves of top ath-letes have attained a level of receptivity, com-munication, and intelligent cooperation that enables them to reach levels of performance most of us only dream about. But there is no magic to it: superior athletes, like creative artists or scientists, know how to observe themselves responding to the situations and materials at hand. In the case of the athlete, he is responding to the workings of his own body. He uses it as a vehicle for problem solv-ing. In the West, we have been conditioned away from believing that the body has its own intelligence, but Soviet-bloc research into athletic physiology as early as the 1970s de-scribed coordination and *athleticism as the body's heightened awareness of itself.* Edwin Moses running hurdles is a good example of an exquisite body "thinking out loud."

Ironically, we admire the intracommun-icative skills within the body of an athlete, or in the makeup of a team, but we rarely appreciate or experience them within our own organism. We write off our own efforts at sports by saying we are too uncoordinated, too fat, too old, or too busy to *practice.* Instead of participating, we become spectators and end up quantifying the performances of ourselves and others. We fall out of the flow. We lose our balance and our sense of harmony.

We quantify our own health in the same way. We tabulate weight, blood pressure, and cholesterol levels as if we were tracking income and net worth; but we don't take the time to *feel* the functioning of our bodies—its joints, muscles, and limbs—any more than we take the time to *feel* the functioning of our relationships. Within the "social body" we men still aspire to impose our wills and egos on those around us; we attempt to *control* rather than to *respond to* others. We impose our control by withholding approval or love or, at best, making it conditional. As a result, we often feel disconnected from friends, spouses, and kids. It is little wonder our society is in conflict with itself—racially, politically, and religiously. A study performed by Redford Williams, M.D., a researcher in behavioral medicine at Duke University Medical Center, identified the emotion of hostility resulting from isolation as a strong contributor to heart disease—the leading killer of men.

Our endless judgment and comparison casts a pall of fear and anxiety over performance. We lose connection to our *being* because we are too much in our *thinking.* We let our competitive natures run to extremes, conditioning even the most intimate relationships with isolation and hostility. It is little wonder men often feel disconnected. We become detached not only from other men and women in our lives, but from our environment—and ultimately from the earth itself.

First as hunters and later as farmers, men identified closely with the cycles and seasons of nature. We were rooted in the soil, and our spirits were attuned to the energy of the elements—earth, air, fire, and water. Today, we are trapped in an experience of the earth filtered through an urbanized, denatured, hypercompetitive consumer consciousness. But we can change, once we apply to others and to our environment the self-acceptance that we create individually by embracing the wisdom of the heart. Harmony embraces both living creatures and living places. When we experience our environment with the wonder of a child, we can begin to experience a degree of bonding and relationship that lies at the very heart of thriving.

Mastering Your Life: The Art of Thriving

In basketball circles, the expression *playing big* refers to the ability to play much larger than one's physical stature. Instead of dominating with sheer size, the guy who "plays big" fills the lane with confidence, with chutzpah, with a passion that has no room for fear. As a result he not only raises the level of his game, but that of his teammates as well. Thriving will help you to play big at whatever game you choose—especially the game of life.

By expanding your concept of health, you

will renew your physical appearance, your energy level, your capacity for healing disease, your enjoyment of sex, and your ability to meet physical challenges. You will become more creative and fulfilled in your work and find ways to become financially healthier. While there is probably no greater reward than that of thriving, there is also no greater challenge. There are no quick fixes. Creating health demands a tough apprenticeship to your own sensibilities and inner self. As your self-awareness develops in stages, your mastery over your life will unfold. Your first step is making a commitment to yourself and affirming your willingness to change. The adventure that follows will be the ultimate treasure hunt. Your body, mind, and spirit will provide the clues as your sense of thriving emerges from unconscious impulses into conscious practice. Additional direction will come from your heightened awareness of emotions, relationships, and your environment. For most men this adventure will mean changing your pace of life and "slowing down" to experience this higher state of energy.

As you learn how to "tune in" to your expanded state of consciousness in the following chapters, you will "turn on" to an optimal state of health. But instead of "dropping out," you will feel more focused and more alive. As you strengthen your *commitment* and release your *fear*, you will experience greater *power* and *harmony* than you ever felt before. Most of us are already familiar with at least one of these four stages, but may have experienced it to excess by being either *overcommitted* to our

work, *painfully self-sacrificing, power hungry* for control, or addicted to the *seductive harmonies* of hedonism. The more you practice to thrive, the easier it will be to balance these stages and experience their natural sequence in every action that we *consciously* undertake. You will learn to value your own readings of how you feel. You will trust your own intuition and find more creative ways of decision making. Yes, your life will change, but don't be intimidated by the prospect. No! . . . you won't end up with a shaved head wearing a dress and selling books at the airport.

Thriving is a transformational journey of rediscovery and re-creation. It leads to a place that you've only briefly known during infrequent moments of peak experience— your heart. Through a series of practical exercises in Part I, this book will bring you "out of your head" and reunite you with your heart and a fuller experience of your body. The ticket for this journey is a growing awareness of life energy in your body, environment, thoughts, emotions, spirit, and relationships. In short, you will learn to nurture your body and mind with life energy and become more aware of how it impacts every facet of your life. To do this, you will learn in depth how to identify and use the four stages of every willful action you undertake. By learning to listen and shifting your awareness more to an innate sense of *being*—instead of *doing*— *commitment, pain, power,* and *harmony* can lead you to thrive.

In Part II, you will find specific holistic medical treatment plans for the most common chronic diseases afflicting men. These treatment plans address the pathology of the body as well as destructive habits of mind. As you learn to address the causes of your disease, you will identify and begin working within the six specific dimensions of your life: *physical, environmental, mental, emotional, spiritual, and social.* Treating the causes of disease requires understanding how each dimension is affected by negative attitudes that cause a deprivation of life energy or love. This creates a corresponding imbalance between body, mind, and spirit. By choosing appropriate therapies, you can change limiting beliefs, renew contact with life energy, and restore balance and harmony.

For example, the treatment plan recommendations for heart disease are designed to reverse this disease on each of six levels. *Physically,* these protocols reduce fat in the diet while prescribing optimal water intake, a full complement of vitamins, minerals, antioxidants, and nutritional supplements, in addition to outlining an exercise program designed for the patient's age and conditioning. *Environmentally,* the heart disease treatment plan includes guidelines for creating healthy indoor air while eliminating toxins from our food and water. *Mentally,* the program prescribes relaxation and stress-reduction techniques that include identifying and changing many of our limiting and self-critical beliefs. *Emotionally,* the recommendations delineate a variety of specific methods for expressing and releasing destructive feelings of rage and hostility. *Spiritually,* the patient will find specific suggestions for learning to listen more attentively to his intuition and developing

trust in his compassionate inner voice. *Socially,* he will learn to enhance intimacy and feel more connected to others. All of the holistic medical treatment plans in *Thriving* are based on the underlying premise that *healing any dis-ease occurs through learning to nurture oneself with unconditional love in all dimensions of life.* Specific dietary, pharmaceutical, herbal, and exercise recommendations for the various chronic diseases are contained in Part II. Underlying principles and practices for the bulk of the mental and spiritual practices are detailed in "Part I: Training to Thrive."

Along this healing path, you will become your own highly skilled and nurturing health care provider. You will become a master in the art of self-nurturing. You will learn to wear many hats: as a compassionate artist, capable of fashioning images and visions into reality; as a consummate tracker, alert to the faintest signs of dis-ease; as a skilled craftsman, who knows his materials, the tolerances, and flexibility of both mind and body. By nature, men were first hunters, but to thrive we must learn to track a different quarry, one that lies deep within our own inner nature. And we must do so by emulating the patience and consistent effort of a master who has learned not only the mechanics but also the spirit of his craft.

The body is constantly changing; almost every one of its atoms is replaced in a year. Thoughts and impressions change in the blink of an eye, and the only constant in the ever-changing stream of energy and consciousness we call our life is *change* itself. We have the capacity to redesign, retool, and reassemble ourselves with far greater speed and precision than the engineers at GM ever dreamed of, but it takes a *conscious* process of harmonizing body and mind with spirit. Once we embrace the power to change and to assume responsibility for directing energy into those nurturing images we actively desire, our thriving will become an ongoing adventure and a celebration of life. Re-creation will become recreation.

Gentlemen, start your engines!

Winning Mind Games:
A Commitment to Peace of Mind

Every idea has within it a motor element. All action proceeds from thought. Every image is an act in a latent state.

Robert Assagioli

All that we are is the result of what we have thought.

Buddha

———————◆———————

Breaking the Rules

Guys like to know exactly how to do things. They like to know how it's been done before. They like to know how long it takes, and what tools they need to do it. We grew up with our fathers telling us this stuff: This is the way you clean a fish. This is the way you change the oil, fix a flat, tie a necktie, shine shoes, throw a football . . . and all the 101 other things guys need to know in order to perform successfully. Most of this "guy stuff gospel" has been passed on father to son through generations without our ever questioning it. Most

of it is common-sense advice that adds up because it works. The problem is we apply this same type of nuts-and-bolts thinking to larger more complex issues where it doesn't always work so well: to attitudes about work, women, family, even the way we think about our bodies, minds, and spirits. We learn about them indirectly through watching our fathers and other important men in our lives. Without our even knowing it, *these beliefs establish the pattern for the way we live.* They seem so normal, we don't even question them.

Here are three simple questions you may never see on *Jeopardy,* but questions that, if you've read this far, probably need your immediate attention. Most men never stop to ask themselves these questions, until it's too late. Why wait until the shit hits the fan. You may as well start questioning the assumptions that frame your life right now.

1. Why do I work sixty-plus hours a week at a job I dislike?
2. Why do I think that I can't have happiness, security, and power without a lot of money?
3. What keeps me thinking this way and playing by rules that don't feel right to me?

If you're like most men who have been led to believe that you don't question these basic assumptions, then you don't want to think about these questions: they are too upsetting and disruptive. But many guys can't help *but* think about them, because they reach a point in their lives where they have invested their heart and soul in "playing the game" but they haven't gotten out of it anywhere close to what they expected. Why wait till forty to start asking? If you honestly think about these questions for a moment, you may find that the messages you've been giving yourself all your life are more limiting, critical, and negative than you may have thought. *Wouldn't it be healthier to consciously choose the positive imagery and messages and simply edit out the negative?* This chapter will show you how to start exercising your free will to do exactly that.

In my own life, I reached a point where I felt I had to change, because I was paying too painful a price. When I was forty, I was a successful physician with the busiest family practice in Denver. Although I administered a large staff, I was physically overworked and emotionally burdened with the responsibility of providing quality health care thirteen hours a day, seven days a week. I was a prisoner to my own success, and it was tearing down my health and my relationships with my wife and daughters. The vision I had seen for myself as a young boy—a family doctor with the power and skill to alleviate the pain and suffering of others—was no longer working. I needed a new vision. Although my ultimate goal would remain to be the best family doc-

tor I could be, I had to change so I could do so without sacrificing my own health in the process. Hippocrates' edict—"Physician, heal thyself"—took on an expanded meaning for me, and I started using it as a daily affirmation for my own healing. I was soon aware that an integral part of that new vision included teaching my patients to heal themselves. Within two years after selling my practice to a local hospital, I had self-published the first edition of a self-help book on the holistic treatment of sinus and respiratory disease, called *Sinus Survival.* My fledgling career as a holistic physician and author had begun.

The challenge of making myself into a new kind of physician was far more difficult than the rigors of medical school had been. I had no guides or models for this process. (My hope is this book will clear a path for you, the reader, in your own journey of self-transformation.) Every aspect of my life was different. My whole routine had changed. Instead of going to the office and managing a busy medical center sixty to seventy hours a week, I was working out of the small study in my home, seeing a handful of private patients, and reading everything I could find about holistic medicine. Every morning I would get up and hear the message "It's time to leave to go to work," but there would be no place to go. Even though I felt that I was working hard at what I was doing, there was nothing tangible to show for it. Most family and friends regarded me as "retired." From my physician father, I received the unspoken message that the only acceptable way for me to make a living was to be seeing patients in a medical office. Being a writer was clearly not approved of, even though the book I was writing might ultimately help more people than I could by seeing individual patients. Furthermore, I was forced to learn skills that I hadn't performed before. With my wife having gone back to graduate school for a degree in social work, I was sharing in the cooking, cleaning, shopping for food, and chauffeuring. I was contending with the negative beliefs associated with this new lifestyle: "These chores are a waste of my valuable time." "Seeing four to five patients a week and spending the rest of my time reading and writing is not real work." After fifteen years of daily positive feedback from grateful patients and colleagues, I was now painfully learning to accept professional rejection on a daily basis. It came from publishing companies, book distributors, and media reporters as I attempted to promote a new and effective treatment for sinus disease. In spite of seeing how well holistic medicine worked on myself and my patients, I still heard, from myself and others, the message that this form of healing was akin to hocus-pocus and charlatanism. From the people closest to me, I received the implicit, and sometimes explicit, message that I was putting my family at great financial risk by chasing windmills. They considered me irrational, stupid, or both to have given up such a good job . . . to do *what?*

All of these critical beliefs and messages made my transition from survival to thriving a relentless uphill struggle. The learning curve was steep, yet the challenge allowed me to learn much more about myself. I discovered

new talents, a greater awareness of what felt good to me and why, and a deeper appreciation for the power of my own intuition. Nonetheless, it was my commitment to an expanded vision of health that enabled me to continue to make this vision become a reality.

What kept me committed was that I was getting results. My sinus infections disappeared, as did those of my patients. Slowly but surely I was encountering commercial success with my book. From this and sporadic speaking engagements, I discovered a sizable audience that was receptive to this new type of medicine. In joining the AHMA (American Holistic Medical Association), I found a group of like-minded physicians, who have provided an invaluable support group, letting me know that I am not the only "outcast" in the medical community. Gradually, I learned to laugh at myself when friends referred to me as a "witch doctor." As I became less critical of myself, I grew more forgiving of those around me. As I started to manifest my short-term goals, taking baby steps, my level of expectation that this vision would come true increased.

The gradual deepening of my commitment encouraged this process of self-transformation. It allowed me to develop a great deal more patience, which had never been my strongest suit. I still work at it. Professionally, I had always operated with a precise game plan and timetable in mind, but my new mode of behavior allowed me to be more open to unexpected possibilities. With a newfound flexibility, I was getting where I wanted to go more quickly and effortlessly. When I started, my objective had been to improve my own health through holistic medicine. I wanted to practice this form of medicine by empowering patients to heal themselves and to put my observations and experience with holistic healing into a book. This way it could benefit as many people as possible. Without my knowing specifically how to accomplish these goals, I focused on a vision of their coming true. Somehow, my focus and commitment to them enabled me to make choices that allowed them to occur. I had discovered the power of the mind in shaping reality. The conscious, disciplined practice of visualization provided the foundation for repatterning my reality and experiencing greater peace of mind than I had ever known. This is how it works.

The mind of a man consists of visions, ideas, thoughts, beliefs, attitudes, and perceptions. Most men structure their lives around the belief that peace of mind derives from financial and professional security. The mental videotapes we see and hear each day reinforce this goal, and they are similar to the messages and self-talk that we unconsciously developed as young boys. Many of the positive impressions and memories from our past can be extremely helpful. For example, if your father enjoyed his job, showed a strong commitment to the family, and talked frequently about a positive sense of responsibility and self-discipline, these associations can inspire you to realize your dreams and reach your goals. However, most of the negative messages from our youth are also still with us, and we repeat them on a daily basis: "I'll

never be able to . . ." "I have no choice but to . . ." "How could I have been so stupid as to . . . ?" "I'm going to have to learn to live with this damn . . . for the rest of my life." Behavioral scientists have found that of the approximately fifty thousand thoughts we have each day, about 95 percent are the same ones we had the day before. These automatic beliefs and attitudes can hold us back from physical well-being, peace of mind, and true happiness.

Beliefs and attitudes are the "software" that we use to program ourselves. The physiological price of these beliefs and attitudes, particularly as they relate to your job and the work place, can be deadly. In the late 1980s, the Massachusetts Department of Health identified the two greatest factors contributing to heart disease in men as unhappiness and job dissatisfaction. High scores for these factors were shown to be more accurate indicators of the likelihood for developing heart disease than conventional indicators such as high cholesterol, high blood pressure, obesity, and sedentary lifestyle. These findings, which underscore the powerful relationship between beliefs and physical health, were further dramatized by the astounding statistic that more men suffered heart attacks on Monday mornings around nine o'clock than at any other time of the week! The only difference between Monday morning and any other time of the week is that negative attitudes and self-talk relating to our jobs are more prevalent then. If you are working at a job that you hate, you could be risking your life.

The path of thriving lies in *consciously*

choosing positive, nurturing images and messages for the mental videotape that governs our actions and behavior. This means deleting the negative messages. For example, the sense of feeling imprisoned by your job is often reinforced by the belief that you have no choice: "How else will I provide for myself or my family?" Not only are there options, but perhaps they would be much better suited to your unique talents and desires, if you could only remove the blinders and escape from your old assumptions and beliefs.

Greater self-awareness starts with knowing the origins of our choices in the past that lead to beliefs and self-talk that influence our behavior in the present. To discover who you really are, start by testing the reality of some of the assumptions that shape your internal dialogue. Your notions of work, money, health, or relationships may include some of the following messages:

- The only way to get ahead in this job is to work seventy to eighty hours a week.
- I hate this job, but I've got to tough it out till retirement.
- I can't get a better job unless I go back and get a degree.
- My clout only extends as far as my net worth.
- The doc says I'm going to have this painful arthritis for the rest of my life, so it's time to give up tennis.
- If she's having an affair, then it's time to find a lawyer.
- If my equipment were bigger, maybe I'd be better in bed.

These messages and their underlying assumptions may not precisely reflect what you want in your own life, but they typify the kinds of choices each of us has made based on beliefs that originally may not have been our own. These beliefs may have been imposed on us by parents, society, physicians, friends, religion, or spouse. If they don't feel nurturing, build confidence, create self-esteem, or regenerate you, then it's time to free yourself from the tyranny of these messages. The first step is to *change the tape.* By rejecting these messages because they create pain, conflict, or even confusion, you can begin the journey of self-discovery and start on your way to peace of mind. Like the food, air, and water that we ingest, like the life energy that we cultivate with exercise and movement, or like the environment that we inhabit, ideas and self-talk are capable of either replenishing or depleting energy. Beliefs are a form of *chi* that can nourish or weaken us. If you don't believe it, just take stock of how you feel after hearing one of these negative messages. Intuitively, we know which beliefs and ideas are toxic to our well-being. We need only clearly identify these poisonous messages and systematically remove them from our lives.

Once you've started to eradicate those messages you *don't* want, how do you know what is going to replace them? How do you know what you really *do* want? Most men have never honestly explored their desires and innate abilities. They have never discovered their full potential. At first, it can be as intimidating as standing at the edge of a frontier without a map. To survive in this wilderness, you'll need to rely on some new tools, to develop different skills, and to create a new map.

The Game Plan— A Different Approach

Your game plan for thriving will bring about a deeper sense of self-awareness and a stronger commitment to caring for yourself, based on your real needs revealed through this new awareness. For the first time in your life, *you* will choose the beliefs and attitudes that are going to shape your life, instead of having them chosen for you by your boss, your wife, or your accountant. Some of the beliefs and self-talk that have brought you to your present condition may still be helpful and worth retaining—you don't have to throw out the baby with the bathwater. But you probably wouldn't have read this far if you weren't looking to make some significant changes in your life. To find out what you really want at this stage of life (and what your particular body, mind, and spirit really need), put aside the rational, judgmental side—the shoulds and supposed to's. Instead, examine your life and goals from the perspective of what will bring passion, life energy, or *chi* into your life. To discover what feels most nurturing to you, start by asking:

1. What am I good at and what do I most appreciate about myself?
2. What do I most enjoy doing?
3. What is most meaningful to me?
4. Where do I see myself five or ten years from now and what am I doing?

What you are *good at*, proud of, and *most enjoy* are usually one and the same. You may be good working with your hands. Perhaps you are a whiz at shuffling numbers. Maybe you're more at home blending colors, or creating designs. You work better with people than by yourself. You are more an effective leader than an enthusiastic follower. You are an idea person instead of an implementer, or vice versa. In other words, what do you do better than others, with less effort and more enjoyment?

The first two questions relate to ability and pleasure. The third question—meaning—is important, because if the activity or pursuit doesn't extend meaningfully to other parts of your life, or benefit others in some way, then it is incomplete and probably not the work that will be your life's passion. By asking yourself the fourth question—Where do I see myself five or ten years from now and what am I doing?—you complete the other three. Visualize yourself in a locale and make that image as detailed as you can. These four questions will outline for you a new belief system—one that reflects your ideal life vision and will provide the foundation for a new set of goals.

The next step in heightening self-awareness is to make a wish list. Identify your goals in each realm of your life: physical, environmental, mental, emotional, spiritual, and social.

For example, physical goals might include healing illnesses or disabilities and accomplishing physical feats. If you're a jogger, you may commit to running a marathon. If you're a golfer, you may set a goal of a ten handicap. If you've been plagued by chronic low-back pain or your activity has been limited by heart disease, you may strive to have a perfectly healthy back or heart.

Environmental goals relate to where you live and work and your connection to your surroundings. You may work in a "sick building," in a dismal office without windows or sunlight, with a coworker who smokes. A likely goal might be to work in a brighter, more well-ventilated, healthier environment.

Mental goals relate to work, career, financial objectives, and limiting beliefs. If you know you don't like your present job but are unclear as to what a new job might be, then your goal might be to find a meaningful job that you enjoy and that utilizes your greatest talents. For instance, if you've recognized that you're a creative guy and find yourself in a monolithic bureaucracy that rewards doing what you are told, then your goal might be to find a job that pays you for your ideas. Your goal may be to start your own business based on an original idea and see it through to acceptance within your field or industry.

Emotional goals have to do with feelings: identifying, expressing, experiencing, or accepting them. Suppose you are aware of feeling increasingly angry at times, so much so that you feel as if you could explode. Your goal may be "to safely release my anger." Or you may be experiencing more stress but aren't sure why or exactly what the specific feelings are. Your goal could be "to better identify what I'm feeling."

Spiritual goals relate to your connection with God or that transcendent power that animates all of life. Your spiritual goal may be to set aside more time for meditation and contemplation, to visit the great cathedrals of Europe to understand the spiritual tradition and expressions of another culture. If you are like most men in this country, your religious upbringing was somewhat devoid of spirituality. Perhaps what you were exposed to had little meaning. You might therefore seek to have a greater awareness or understanding of God, and a greater sense of spirituality in your everyday life. You may resolve to have a more open mind on the subject of spirituality itself.

Social goals have to do with relationships and intimacy. If you want to live in a committed relationship and you are not, that could be your objective. Not long ago, I worked with a patient who had this same goal. He was very specific in what he was looking for: an attractive woman who was independent, caring, sensitive, interested in good health and the outdoors, and liked to travel. Within three months he met and, soon thereafter, married the woman he had envisioned. It goes to show that the more specific you can be, the more likely you are to get what you want.

To create physical fitness, we will learn in chapter 3 to appreciate our bodies by becoming more sensitized to them and thus become better caretakers. We will commit to specific goals and follow through. To experience greater mental fitness, you'll learn to create a new set of beliefs and messages based on positive mental imagery. Just by taking a few seconds to hear the message and focus on its image, you can trigger a smile, induce a state of tranquillity or even a state of exhilaration. Just as you will improve physical fitness by learning to heighten reflexes, muscular response, and aerobic capacity, you can increase your mental fitness by strengthening your grip on positive images and beliefs. Consciously focusing on them with a clarity and intensity that bring them to life will enable you to quickly make them a reality.

Affirmations provide the most effective method I have found for generating positive mental imagery. Affirmations allow you to direct patterns of action by first shaping patterns of thought. In communicating directly with the subconscious, affirmations use an internal language of thought and imagery to tap in new and powerfully creative ways the healing energy stored in positive feelings and sensations. In the simplest sense, affirmations help you to change your behavior. If you are recovering from your first heart attack, and you are affirming, "My heart is getting stronger every day," this affirmation will facilitate dramatic lifestyle changes in diet, exercise, and attitude that will in fact strengthen your heart. It will do so by redirecting the thousands of thoughts and decisions made each day that affect your behavior, often without your even knowing it.

Affirmations also work by infusing the immune system with the life energy of *hope.* Whether the problem is chronic fatigue, chronic prostatitis, or chronic sinusitis, I've seen hundreds of patients who made steady progress after they began affirming, "My prostate, sinuses, or ____ is/are getting better every day." Or "I am getting stronger and

feeling more energized daily." These were all patients who had been led to believe they would have to learn to live with their condition. They were, in fact, using other therapies as well. Medical science is beginning to prove the value of affirmations in the treatment of a number of chronic diseases. The NIH Office of Alternative Medicine is funding one such study. Affirmations have played an integral role in PNI (psychoneuroimmunology), described in chapter 1. When practiced consistently, they provide the trigger for the secretion of health-enhancing neuropeptides.

As for the power of affirmations to change aspects of our lives other than disease, I have witnessed numerous examples of this too. The aforementioned patient who met the woman of his dreams was a regular practitioner of affirmations. Another patient who ran his own successful advertising agency had for years been overwhelmed with stress and terrible sinusitis. Furthermore, he was overworked and disliked his job mostly as a result of his belief that he had to be deeply involved with the administration of every department. He started to recite the affirmation "My business is thriving as I release my need to control, and I am happily delegating responsibility to others." Within weeks, his business was running more efficiently and he was enjoying his job more than he had in years.

My favorite example is a woman from North Carolina whom I was treating for chronic fatigue, allergies, and sinusitis. In the early years of my holistic practice, I worked with a number of patients long-distance over the phone, never actually meeting them in person. An RN in her fifties, she taught in a nursing school in a small town and had never married, although she wanted to. She had resisted putting marriage on her goal list because, as she explained to me, "I know all of the eligible men in town and in my church, and there aren't any possible candidates." I convinced her to include it on her goal list, and her affirmation read simply, "I am happily married." Within a few months, she received a letter from a former professor of hers with whom she'd had a friendship years earlier. His wife had died the year before, and he wanted to visit his former student. Within months they were engaged, and a year after beginning her affirmation she was happily married. Her tears of joy over the phone and her gratitude left me in tears as well. We both felt as if we had experienced a miracle.

I must admit that when I first started using affirmations ten years ago, I was more than a little skeptical. At the time, they seemed too simple and effortless. But I didn't realize their ability to reshape the unconscious mind. And now, having seen them work in my own life—with family, friends, and patients—I'm convinced they may be the most powerful transformational tool we have at our disposal.

The greatest challenge to using affirmations is to suspend judgment long enough to make them as vivid as possible. Instead of letting your goals and affirmations be limited by criticisms and judgments based on your *past*, try to *directly experience* your affirmation in a more energetic way—solely in the *present*. Think of an affirmation as the last minute in the final scene of a two-hour movie. Make that final minute as vivid and real as possible, engaging every sensory detail you can in placing yourself within it. Don't worry about the previous one hour and fifty-nine minutes. Your subconscious will plot what needs to happen to bring you into the realization of that final scene. As it happened to me, you too may at first feel this sounds oversimplistic, too easy; but if you commit to your visualization, you will be astonished by its power. You are using compassion to program your mind and to bring yourself into a reality of *your* choosing. This process first takes place on a level of reality that is more *energetic* than *material*. Merely by envisioning this reality, you can begin to taste the sweetness of thriving.

In Frederick Lenz's novel *Surfing the Himalayas*, a young snowboarder meets a Tibetan Buddhist monk who initiates him into the mystery of enlightenment. The young man learns to explore life and snowboarding as actions occurring on a level of energy that most of us don't allow ourselves to experience. The monk explains:

> Once you get beyond your conception of what reality is . . . you will transcend the words and concepts you have already developed of reality. It's really that easy. But as long as you continue to "think" life, instead of directly experiencing it in a nonconceptual way, you will not understand any more about reality than you do today.

Affirmations demand the same suspension of conceptual thinking. They *provide an imaginative experience of a consciously expressed desire.* What usually prevents us from attaining our desires is fear, which limits our experience of the present to the painful feelings associated with the consequences of past actions. For example, the inability to leave a job in which you feel imprisoned may derive from traumatic memories of your father's being laid off and unemployed for an extended time. Instead of consciously and compassionately directing our experience of life, we allow ourselves to be victimized by seemingly inescapable feelings of fear that control our thinking. Too often the message we give ourselves is "I have no choice."

Affirmations consist of positive statements, always expressed in the present tense and devoid of negative words, which powerfully convey and express an image either directly or indirectly. Affirmations should be kept short and simple, no longer than two brief sentences. As you practice using affirmations, your images will become clearer, their details more precise. The clearer and more focused these images become, the sooner they will be realized. For instance, if one of your goals is to make money, a corresponding affirmation might be stated: "I am earning enough money to satisfy all of my needs and desires." If you are trying to lose weight, then your affirmation might say: "I am losing weight steadily and comfortably." If your goal is to have more energy, you might affirm: "I have a limitless supply of vitality and life energy."

In constructing your affirmations, use declarative statements in the present tense that convey a decisive action and imagery that clearly shows what you want to occur. A negatively expressed command only confuses the imagery. For example, if your goal is to lose weight and your affirmation reads "I am not going to eat sweets," the subconscious mind focuses on the concrete image of sweets—candy, ice cream, and cookies. Instead, formulate this affirmation using images that clearly picture the intended action: "I am enjoying only those foods that are low in calories yet nurturing to my body." Use of the present tense also adds more immediacy and hence has a stronger impact on your behavior.

Now that you know how to create powerful affirmations, return to your list of physical, environmental, mental, emotional, spiritual, and social goals, and rewrite each one into the form of an affirmation. Here are some sample goals and possible affirmations. Keep in mind that we're not looking for great poetry, just effective communication with the subconscious. Content here is more important than form. The affirmation should stimulate a state of mind akin to a waking dream.

PHYSICAL HEALTH

- **Goal:** To cure my arthritis.
  Affirmation: *"My knees are flexible, strong, and free of pain. They move easily and allow me to enjoy playing tennis."*
- **Goal:** To improve my golf game.
  Affirmation: *"I am unhurried, focused, and completely relaxed on every stroke."*

ENVIRONMENTAL

- **Goal:** To live and work in a healthier environment.
  Affirmation: *"I am nourished by the pure air and tranquil beauty that surround me."*
- **Goal:** To spend more time outdoors.
  Affirmation: *"I am empowered by nature and spend some time outdoors every day."*

MENTAL

- **Goal:** To work at a job that doesn't make me anxious and irritable at home.
  Affirmation: *"I eagerly look forward to arriving at work, and I feel fulfilled when I leave at the end of the day."*
  Affirmation: *"My job is a stimulating challenge that brings out all of my best talents."*
- **Goal:** To make a lot of money and feel financially secure.
  Affirmation: *"I am making more than enough money to satisfy all of my needs and desires."*
  Affirmation: *"I am thriving financially, and the power and energy of money flow freely into my life."*

EMOTIONAL

- **Goal:** To stop denying fear and sadness.
  Affirmation: *"I am safely expressing all of my fears and sadness."*
- **Goal:** Not to use alcohol and drugs to escape painful feelings.
  Affirmation: *"I am allowing myself the gift of fully experiencing my feelings."*

SOCIAL

- **Goal:** To have more intimacy in my marriage.
  Affirmation: *"I am affectionate to my wife. I respect and understand her needs and desires."*
- **Goal:** To improve my relationship with my father.
  Affirmation: *"I am accepting and forgiving of my father. I enjoy our time together."*

SPIRITUAL

- **Goal:** To add more spirit and dimension to my everyday life.
  Affirmation: *"Every day I encounter God in unexpected ways."*
- **Goal:** To have greater appreciation of life.
  Affirmation: *"I recognize a multitude of blessings in my life."*

To conveniently carry your own list of affirmations, photocopy the form opposite and fill it in with your own affirmations. Use as many copies as you need. Before you know it, you will have memorized your affirmations and you will be able to use them anytime during the day.

Since your affirmation speaks directly to your subconscious, express it in a way that feels convincing to you. *Experience* your affirmation. When choosing a goal, remember that you don't need a definitive plan for reaching it. Most men resist the notion of desiring something that they don't know how to achieve. Don't let this stop you. Instead, take

Daily Affirmations:
Do one or two for each component of health.

Physical
Goal:
Affirmation:

Environmental
Goal:
Affirmation:

Mental
Goal:
Affirmation:

Emotional
Goal:
Affirmation:

Social
Goal:
Affirmation:

Spiritual
Goal:
Affirmation:

Use positive statements only, no negative words. Write everything in the present tense, using no more than two short sentences. Write and vocalize each affirmation at least once in a soothing, confident voice, followed by visualization.

a risk, make this commitment, and let the power of the affirmation unfold before you. Allow the 95 percent of your brain that you haven't used to reveal some of its unlimited capacity. Don't resist using affirmations because you feel as if you're lying to yourself. You're lying to yourself only as much as the architect at his drafting table sketching preliminary drawings for a stunning office building. His intent, like yours, is for the sketch to become reality. He too is able to transport himself through time, to bring the future into a present vision.

The practice of affirmations can take many forms: reciting them out loud, writing them down, visualizing them, typing them on a computer keyboard, recording them on a cassette and listening to them. Schedule ten minutes each day, preferably in the morning, to work with your affirmations. Ideally, you should be in a quiet place where you will not be interrupted. Sit in the same position described for the One-Minute Drill (see page 58): feet flat on the floor, hands on your thighs, back straight. If you are reciting your affirmations, voice them in a soothing and confident tone. Express each affirmation once as you go down the list. (Limit your list to ten to twelve affirmations.) If you want to concentrate on one affirmation in particular, rewriting it many times over so that it fills one side of a sheet of 8½-by-11-inch paper is effective. Although listening to affirmations is usually less effective than reciting or writing, if you want to record them on a cassette and listen to them as you drive to work you can derive some added benefit. Possibly, the most pow-

erful method may be *the combination of writing, reciting, and visualizing.* For example, as you write down the affirmation, recite it out loud. When you have finished each one, close your eyes and picture what that affirmation looks like or feels like for twenty to thirty seconds. Try to engage every sense in creating the experience of this affirmation.

Although it may have taken you several hours, or even days, to establish your list of goals and affirmations, it shouldn't take more than ten to twenty minutes a day to experience them. You might be amazed, as I was, to find that it took a relatively short time— sometimes only days or weeks—to watch them become reality. Within two months of using these techniques, some of my patients have realized nearly half of their goals—a new job, home, partner, reconciliation of a rift in a relationship, realization of a long-standing professional goal, significant weight loss, or achievement of physical feats. Practice daily for at least sixty consecutive days. Before you know it, your dreams will start to come true.

During the day, whenever you are confronted with a negative or limiting belief, use your corresponding affirmation to loosen its hold. For example, if you are chronically late or always feeling pressed for time, you may hear the negative message, "I'll never have enough time to . . ." Your corresponding affirmation might be "Everything is happening at just the right time." Or if you're a perfectionist, you may hear yourself say, "Why can't you ever get it right?" The majority of us tend to be perfectionists and beat ourselves up when we make mistakes. Making mistakes may, in fact, be our greatest fear. But we can always choose to believe "there are no mistakes—only lessons." There's something we can learn from every so-called mistake. Although many men might initially reject it, I have found the affirmation "I am always doing the best I can" to be the most helpful one I've ever used. This affirmation can be an intermediate step to getting beyond the self-criticism of the ego. Its message of forgiveness allows us to be more accepting of ourselves and to maintain our confidence and high performance levels. Top athletes and high achievers both share this ability to quickly forgive themselves and stay focused in the moment. If you think of the present moment as the sum of all of your life experiences and influences—parents, education, the particular stresses of that day—then at every moment of every day you are always doing the best you can. This practice of self-acceptance and forgiveness is crucial to creating peace of mind and for men to thrive. In chapter 6, there is a "forgiveness meditation."

Playing the Game of Self-Realization ("Re-creating" Yourself)

Having created a new set of goals and the ground rules for their realization, let's look more closely at the playing of the game. The actual attainment of a goal, or the momentary thrill of victory, comprises only a small fraction of our lives. Most of our lives are spent working toward our goals. *Thriving is all about enjoying the process as much as the result.* This redirecting of your life to achieve a state of thriving is based on seeing that new life so intensely that you feel as though you are actually living it. Do this long enough and you will. This concentration of energy on a specific image is the heart and soul of *re-creating* yourself. We can do this in part through affirmations, but we can also shape our lives through the practice of more extended **visualizations.** These visualizations consist of more detailed scene-setting that uses all of the senses to literally create a new reality as vividly as possible. What would a typical visualization look like?

Let's say you have entrepreneurial aspirations, and you're presently feeling stuck in a nine-to-five job. You're excited about an idea for a unique air-cleaner but are afraid to risk leaving your present job to launch this new project. You have two kids, a nice home, but your wife's income alone can't maintain your cost of living. You do have some money in savings and some conservative investments, but even though you're convinced that this new air-cleaner has the potential to be incredibly successful, you're still too insecure to use any of your savings to give yourself a jump start. To clear this hurdle of fear, you need a powerful combination of affirmation and visualization. After affirming, "My air-cleaner business is a smashing success," here's what your visualization might look like.

You picture yourself
• finding a manufacturer
• completing a comprehensive business plan

- successfully meeting with venture capitalists
- signing contracts with the largest distributors, or with Wal-Mart or Sears
- enjoying the results of such successful marketing that your cleaner becomes a household name—in fact, everyone wants one
- observing people buying your air-cleaner in droves and walking out of the stores with looks of satisfaction
- enjoying a flow of monthly commission checks that steadily increases—more money than you'd ever imagined before— but now you can see it clearly
- buying a Mercedes-Benz, a country estate, your kids going to private schools, and you and your wife enjoying regular vacations at exotic places all over the world

This could be the start of a new business, a new product, a new foundation, or a new job. It can take place in any "arena" where you have committed to playing the game of life at your highest level. *Thriving is about the joy of playing the game, whatever game you've chosen.* We all know that winning feels better than losing, but the more you enjoy the game, the greater your chances of victory. This is because the more you enjoy the game, the more fully you participate in the deeper rhythms and dimensions of its unfolding. Through affirmations and extended visualizations, you create a sense of participation that releases you from the constraints of the mind, its judgments—and the need to win—into a realm of pure joy and creativity. Ironically, the mind's ability to direct the resources of body and

spirit brings these guided daydreams to this exquisite moment of exhilaration and focuses you in the present. By escaping the constraints of the past to create a new reality, we not only enjoy whatever we are doing, but we start to "win" on a daily basis. Through this reinforcement, thriving becomes a way of life.

Commitment is the single most important ingredient that will allow you to play your game at your highest level. By using the goal-affirmation list and extended visualizations, you give shape and focus to your commitments. The strength of those commitments will be determined by the time and discipline you devote to realizing those visions. There are four practical consequences of working with affirmations. As with anything else that you practice, (1) you *will* see results; (2) these results may not be exactly what you had anticipated (make sure your affirmations accurately reflect your needs and desires—who you are); (3) with practice, as you become more aware of both your conscious and unconscious desires, you will continue to modify your list of affirmations; (4) you will find yourself moving out of old ruts and exploring new options.

Your commitment to realizing goals through affirmations and visualization is like planting seeds. You water and nurture the seeds with your attention and energy. Though they remain invisible in the ground, they are quietly germinating and preparing to sprout. To realize the full power of affirmations, you must understand the three stages of this "growing" process: desire, belief, and expectation. Think of your *desire* as a goal existing in the future. Your *belief* in that goal's becoming a reality exists in the present as an affirmation. Your *expectation* that your desire will occur is based in part on the clarity of your vision and previous success in having manifested other goals in the past.

In a way you are creating a new pattern of energy that will change your experience of time. Conventionally, we think of events in the present as having been conditioned by events in the past, which will in turn be reflected in our future. However, by imagining the future, or goal, in the present through the power of affirmation, we absorb its image with all the certainty as if it had already occurred in the past. You might even say we have used this new pattern of energy to dissolve the old demarcations between past, present, and future. In so doing, we create a new reality in a new "present."

The fuel for this new sense of reality is the imaginative energy we bring to this process, the energy contained in our commitment—or *will*—"to see it through." Just as seeds need life energy, or *chi*, contained in earth, sunlight, water, and air, we too need to feed our visions or affirmations with the power of *chi* in the form of unconditional love. We nourish our commitment to these goals with beliefs predicated on a sense of what feels most loving to us, regardless of what society, parents, or even our spouse might say. *Just as you will learn to love your body in chapter 3, here you are learning to create a loving mind filled with nurturing messages and images.* A mind infused with the power of unconditional love can transform old patterns of energy and un-

healthy behavior into a new thriving reality. This is the core of self-realization.

Staying in the Game: The Importance of Character

The difference between sports in this country and martial arts as practiced in the East is what I call the character factor. In this country when the baseball season is over, major league players retire to their homes and take time off for an extended period. Some play winter ball to improve their skills, but most simply relax. When martial artists finish competing, they go back into the dojo and resume their training. For martial artists, training is a test of character that is never complete. *The discipline of their art extends to every facet of their lives.* Every moment is an opportunity to display character, and it imbues even the smallest gesture.

In our culture, Cal Ripken Jr. is an exception to the rule. All accounts describe him as training as hard in the off-season as he plays during the regular season. As a result, his total commitment to his craft has allowed him literally to stay in every game over a span of fourteen seasons: 2,153 games. To accomplish this, he clearly developed a different vision of himself from most other athletes and probably reinforced that vision with his own type of affirmation that expressed a fundamental joy in the game. As Ripken explained in the December 1995 *Sports Illustrated* naming him Sportsman of the Year, "If you could play baseball every day, wouldn't you?" The question reflects a basic message Ripken has probably given himself every day of his career.

The art of thriving is a lifelong commitment to changing behavior. Like martial arts, thriving entails a transformation of character that doesn't end with achieving your goals— even a World Series or Super Bowl victory. Only with time, your thriving skills improve, the challenge becomes less of a struggle, and the process grows more enjoyable. The Japanese word for the efficiency and ease that comes with the mastery of technique is *jissen.* The judo master who effortlessly sweeps a larger, younger opponent to the mat displays *jissen.* Rather than putting in sixty-hour weeks to keep up in the workplace, the thriving executive has learned to put in fewer hours of "conscious" creativity and has far more to show for it. This too is *jissen.* The path to this level of mastery is not easy. The most important part is to stay in the game: to stay engaged, focused, and committed.

Some of the qualities that enable you to strengthen commitment are patience, courage, discipline, flexibility, forgiveness, humility, and humor. Each quality helps you to face the stress that is part of playing your game at its highest level. Together they determine that measure of a man that we call *character.* Typically a man demonstrates that character through his ability to stay in the game. By staying committed, even in the face of great odds, he transforms himself.

As a neophyte on the road to thriving, you will take your share of losses, but they do not necessarily signify a regression, simply a part of changing. There is no universal formula or

timetable to guide us through this process. For most men, the opportunity for greatest change occurs in their late thirties and early forties. Since each of us is unique—a blend of genetic, environmental, social, and spiritual ingredients—no two of us have the exact same needs and desires, nor the same path to thriving.

However, the practice of thriving must go further than mental imagery alone. Commitment means vision and practice. And if you look at any of the books on inner golf, skiing, or tennis, the techniques are the same: first you visualize, then you practice to physically emulate that inner vision of how your stroke should feel or how your turns should be carved. Unless you're actively engaged and grounded in doing those things in the material realm that you have visualized and affirmed mentally, you'll be unable to progress. If I had not taken the risk of changing my approach to medicine by treating more challenging patients holistically, speaking out publicly, becoming more actively involved in the leadership of the AHMA, and thereby playing a role in shaping medicine's newest specialty, my vision would never have materialized.

The most difficult part of making your vision a physical reality is precisely this risk factor. Not knowing how you will achieve your goal, how long it will take, or what it will actually feel like once you get there engenders a tremendous sense of risk. This fear of the unknown knocks most men out of the game; instead, they opt for secure and known pathways, even if in the long run those "easier" choices prove more painful or self-destructive.

The greater your *involvement* in your self-transformation—in the behavior and actions that realize that vision—the more information and feedback you will have, and the less fearful you will be. Information is power. The more experience and feedback you derive from staying in the game and taking risks, the better prepared you are to react. *The less your fear factor, the greater is your peace of mind and level of performance.*

The driving force behind creating your ideal life and fulfilling your greatest potential is commitment. To begin to change your life, start by looking at your body and choose what you'd like to change. Would you like to heal a disease, to lose weight, increase energy, or rehabilitate an old injury? As you will see in the next chapter, *the body provides the clearest evidence of the quality of your commitment.* If you have committed to losing weight or to eating more intelligently, you will see results in a matter of days. If you commit to exercising regularly, you will feel a difference in your energy level within a week. Remember, the only limit to the changes you can make lies in the scope of your imagination and in your commitment to practice. The experience of this fundamental truth is the key to peace of mind.

T h e   P h y s i c a l l y   F i t   M a l e

The body is a machine made for living.

Tolstoy

———————————•———————————

In the days of vaudeville, a familiar comedic sketch featured a male patient sitting in a doctor's office with his shirt off, undergoing a physical exam. The doctor was usually an older man with a stethoscope and a nose-and-throat mirror around his head. As he grilled the patient with a series of diagnostic questions, he thumped the patient's chest, listened to his heart, and hammered his knee with a rubber mallet. Inevitably, the examination was interrupted by a bleached-blond, buxom nurse in a tight-fitting uniform. She would sashay in and out of the office, assisting the doctor through a series of exaggerated postures that required increasingly more physical contact with the patient. By the end of his examination, the patient was so aroused that he was focusing his attention more on the voluptuous nurse than on his own physical problem. Burlesque though this skit may be, it is probably a fairly accurate depiction of how most men will pay more attention to the nearest female body than they do to their own.

The fact is we men live so much in our heads that we hardly inhabit our bodies. Appearance is everything. We will enlarge our pecs, flatten our stomachs, and build our biceps, but we rarely pay attention to what goes on inside. Other than noticing the flavor, we seldom give a thought to what we are eating, drinking, or breathing. Not only don't we know how these factors affect our bodies, we've become desensitized to most physical dysfunction. It takes a medical crisis to get our attention, and then we tend to rely too much on the detached evaluation of doctors to describe our condition. In so doing, we relinquish our responsibility for caring for ourselves and distance ourselves even further from our physical condition. We may believe we are maintaining good health by undergoing annual physicals, but these exams are of limited value. Several good preventive tests—PSA (prostate), cholesterol, and a stress EKG (treadmill)—do provide helpful information and early detection. However, if the results are good, most men will use these annual physicals as a rationalization for not paying attention to their bodies the rest of the year.

The purpose of this chapter is to help you heighten your awareness of your body so that you become tuned in to the slightest aberration and dysfunction *before* it reaches crisis proportions, while learning effective methods for *maintaining* optimal physical health. This tendency in men to wait too long to address both physical and emotional discomfort might well be the single most important factor in contributing to men's poor health and their high rate of suicide and drug addiction. It explains why men are in the habit of surviving, or "just hanging in there," instead of thriving.

When you are in pain or have a chronic disease and drag yourself to the doctor, he starts by taking a history to identify the major symptoms that characterize a particular disease. The physician reviews these symptoms to make a diagnosis so he can prescribe a treatment. Some doctors even feed symptoms into a computer and let the machine make a diagnosis. This mechanical methodology cannot possibly match an individual's heightened awareness of and sensitivity to his own body. In reality, you don't need seven years of medical training to take your own medical history, and you don't have to rely on a doctor to provide a comprehensive evaluation of your own physical condition. He might be able to provide you with a medical diagnosis and treatment plan using drugs or possibly surgery, but he can't tell you how your body *feels*. Only you can know that, and developing this knowledge and awareness is a skill that takes practice. This ability is an integral part of training to thrive. You have an array of built-in sensors and an onboard "computer" that can be ex-

quisitely precise in giving you feedback on your condition and guidance on how to program your body for better health. If you ignore that awareness and relinquish responsibility for your health to doctors, you will limit your ability to experience optimal health.

The first step in building this sensitivity is to establish an ongoing dialogue with your body. In this and the following chapter, you will learn to hear what your body has been trying to tell you all these years, primarily through pain and dysfunction. You will learn to apply a simple method to scan the body for early signs of tension and discomfort while fine-tuning it as well. For example, the body scan will make you more aware of your energy level at any given moment, the muscle tension in your upper back and shoulders, the constriction of your bowel, the volume of your air intake, your level of hydration and its corresponding effect on a multitude of functions. This flow of information is an integral part of your body's operating system. The greater your awareness of this stream of information as it manifests within the body, the greater will be your potential for achieving optimal physical well-being. If you already have a diagnosed disease, you will learn to understand its physical pathology, the imbalance it has created in your body, and how to restore the balance. This "body scan" will develop into an ongoing dialogue and will become a part of your daily regimen. You will probably be surprised at the depth and *intelligence* of your body's communications with you and more fully appreciate its capacity to heal itself, with your cooperation.

The "Body" portion of the Thriving Self-Test at the beginning of this book should provide a starting point for you to evaluate your present physical status. In addition to measuring your level of thriving, the self-test will identify specific pain and problem areas, while providing parameters to help you set goals and to program your system to thrive. If you have not done so already, take the entire Thriving Self-Test. Answer the questions as honestly as you can, and total your score. Try not to judge the questions as you go through them; simply respond to all of them objectively. Although you will grade yourself, your score will not prevent you from thriving . . . or disqualify you from obtaining life insurance. When you have finished, take note of which section scored lowest: body, mind, or spirit. Are there specific questions that you don't understand or perhaps feel do not apply to you? Were there specific questions you found difficult to score because you felt that you lacked an adequate standard against which to measure yourself? Circle these specific questions and put the self-test aside. We'll return to the results throughout Part I of this book.

When Henry Ford rolled out the first automobiles, they were simple mechanisms with an operating system consisting of a steering wheel, gas pedal, brake, and clutch. As time went on, engineering grew more sophisticated. In the last fifteen years, the automobile's range of function has expanded geometrically. Computerized climate control, fuel injection, braking function, and warning systems are now commonplace. In short, the operating system of the automobile has grown in step with *the expanded awareness of what an automobile could be.* By building intelligence into the automobile, man has greatly expanded its performance potential. On the other hand, the human body is an organic mechanism, possessing a built-in intelligence that we have only begun to explore. Each of us has a unique body with its own particular programming, the intelligence of which extends to every single cell. The potential for shaping or reconfiguring this body is almost unlimited, as long as we understand the body's operating system that enables us to cooperate with it. If we don't make the effort, it's like having an IBM supercomputer in the basement, but forgetting to read the instruction manual. Think of this chapter as your instruction manual to that unique supercomputer we call the body.

Conventionally, we believed that all intelligence was located in and directed by the brain. Thanks to PNI research, we now know that intelligence resides not only in the brain, but throughout the body—in fact in every cell. This intelligence is transmitted through three of the body's regulatory systems—the central nervous system, the immune system, and the endocrine system. Together they constitute an intricately complex and sensitive network that not only protects us from disease but provides the key to thriving and optimal physical health.

Let's look more closely at the three parts of this network. The first component, the *central nervous system,* consists of the brain, spinal cord, and neurons. (Neurons are nerve cells located in the brain, spinal cord, and throughout the body. Like microscopic processors, their function is to store and transmit information.) The *immune system* consists of white blood cells and unique proteins called immunoglobulins, which circulate throughout the body attacking and eliminating potentially harmful antigens (foreign substances), such as bacteria, viruses, pollen, toxins, chemicals, and cancer cells. Also included in the immune system are those organs involved in generating and storing, and destroying old and defective, white blood cells: bone marrow, thymus gland, spleen, liver, and lymph nodes. The *endocrine system* consists of organs that secrete hormones into the blood, triggering a response in other organs and affecting bodily function. The endocrine organs include the pituitary, pineal, thyroid, parathyroid, and adrenal glands, along with the pancreas and testicles. (In women, these would include the ovaries.)

Science has just begun to reveal the complex and intimate connection among these three regulatory systems that transmit the body's intelligence and direct its defense system. For example, consider the function of natural opioids, chemicals that are produced by neurons in the central nervous system and by some white blood cells. In addition to serving as immune regulators, opioids induce a feeling of well-being. Opioids directly affect the immune system because, as PNI research has shown, natural opioid receptors appear on monocytes—scavenger white blood cells that destroy viruses. On an emotional level, this means that if you are feeling particularly euphoric because you

just learned that you got a substantial raise, you are probably secreting natural opioids. On a cellular level, these opioids are traveling from your brain throughout your body in a matter of seconds and connecting with monocytes in the bloodstream, like satellites docking in space. The monocytes receive messages from the opioids that trigger a Pac-Man–like response, and together the opioid-monocyte tag team sets to work, cleansing your entire bloodstream of potential infection in a matter of minutes. Although this process of monocytes removing bacteria or viruses is an integral aspect of daily immune function, it is certainly enhanced by opioid stimulation. Conversely, if you hate your job and you are chronically depressed, you are not secreting opioids into the bloodstream, and your monocyte function is also depressed. As a result, the potential for developing a viral infection such as a cold greatly increases.

As you can see, a very real connection exists between our emotional experience and our cellular function. Mind and body are one and the same. Because physical fitness ultimately reflects mental well-being, staying healthy depends on making life-enhancing choices. This chapter will present a variety of healthy options, all of which, if put into practice, guarantee to improve your physical well-being. If you commit to practicing all of them for at least three months, you will experience dramatic improvement in your condition. You will allow your body to function in the way nature intended.

The body has the capacity to regenerate almost every one of its cells each year. It also has the capacity to maintain homeostasis—a steady state of function—in fairly extreme conditions. However, the body can derail itself in an instant if you feed it the wrong information or attitude. The body's condition is a reflection of the messages that it receives from the mind, and conversely the mind—if left to its own devices—reflects the condition of the body. What we have is an exquisitely sensitive marriage between two partners who want only to accommodate one another. At best this marriage can provide a wonderfully cooperative relationship that achieves goals far beyond the potential of either partner alone. At worst, it can degenerate into a nagging conflict in which each partner mirrors the other's misery. To succeed, mind and body need conscious direction to keep both partners on task. As an operating system, body and mind work together only as well as the nourishment, information, and instructions fed into them. The caveat to computer programmers—GIGO—is particularly apt for developing a cooperative relationship between mind and body: "Garbage in—garbage out."

Let's take a look at your body's "owner's manual" and see what its basic components are and how they work.

Breathing

To the extent that you breathe is the extent that you experience life.

Anonymous

The most vital function of the body is respiration—breathing. Whereas you can survive a month without food, and about one week without water, most of us cannot survive more than a few minutes without air. Breathing originates traumatically at birth and for the majority of us continues unconsciously and inefficiently until death.

The primary purpose of breathing is to carry oxygen *to,* and to remove carbon dioxide *from,* every cell and tissue in the body. Every cell in the body requires an ample supply of oxygen. The greater the supply of oxygen, the less the risk of disease and the greater the opportunity for optimal functioning. Conversely, the damage resulting from oxygen deprivation can weaken any tissue or organ in the body. Specifically, oxygen is responsible for the production of the energy required for every basic bodily function. The essence of this chemical energy on a cellular level is ATP (adenosine triphosphate)—the result of the enzymatic reduction of proteins, fats, and carbohydrates in the presence of oxygen. The other by-products of this energy production are heat, water, and carbon dioxide.

The cellular content of ATP throughout the body is responsible for the body's total energy level and its subsequent ability to perform all of its vital functions. Reduce the oxygen content of the ATP and you will diminish the body's ability to function. One well-documented cause of reduced oxygen supply is an environmental deficiency, such as high carbon monoxide and smoke pollution, or high altitude (for every thousand feet above sea level, the oxygen content diminishes by more than 3 percent).

However, aware as we may be of the environmental causes for reduced oxygen content in the body, the main cause of chronic oxygen depletion is shallow, inefficient chest breathing. We may be somewhat limited in our ability to change atmospheric or environmental conditions, but we can certainly change the way we breathe. The poor mechanics of our breathing are significantly responsible for reducing oxygen supply. By improving the way we breathe, we can provide considerably more oxygen to every cell in our body.

The primary job of the heart and lungs is to pump oxygen, which is carried by red blood cells through arteries to reach every cell in your body. To provide the body an optimal oxygen supply (1) the heart's pumping action must be strong, (2) the arteries must be free of any constriction or obstruction, and (3) the lungs must function near full capacity. The greatest impediment to an optimal oxygen supply and the prospect of thriving is cigarette smoking. (If you intend to thrive but still have your pack-a-day habit, you need to commit to getting rid of it right now.)

Any type of heart disease will decrease the efficiency and strength of the heart's pumping action. This may be caused by the scarring of a previous heart attack, diminished coronary artery blood flow resulting in angina, abnormal heart rhythm, or by a variety of other heart problems. *Constricted* arteries can result from high blood pressure, which causes a chronic contraction of the muscles lining the arterial walls. *Blocked* arteries can be pro-

duced by fatty deposits or plaques on the inner lining of the arterial wall, which impede the flow of blood—a condition called arteriosclerosis (hardening of the arteries). When a coronary artery supplying the heart muscle with oxygen is completely cut off, it results in a heart attack—the death of a portion of the heart. If the damage to the heart is extensive, it will result in death. If an artery to the brain is obstructed, cutting off oxygen, it results in a stroke—the death of a piece of the brain. Diseases of the lungs that reduce oxygen supply in men are usually chronic obstructive pulmonary diseases (COPD). These include emphysema, which results in scarring and destruction of the small air sacs (alveoli), and chronic bronchitis, which consists of chronic inflammation that narrows the large airways (bronchi). This latter condition is most often seen in cigarette smokers and can lead to emphysema. These three physical crises—heart attacks, strokes, and lung disease—are three of the leading causes of death among men.

The heart is generally recognized as the most important muscle in the body. However, the most overlooked—in its contribution to respiration, to the function of the heart, and to optimal health—is the *diaphragm*, the muscle that controls the lungs. The diaphragm is a thin, dome-shaped muscle connected to the ribs, breastbone (sternum), and spine. It separates the chest (thoracic) cavity from the abdominal cavity. During restful inhalation in a healthy individual, the diaphragm contracts, pulling downward pressure on the abdominal cavity and creating expanded capacity in the chest, as the resulting vacuum draws air into the lungs. During exhalation, the diaphragm relaxes and the passive recoil of the elastic structure of the lungs, chest, and abdomen expels carbon dioxide.

Most people breathe inefficiently by using their chest muscles instead of the diaphragm to drive respiration. The chest muscles expand the chest cavity front to back but do not fully engage the diaphragm. As a result, the lower lungs do not fill with fresh air and the body receives only a partial supply of oxygen.

Poor posture can also diminish lung capacity by compressing the chest cavity against the diaphragm and preventing its full contraction. *"Abdominal breathing" is the method of respiration that uses full contraction of the diaphragm.* Developing the habit of breathing abdominally *provides the physical foundation on which thriving is built.* There is probably no single step you can take in training to thrive that will so profoundly and positively affect body, mind, and spirit.

You can learn abdominal breathing in less than a minute. You can practice it anywhere, even right now as you read this book. It costs nothing, and since you're already breathing twelve to sixteen times per minute (about twenty-three thousand times a day), you may as well be doing it right. Here's how.

Standing in profile in front of a mirror with your shirt off, inhale through your nose and observe how your torso fills with air. If the chest alone expands, you are using only the chest muscles. You are breathing inefficiently because you are limiting your lung capacity. On the other hand, if you inhale and your belly expands, you are breathing abdominally.

For maximum oxygen intake, expand the belly first and then the chest.

Another way to physically experience the abdominal breath is to lie on your back with your fingers lightly interlaced over your belly. As you inhale, contract the diaphragm. This expands the abdominal cavity, and your fingers on each hand should part approximately one inch. If your fingers do not part, you are still using your chest muscles alone instead of your diaphragm.

Once you have experienced the basic abdominal breath, you are now ready to practice a series of four exercises that will help instill the habit of abdominal breathing. The One-Minute Drill and the Quiet Five can reduce heart rate, blood pressure, emotional stress, and headache, while providing a greater supply of oxygen along with a heightened sense of well-being. The Brain Booster can strengthen focus and concentration on specific tasks. The Body Scan can help build body awareness by identifying areas of tension and discomfort. All of these exercises will help to make abdominal breathing a habit.

One-Minute Drill

Sit in a chair without armrests, feet flat on the floor, and thighs parallel to the floor. Your back is straight, either supported or unsupported by the chair back. Lay one hand on top of the other, or place your palms on your thighs slightly above the knee. If you prefer to use your hands to monitor the contractions of your diaphragm, then lightly lace your fingers over your abdomen. To reduce visual stimulation, close your eyes halfway (or entirely). Abdominally inhale and exhale slowly through the nose for one minute. The breath should originate in the diaphragm, first expanding the abdominal cavity, then filling the chest. To stay focused on your breath, count each cycle of inhalation and exhalation as one full breath. Make a mental note of how many breaths you take in a minute. Over a period of weeks, you will find that you can comfortably reduce your breaths to three or four per minute. Stay in a comfortable rhythm and don't strain. Feel your body relaxing and releasing tension with each exhalation, and note the areas of greatest tension. Maintain this rhythm for about one minute, although you can certainly go longer if you have the time. At first, it may be helpful to use a kitchen timer so you are not distracted keeping track of the time. Do the One-Minute Drill at least once a day for twenty-one days, or if you are willing to commit a little more time for increased benefits, then try the Quiet Five.

Quiet Five

Seated as in the One-Minute Drill, you again breathe abdominally, but this time for five minutes and in a different rhythm. Inhale through the nose for a count of eight ("one thousand one, one thousand two"). Hold the breath for a count of four. Exhale through the nose for a count of eight. Then hold the breath for a count of four before beginning the cycle again. Continue to breathe in this rhythm for five minutes. If you interrupt your rhythm or lose track of where you are in the cycle, simply start over and reestablish your rhythm. It's best to do this in a quiet place, where you will be undisturbed. Practice the Quiet Five daily for twenty-one days.

In just five minutes, you will experience a deep sense of relaxation and peace of mind. By focusing on your count, you can more easily let go of thoughts and concerns that may interrupt your concentration. Try to become a detached observer of your thoughts as you breathe through this exercise, while also paying attention to areas of tightness or discomfort. On a cellular level, the Quiet Five will oxygenate and recharge your entire body. It will pay dividends in both greater relaxation and in higher performance: increased clarity, concentration, and creativity.

Shoshin is a Japanese word that literally means "beginner's mind." It refers to the open awareness that often precedes our first experience of an activity, which by repetition may become routine or commonplace. Whether in martial arts or meditation, awareness of your breathing is a way to bring yourself back into the present moment. Focusing on your breathing clears the mind and can be the most easily accessible harmonizer that we have. In addition to slowing the heart rate and metabolism, the breathing exercises in this chapter can reduce levels of adrenaline. They will diminish anxious imagery, reduce brain wave activity, and create a sense of harmony and peace.

Brain Booster

After practicing the One-Minute Drill or Quiet Five exercises for twenty-one days, you can supplement this regimen with the Brain

Booster. This exercise involves alternately breathing through one nostril at a time while pressing the other one closed. Although science cannot explain how it happens, the benefit from the Brain Booster include greater capacity for either the right or left hemispheres of the brain. If you are faced with a task specific to the right or left hemisphere, you can modify the Brain Booster to cycle through the nostril that activates its related hemisphere. For example, if you are writing a speech or solving complex mathematical computations involving the left brain, you would perform the Brain Booster, inhaling and exhaling through the right nostril only. For artistic or creative tasks engaging the right brain, breathe only through the left nostril. Studies done at the Salk Institute for Biological Sciences in San Diego have shown that breathing through one nostril for up to ten to fifteen minutes can greatly enhance the performance of the opposite brain hemisphere.

To stimulate both hemispheres equally, sit with feet flat on the floor and the right palm in your lap. Begin by closing the left nostril with your left thumb as you inhale through the right nostril to a count of eight. Press the right nostril closed with your left forefinger, as you hold your breath for a count of four. Release the left forefinger and exhale for a count of eight. Close the right nostril with your left forefinger and hold your breath for a count of four. Reverse the cycle by releasing the thumb and inhaling through the left nostril for a count of eight. Close the left nostril with the thumb, and hold the breath for a count of four. Lift the thumb and exhale through the left

nostril for a count of eight. Close the left nostril and hold the breath for four counts. This completes one cycle of the Brain Booster. Do four cycles each morning for one week. The next week add one more cycle, and continue to add one cycle per week until you are doing seven cycles per session.

If you experience nasal congestion and are unable to perform any of these three exercises, don't be discouraged. Try breathing partially through the mouth or shorten the count. Better yet, see the natural remedies for nasal congestion in chapter 10.

Body Scan

The Body Scan is a method of using abdominal breath to identify and release tension areas within the body. Assume a seated position as you would for the One-Minute Drill. As you breathe abdominally, mentally scan your body slowly from head to toe, identifying areas of tightness or pain. As you locate each problem, think of the breath as a charge of healing energy that you direct into the constriction to relieve the tension and promote relaxation. When you have completed the total body scan, return your attention to the lower abdomen and finish with the One-Minute Drill. With the Body Scan, there is no counting or timing of breaths. But if you do a thorough job and focus on every part of your body for at least two or three breaths (more if you encounter tension), then you might spend thirty to forty minutes on this exercise. The relaxation rewards can be profound. It can be especially beneficial helping you get to sleep. It doesn't matter whether you start from the head or the toes; work your way methodically from one end of the body to the other, paying close attention to muscles, joints, and even organs.

To create the habit of abdominal breathing, adapt the One-Minute Drill to everyday situations. For example, if you are sitting on the bus or are caught in traffic, take a minute to breath abdominally, even if you can't half-close your eyes and sit with your hands in your lap. Create instances in which you automatically remember to use the One-Minute Drill. For example, every time you stop at a traffic light, begin the One-Minute Drill. You might also apply the same association to the stopping or completion of any task, no matter how small. For example, completing a phone conversation, finishing brushing your teeth, or closing the newspaper would trigger the One-Minute Drill. By association, the act of abdominal breathing will work backward to the beginning of each activity and can eventually accompany it from beginning to end. For example, you will soon find yourself breathing abdominally throughout the phone conversation. It may even make you a better listener.

The physiological effects of abdominal breathing are apparent in conscious and unconscious ways, while affecting every cell and tissue in the body. One of the unmistakable effects of abdominal breathing is that it will bring you into the present moment and help you to stay centered in the most stressful situations. If you take nothing else from this book except this simple technique, and practice it on a daily basis, I guarantee you will feel better. You will also be well on your way to thriving.

Air Quality

Now that you have a better idea of *how* to breathe, I'd like you to begin paying more attention to *what* you're breathing. As a result of the environmental plague of air pollution, most urban dwellers are breathing unhealthy air. The EPA says that 60 percent of Americans live in areas where breathing is a risk to one's health, and that indoor air is often far more polluted than outdoor air. At least sixty thousand of us will die every year from air pollution, and its effects are responsible for respiratory disease becoming our *first environmental epidemic.* Four of America's most common chronic diseases are now respiratory ailments: chronic sinusitis (#1), allergies (#5), chronic bronchitis (#8), and asthma (#9). More than 92 million people, one out of every three, are afflicted with one or more of these four conditions.

By far, the greatest health hazard of the indoor air pollutants is tobacco smoke—even if you're a nonsmoker. The American Heart Association estimates that, in addition to its effects on lungs, secondhand smoke could be a contributing factor in the heart-disease deaths of forty thousand nonsmoking Americans every year.

In 1992, a Harvard research team reported the first direct medical evidence that secondhand smoke can damage the lungs of nonsmokers. The study reported that secondhand smoke

- kills at least four thousand people annually from lung cancer
- increases the risk of respiratory infections in children
- aggravates the symptoms of asthma in children

In addition to tobacco smoke, we are regularly exposed to so many other indoor air pollutants (see table below) that the EPA considers indoor air to be our most critical environmental health risk. Millions of buildings—office buildings, schools, factories, apartments, even hospitals—suffer from "sick building syndrome." A "sick" building is one in which at least 20 percent of the occupants experience discomfort that is suspected (it need not be proven) to be caused by contaminated indoor air. These ailments usually range from headaches and fatigue to colds, influenza, and chronic respiratory illnesses (e.g., chronic sinusitis and chronic bronchitis).

In most cities, going outside or opening the windows for fresh air usually doesn't work. There is often some degree of visible oxides of sulfur, oxides of nitrogen, hydrocarbons, and ozone. Scientists have already proven that every one of these pollutants is harmful to the respiratory tract. In 1993, calculations emerging from studies at the Environmental Protection Agency and the Harvard School of Public Health estimated that fifty thousand to sixty thousand deaths a year are caused by particulate pollution. This number far surpasses that of any other pollutant and is one that rivals the death toll from some cancers. The most harmful particles are small—less than ten microns

in diameter—and are produced chiefly from industrial plants and to a lesser extent from the exhaust of diesel vehicles.

In my book *Sinus Survival: The Holistic Medical Treatment for Allergies, Asthma, Bronchitis, Colds, and Sinusitis* (Tarcher/Putnam, 1995), I list the cities that have the highest concentrations of each of these pollutants. If you're looking for healthier air and have the freedom to move, avoid the following regions: southern California, the Northeast, and the Texas Gulf Coast. The healthiest air can usually be found along the West Coast (with the distinct exception of the Los Angeles metropolitan area and southward), rural areas along the Gulf Coast (other than Texas), the west coast of Florida, and most of Hawaii (other than Honolulu, plagued by automobile emissions, and the big island of Hawaii, which has been polluted for the last ten years by a stream of ash from active volcanoes).

Healthy air is clean (free of pollutants), moist (humidity between 35 and 50 percent), warm (between 65 and 85 degrees Fahrenheit), oxygen rich (21 percent of total volume and 100 percent saturation), and high in negative ions (3,000–6,000 .001-micron ions per cubic centimeter). Fortunately, technology has made it possible for us to create these optimum air conditions indoors through the use of negative-ion generators, air-cleaners, humidifiers, highly efficient furnace filters, air-duct cleaning, good ventilation, and "air-cleaning plants." For more information on creating a healthy home or work environment, see chapter 10 in Part II.

Indoor Air Pollutants

Automotive Fumes
Sources include outdoor traffic, outdoor parking lots, and outdoor loading and unloading spaces, as well as indoor garages

Chemicals and Chemical Solutions (chemicals that affect indoor air quality are those associated with architecture, the interior, artifacts, and maintenance)
Fungicides and pesticides in carpet-cleaning residues and sprays; formaldehyde used in the manufacture of insulation, plywood, fiberboard, furniture, and wood paneling; toxic solvents in oil-based paints, finishes, and wall sealants; aerosol sprays; office equipment chemicals, especially photocopiers and computers; and chemicals from dry cleaning

Combustion Products
Tobacco smoke (from all of the available scientific data, tobacco smoke is the most unhealthy indoor air pollutant)
Coal- or wood-burning fireplaces and stoves
Fuel-combustion gases from gas-fired appliances such as ranges, clothes dryers, water heaters, and fireplaces (they produce nitrogen dioxide, carbon monoxide, nitrous oxides, sulfur oxides, hydrocarbons, and formaldehyde)

Ion Depletion or Imbalance
Too few negative ions, especially in airplanes and in sealed buildings
Excess of positive ions over negative ions (primarily from computer and TV screens)

Microorganisms (primarily from humidifiers, air conditioners, and any other building components affected by excessive moisture)
Bacteria
Viruses
Molds
Dust mites (usually found in humid areas)

Particulates
Dust
Pollen
Animal dander
Particles (frayed materials)
Asbestos

Radionuclides
Radon, a radioactive gas emitted from the earth that enters homes primarily through basements, crawl spaces, and water supply, especially from wells (it can attach to the particulates of cigarette smoke, dust particles, and natural aerosols)

Drinking

After oxygen, the second most vital nutrient is water. At birth, a human infant is composed of 75–80 percent water. As an adult, we are 60–70 percent water. It is the basis of all body fluids, including blood, digestive juices, urine, lymph, and perspiration. We can survive no more than a few days without water. We have already seen the importance of breath in providing oxygen to every cell and tissue in the body. Before oxygen even enters the bloodstream, the surface of the lungs must be moistened with water to facilitate the intake of oxygen and the excretion of carbon dioxide. Only then can that oxygen be transported through the bloodstream, which is composed almost totally of water. In fact, every vital and nonvital physiological function in our bodies occurs through the medium of water.

- Water is responsible for cleansing the blood by removing waste through the kidneys. It helps to prevent kidney stones and urinary tract infections.
- Water regulates the body's temperature through perspiration.
- Water increases the health of the skin.
- Water is vital to metabolism and digestion and helps prevent constipation.
- Water lubricates the joints and enhances muscular function (especially during and after exercise).
- Water moistens the mucous membranes of the respiratory tract and consequently increases resistance to infection.
- Water is critical to healthy nerve-impulse conduction and brain function.

We must make a conscious effort to stay well hydrated because most of us are losing water faster than we replace it. For example, during normal restful breathing, exhalation alone accounts for a loss of one pint of water per day. In addition to the water lost through breathing, we lose one pint per day through perspiration and three pints per day through urination and bowel movements. Both exercise and heat will increase water loss, especially if you work out on a hot day or live in a dry climate. If you add up the different ways that we can lose water, you'll find that on average, under normal conditions, the body loses two and one-half quarts (eighty ounces) of water per day.

Vital as water is, most people don't drink enough. In fact, many American men are chronically dehydrated. Typically, our image of dehydration is an emaciated prospector crawling across a salt flat with a dry canteen. But an office worker drinking his third cup of coffee in a centrally heated high-rise is also probably dehydrated. His dehydration, though much less dramatic, has a widespread and insidious impact *on every bodily function.* By reducing blood volume, even minimal dehydration creates thicker, more concentrated blood. This overworks the heart, undersupplies all of the body's tissues with oxygen and nutrients, and impairs elimination of accumulated waste.

This shows up most dramatically in athletic performance. According to nutritional researchers and sports physiologists, water balance is the single most important factor in top performance. Muscle dehydration of only

3 percent can cause a 10 percent loss of strength and 8 percent loss of speed.

Dehydration is so deceptive, it can happen without your even being thirsty. It takes only 1 percent of fluid loss to become clinically dehydrated, and you needn't be perspiring profusely or urinating frequently for this to occur. Alcohol and caffeine are both diuretics that increase the body's loss of fluid and, for this reason, are not acceptable substitutes for water. Stress can have the same dehydrating effect. Soft drinks, with a high concentration of sugar, can raise heart rate, thus contributing to water loss. Besides heat, environmental factors can also cause water loss; stuffy, dry buildings and airplanes are common culprits. A three-to-four-hour flight can result in a loss of as much as two pounds of water, the equivalent of two pints.

The signs of chronic dehydration can include dry skin, constipation, increased upper-respiratory-tract infection, fatigue, kidney stones, urinary tract infections, and elevated blood pressure. Another consequence of dehydration is water retention—or edema—which might show up as excess fluid in the ankles, feet, lower legs, and hands. This results from the body's retaining water to compensate for a chronic shortage of fluid. This seemingly contradictory response is in reality another example of the body's intelligence. Sensing that the body's water level is low, its survival instinct causes the cells to retain fluid. This is why proper water intake is important in weight loss programs. Studies have found that a minimal level of dehydration in the body can reduce the size of the brain and

impair neuromuscular coordination, concentration, and thinking. Clearly dehydration creates a state of health that is far less than optimal. But how much water is enough?

Although there are many differing views on acceptable levels of water intake, most experts agree we need to drink more than our thirst requires. The exact amount depends on body weight, diet, metabolic rate, climate, physical activity level, and stress factors. We know we need to replace at least eighty ounces lost through normal breathing, perspiration, urination, and bowel movements. Although some nutritionists recommend eight glasses of water per day, a more accurate guideline would prescribe one-half to two-thirds ounce of water per pound of body weight, depending on your level and intensity of exercise. For a 160-pound male, this is equivalent to 80 to 110 ounces (ten to fourteen eight-ounce glasses) of water per day.

The foods you eat can help restore lost fluids. Fruits and vegetables have the highest water content (85–90 percent), whereas meats and bread are low in water. Another often overlooked source of hydration is the absorption of water through bathing and showering. However, none of these secondary sources can adequately replace drinking one-half to two-thirds ounce of water per pound of body weight.

Almost as important as *quantity* is the *quality* of your water. If you aren't drinking filtered water, then your body becomes the filter. Government guidelines are very specific about limiting the number of microorganisms and contaminants in public drinking water.

Although testing for 89 contaminants is mandated by law, a report commissioned by Ralph Nader stated that at least 2,110 contaminants have been identified in the nation's drinking water supplies.

Since chlorinating of water was first introduced in this country in 1908, it has eliminated epidemics of cholera, dysentery, and typhoid. However, multiple studies have suggested an association between chlorine and diminished immune function, possibly contributing to a higher incidence of cancer. One study done in 1995 suggested that long-term drinking of chlorinated water caused a 35 percent increase in the incidence of bladder and colon cancers. Dangerous levels of toxic heavy metals (lead, cadmium, mercury, cobalt, and copper) have been measured in drinking water supplies across the United States. Lead is considered the greatest health risk to children, and the effects of lead poisoning can last a lifetime. It not only stunts growth and damages the nervous system, but it has now been linked to crime and antisocial behavior in children. The majority of health-related risks that are present in drinking water are the result of the contamination added *after* the water leaves the treatment and distribution plant. This includes pipes that run from municipal systems into your house, lead-soldered pipes, and fixtures that contain lead and may leach lead or other toxic metals into your tap water.

Although chlorine does a good job of eliminating most microorganisms from our drinking water, the parasite known as *Cryptosporidium* is resistant to chlorine disinfection, and over 45 million Americans drink water from treatment plants that have been found to contain *Cryptosporidium*. In 1993 this protozoan infected an estimated four hundred thousand people in Milwaukee, where it killed over one hundred people with compromised immune systems. Healthy individuals infected by these parasites experience diarrhea, vomiting, headache, and mild fevers. The only effective solutions to remove *Cryptosporidium* are either to boil your tap water, invest in bottled water, or purchase a filter that is certified to remove *Cryptosporidium* or cysts.

Bottled water is often the first choice for those seeking to improve their quality of drinking water. This can prove to be an expensive proposition, however, with bottled water costing anywhere from sixty cents to six dollars per gallon. Bottled-water regulations are similar to those that must be followed by the public water treatment industry, and they are currently not required to test for *Cryptosporidium* or many other contaminants. According to the March 1996 *Parents* magazine, "a quarter of bottled waters sold comes from filtered municipal water that is then treated."

An excellent way to obtain high-quality drinking water is to invest in a point-of-use water filter (usually installed under the sink or on the kitchen counter). The market is flooded with numerous brands of filters, many of questionable effectiveness. Fortunately for consumers, there is help in the form of an independent testing organization called the National Sanitation Foundation (NSF), a non-profit, internationally recognized authority for testing water and certifying products to ensure that they meet strict public health standards. Contact NSF at 1-800-673-6275 for a free brochure and listing of certified water treatment units and certified water bottlers. There are several different brands of carbon or solid carbon block type filters that not only remove chlorine, lead, volatile organic compounds, and asbestos, but also *Cryptosporidium* and particulate matter to .5 microns. A good filter will cost from $250 to $600 and should last a lifetime (with filter cartridges replaced periodically at a cost from $20 to $100). When shopping for a water filter, compare models for contaminants removed, initial cost, and ongoing cost as well as warranties, to find the best unit for your situation. Good-quality filtered water will end up costing only pennies per gallon, with the added advantage of having plenty available for cooking, juices, teas, etc. Look for a filter that does not remove dissolved minerals such as iron, calcium, or especially magnesium, as these are considered beneficial and may reduce the risk of heart disease (according to a 1994 study in the *Journal of the American Dietetic Association*). Reverse-osmosis filters remove minerals, require electricity, and waste water, but are effective filters in certain situations. Whole-house filters will remove some chlorine, but may not be effective in removing other possible contaminants. After choosing and installing a filter, drinking more water comes naturally as you experience the improved taste of pure water.

To get in the habit of drinking enough water, spread your intake throughout the day (it's best to drink between meals), and don't drink more than four eight-ounce glasses in any given hour. Don't substitute beer, coffee, tea, soft drinks, milk, or processed fruit juice for pure water. Although they all contain water, they also have other ingredients, especially caffeine and sugar, that can negate the benefits of pure water. If you engage in heavy exercise, a sports drink containing sugar is fine. Alcohol and caffeine are diuretics that increase urination and can contribute to dehydration. Decaffeinated coffee is less of a diuretic. Nonorganic juices may contain pesticides; commercial milk is laced with hormones and antibiotics. Herbal tea, natural fruit juices (without sugar and diluted 50 percent with water), and some soups (low salt, no sugar, the clearer and thinner the better) can substitute for a portion of your daily water requirement. Frequent trips to the bathroom and urine the color of pale lemon juice are two positive signs that you are probably drinking enough water.

Unfortunately, it is a fact of life in America today that we can never know for sure if our water is completely safe. A quality water filter or quality bottled water can provide excellent insurance. Do the best you can. To drink more healthy water, make it convenient. Keep a water container at hand, in the car or at your desk. Don't wait until you're thirsty to drink. And by the way, always know where the nearest men's room is.

Eating

Thy food shall be thy remedy.

Hippocrates

It takes five to seven times the normal amount of nutrition to build and repair than it does to maintain.

The Journal of the Certified Natural Health Professional

————————————————◆————————————————

Food is one of men's greatest pleasures, but we consume far more than we need and often too much of the wrong kind. The kinds of foods that we most require are those that enhance life force energy; the wrong kinds are those that deplete the body's energy. The typical male diet consists largely of lifeless "empty" foods that overstimulate and congest our bodies. In a culture that encourages over-consumption of everything from energy to consumer goods and information, it's no wonder that one-third of adult Americans are obese. Not just overweight, but obese, which, according to the medical definition, means at least 20 percent above ideal body weight. Are you part of this "expanding" population?

To find out, determine your weight as measured against the ideal corresponding weight for your height (without shoes) in the table below. This assumes you have a medium frame, and that you are not an NFL running back or body builder (muscle weighs more than fat). To determine if you have an average-size frame, wrap your thumb and forefinger around your wrist, over the bony prominence. If they touch, or are close to touching, you have a medium frame. If there is a significant gap, you have a large frame,

and if they overlap, you have a small frame. For example, if you are six feet tall with an average frame, your upper limit is 169 pounds. If you actually weigh more than 203, then you are obese. If you thought you were just carrying a little extra weight, the fact is you're fat. You can either get used to a diminished life expectancy, increased health risks, and fat-man jokes or start to do something about it.

If you are not happy with how you fared on the Met Life weight table, Barry Eckel, M.D.—professor of medicine in the division of endocrinology, metabolism, and diabetes at the University of Colorado—offers a different way of determining if your weight falls within an ideal range. Here is the formula for Dr. Eckel's body-mass index (BMI):

$$\textbf{BMI} = \frac{\textbf{weight in kilograms}}{\textbf{(height in meters)}^2}$$

To find your weight in kilograms, multiply your weight in pounds by 0.455

To find your height in meters, multiply your height in inches by 0.0254

From the Fall 1996 University Health Report, *University of Colorado Health Sciences Center*

According to Dr. Eckel, normal-weight people score in the 20s. A number under 27 is felt to be acceptable, although a score between 27

Metropolitan Life Insurance Company
Table for Ideal Body Weight for Men Revised (1983)

Height	Men		
	Small Frame	Medium Frame	Large Frame
5'1''	123–134	126–136	133–145
5'2''	125–131	128–138	135–148
5'3''	127–133	130–140	137–151
5'4''	129–135	132–143	139–155
5'5''	131–137	134–146	141–159
5'6''	133–140	137–149	145–163
5'7''	135–143	140–152	147–167
5'8''	137–145	143–155	150–171
5'9''	139–149	146–158	153–175
5'10''	141–152	149–161	156–179
5'11''	144–155	152–165	159–183
6'	147–159	155–169	163–187
6'1''	150–163	159–173	167–192
6'2''	153–167	162–177	171–197
6'3''	157–171	166–182	176–202
6'4''	161–175	169–187	179–207
6'5''	165–179	172–192	182–212

and 30 is considered borderline and suggests increased risks. Any score over 30 is considered "medically significant obesity."

We all think we know something about eating well, but for most of us it is largely an "unconscious" process just like breathing and drinking. To find out just exactly what this process consists of, let's follow a typical bite of dinner on its alimentary odyssey from lips to anus. Even before you take your first bite, anticipation triggers the secretion of saliva, which contains a digestive enzyme to begin breaking down carbohydrates. Once the morsel finds its way past the lips, the cutting and grinding action of the teeth breaks down the food into smaller digestible pieces. Unfortunately, most of us shortchange this part of digestion. A recent Gallup poll revealed that among those who dined at home in the company of others, 40 percent watched TV, studied, worked, or read while eating. It's no secret that men tend to be in a hurry, and when we are distracted, we eat even faster. Ideally, we should chew each mouthful about twenty times to prepare the food for optimal digestion. If we don't, we place an even greater burden on the stomach and small intestine.

After leaving the mouth, food travels down the esophagus and into the stomach, where it is greeted by hydrochloric acid and several digestive enzymes that break down both proteins and carbohydrates. Fats, conversely, are digested in the small intestine through a combination of bile from the liver and enzymes from the pancreas and from the wall of the small intestine. In the small intestine, a different blend of digestive juices along with

those from the pancreas mix with this thick, syrupy mass. The peristaltic waves of the gastrointestinal tract propel the digesting food through the twenty-six-foot length of the small intestine. Here the body absorbs most of the food's nutrients and water through the intestinal walls. When the digestive mass enters the large intestine, or colon, most of the remaining water and nutrients are absorbed through the walls of the colon into the bloodstream, leaving a thicker, pastelike substance devoid of most of its nutritive value. What may have started as $26-a-plate chateaubriand has gradually been transformed into "some really good shit."

Now that you know how food is digested and absorbed, you won't be surprised to learn that the foods that the body needs most are those that are most easily digested.

The Thriving Food Pyramid places those foods containing the highest nutritional value

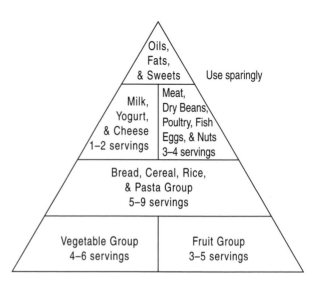

Thriving Food Pyramid Based on the USDA Model

at the base of the pyramid, and those that are the least nutritious and digestible at the apex. According to this diet pyramid, which is a significantly modified version of the U.S. Department of Agriculture Food Pyramid, our daily diet should consist of seven to eleven servings of fruit and vegetables, and between five to nine servings of bread, cereal, rice, and pasta. Although the USDA recommends more servings of bread, cereal, and pasta than fruits and vegetables, recent studies are showing that carbohydrates are not as essential as was once thought. Additionally, I've eliminated all milk, other than 1% or skim, while drastically reducing butter, margarine, and cheese. Similarly, limit your daily number of dairy servings to one or two. Limit your intake of red meat (eat only the leanest cuts) but maintain two to three servings per day of poultry, fish, dry beans, and nuts. As for fats, oils, and sweets at the top of the pyramid, eliminate all cooking fats and oils from animal derivatives, especially hydrogenated fats such as margarine, and hydrogenated peanut butter. Instead, use vegetable oils (olive, canola, safflower). Either cut out all added sugar or substitute honey.

The USDA recommends about 2,200 calories per day for sedentary men, 2,800 calories for active men (who exercise regularly) and teenage boys. To give a clear picture of what constitutes a serving size, refer to the following chart from the USDA.

The primary reason for restructuring the USDA pyramid is to substantially eliminate from men's diets those foods or substances that become unhealthy when consumed to *excess*—sugar, fat, caffeine, salt, refined

What Counts as a Serving?

Food Groups

Bread, Cereal, Rice, and Pasta

1 slice of bread
1 ounce of ready-to-eat cereal
$\frac{1}{2}$ cup of cooked cereal, rice, or pasta

Vegetable

1 cup of raw leafy vegetables
$\frac{1}{2}$ cup of other vegetables, cooked or chopped raw
$\frac{3}{4}$ cup of vegetable juice

Milk, Yogurt, and Cheese

1 cup of milk or yogurt
$1\frac{1}{2}$ ounces of natural cheese
2 ounces of process cheese

Meat, Poultry, Fish, Dry Beans, Eggs, and Nuts

2-3 ounces of cooked lean meat, poultry, or fish
$\frac{1}{2}$ cup of cooked dry beans, 1 egg, or 2 tablespoons of peanut butter count as 1 ounce of lean meat

From The Food Guide Pyramid, United States Department of Agriculture Human Information Service Home & Garden Bulletin Number 252

carbohydrates, and alcohol—*"**the sickening six**."* The axiom I live and eat by is "Everything in moderation, including moderation." We are presenting you with the ideal thriving diet, but that doesn't mean you can't have "a little play in the wheel." Don't be so fanatical that you take all the joy out of eating.

Sugar may prove to be the greatest health hazard in our diet. Sugar is everywhere, added to almost everything we eat, from nearly every breakfast cereal to—believe it or not—even 50 percent of our table salt. Not only do Americans consume an average of forty-one teaspoons per day (or 150 pounds per person, per year), but some studies indicate that *sugar is probably a greater risk factor for heart disease than cholesterol.* Although there is no conclusive evidence of dietary fat or cholesterol as causes of coronary artery disease, there is stronger evidence of sucrose (refined sugar) as a cause. A study cited in a 1992 edition of the *Journal of the Royal Society of Medicine* showed that in 30 percent of the studied men, an experimental increase in dietary sucrose produced all the same increases in blood chemistry that typically occur in coronary artery disease: higher cholesterol and lipids, uric acid, insulin, insulin resistance, platelet adhesiveness, and lower HDL (the good cholesterol). Furthermore, scientific evidence has shown that *sugar weakens the immune system,* making us more susceptible to both infection and allergy. Two studies in the *American Journal of Clinical Nutrition* (April 1977 and November 1973) showed an acute depression of white blood cell activity immediately following high sucrose ingestion. This diminished white-blood-cell function persisted for two hours in one study and six hours in the other.

Most men know that insulin metabolizes (breaks down into usable energy) sugar. Insulin also metabolizes other carbohydrates, fats, and proteins. However, when an excess of sugar overstimulates insulin secretion, (1) more fat is metabolized and stored in the body, while HDL cholesterol (the good cholesterol) is lowered, (2) triglycerides (the other fat component in the blood) increase, and (3) the risk of arteriosclerosis (hardening of the arteries) is heightened.

The media has done a good job of alerting men to the dangers of **red meat** and **fat** and their relationship to heart disease. We know how fatty deposits, or plaques, can build up on the inner lining of arterial walls, either diminishing or completely obstructing blood flow and its corresponding transport of oxygen and nutrients. Those fats identified as most harmful are called trans-fats or hydrogenated fats, which are predominantly found in margarine, cooking fats, and some peanut butters. They are easily identifiable, because they become solid, or semi-solid, at room temperature. These fats are worse than those found in red meat. "Good" fats, which include olive oil, canola, or safflower oil are liquid at room temperature.

Although many men monitor their cholesterol levels and restrict their intake of fat accordingly, they have developed a false sense of security about sugar and **refined carbohydrates,** believing they are harmless and overindulging in both. Refined carbohydrates consist of white rice, products made with white flour from which the germ and the bran (the healthy components) have been extracted, and sugar. To avoid red meat and fat, many men tend to fill up on refined carbohydrates (rice, bread, and pasta). But refined carbohydrates, such as white bread or white rice, when eaten to excess, also overstimulate insulin production and produce the same excessive fat storage in the body. With the popularity of pasta and high-carbohydrate diets over the last decade, fat intake has declined by 10 percent, with a corresponding improvement in cholesterol levels. However, in this same ten-year period, obesity has increased by 33 percent. Unfortunately, although carbohydrates certainly contain less fat than red meat, they have an abundance of calories that can turn into fat. What's more, the excessive consumption of carbohydrates—as with sugar—can stimulate an erratic fluctuation of insulin that can eventually lead to diabetes, one of the most common chronic diseases among men.

Research by Dr. Barry Sears, Ph.D., a pioneer in biotechnology and author of *The Zone*, describes the harmful effects of excessive carbohydrates. In addition to diabetes, they include several chronic diseases, such as heart disease, arthritis, and skin disorders; and they can account for diminished physical and mental capacity. Sears's research also indicates that excessive consumption of carbohydrates inhibits the body's ability to burn fat. He recommends balancing consumption of protein, carbohydrates, and fat in a nearly 1:1:1 ratio (with fat quantities slightly less than protein or carbohydrates). Sears encourages intake of

healthy carbohydrates (unrefined), substituting fruits and vegetables for rice, pasta, and bread. He prefers those fruits and vegetables that have a low glycemic index—less sugar—such as asparagus, black beans, green beans, broccoli, cabbage, chickpeas, kale, onions, spinach, and zucchini. With the recent emphasis on high carbohydrate diets, it is no wonder that one American in three is obese. Restrict your consumption of healthy carbos (fruits, vegetables, and whole grains) to five to nine servings per day, and balance them with protein and healthy fats.

Caffeine is a drug to which the majority of men are addicted, drinking an average of two to three cups of coffee per day. When its stimulation wears off, the quick fix is usually another cup of coffee or a bottle of caffeine-rich soda pop. Unfortunately, our quest for the quick energy that enables us to compete effectively in the workplace has a steep price tag. Even two cups of coffee a day can contribute to a multitude of harmful health effects. Here are some of caffeine's other effects.

CAFFEINE

Use

More than 50% of Americans drink coffee daily. Average daily caffeine consumption by those who drink is 400 mg.

Hazardous Effects

BLOOD PRESSURE
200–400 mg ($1\frac{1}{2}$ to $2\frac{1}{2}$ cups of coffee) increases adrenaline 200%, noradrenaline

75%, renin 60%, systolic blood pressure, 14 mmHg, diastolic blood pressure 10 mmHg, and respiratory rate 20%.

CANCER

Some (not all) reports relate coffee to a higher incidence of pancreatic cancer; mutagens have been found in coffee.

CARDIAC EFFECTS

Contributes to heart-rhythm disturbances. Four or more cups of coffee/day (decaf or not) increases men's rate of heart disease 3% (and women's 60%!).

CENTRAL NERVOUS SYSTEM

Stimulates the central nervous system.

CIRCULATION

Causes local vasoconstriction by blocking adenosine release; causes dizziness.

CLOTTING

Decreases platelet stickiness.

DEGENERATIVE DISEASE AND FREE RADICALS

Increases adrenaline; adrenaline metabolites increase free radicals and risks of degenerative diseases.

GASTROINTESTINAL EFFECTS

Stimulates gastric acid secretion.

INTERACTION WITH DRUGS

Interacts and/or competes with prescription drugs.

MUSCULAR EFFECTS

Is a major factor in restless-leg syndrome; contributes to muscle-tension syndromes by promoting calcium loss from muscle cells.

OSTEOPOROSIS

Contributes to osteoporosis by increasing calcium loss; one cup of coffee raises calcium requirements 30–50 mg.

PAIN

Coffee contains a narcotic antagonist and may decrease pain tolerance.

PREGNANCY

Can contribute to certain problems in pregnancy.

PSYCHOACTIVE EFFECTS

Causes anxiety and irritability; large amounts can precipitate psychosis and acute schizophrenia; can precipitate agoraphobia in susceptible persons; affects adenosine and beta-adrenergic receptors causing euphoria, tolerance, dependence, addiction, and symptoms of physical withdrawal.

SLEEP

Caffeine reduces the depth of sleep.

URINARY TRACT

Increases urinary frequency.

Beneficial Effects

Caffeine and coffee act as a stimulant, can lengthen sleep latency, thus keeping people awake.

The best way to break the caffeine addiction is to do it gradually over a couple of weeks or even months. If you drink four to five cups per day of coffee, hot chocolate, soft drinks, or black tea, start by cutting down your intake to three cups, then to one cup per day. (To get a better idea of how much caffeine you are consuming, see the table below.) Once you reach this level of one cup per day, substitute over a couple of weeks, or even months, noncaffeinated beverages such as an herb tea or a roasted-grain beverage (if you can stand the taste). Be aware of the possible withdrawal symptoms of headache, nervousness, and irritability.

CAFFEINE AMOUNTS (MG)

Coffee, 5-Ounce Cup
Decaffeinated instant: 2
Decaffeinated brewed: 2–5
Instant: 40–108
Percolated: 64–124
Drip: 110–150

Tea, 5-Ounce Cup
Bag, brewed for five minutes: 20–50
Bag, brewed for one minute: 9–33
Loose, black, five-minute brew: 20–85
Loose, green, five-minute brew: 15–80
Iced: 22–36

Soft Drinks, 12-Ounce Glass
Cola: 44–46

Chocolate
Cocoa, 5-ounce cup: 4–6
Milk chocolate, 1 ounce: 3–6
Bittersweet chocolate, 1 ounce: 25–35

Men with high blood pressure problems are aware of the dangers of too much **salt.** But many of us have been conditioned since childhood to crave salt. Its overuse draws water into the blood vessels, thereby increasing blood volume and contributing to higher blood pressure. Although some salt can be used in cooking, it is best to avoid adding salt to your food once it reaches the table.

The sixth nutritional excess happens to be one of men's greatest pleasures and our most popular social lubricant. However, **alcohol** (like refined carbohydrates) contributes significantly to obesity. In addition to building beer bellies, it contributes to increased blood pressure; diabetes; colon, stomach, and pancreatic cancer; and gastrointestinal and liver problems. As a depressant, alcohol can be associated with a host of emotional and behavioral dysfunctions. As with everything else in the *Thriving* diet, moderation should prevail: if you feel like having a drink, go ahead and enjoy. Sometimes the benefits of stress reduction can outweigh other health concerns . . . but again, not to excess. Try to limit yourself to no more than two servings of alcohol— approximately two beers or two glasses of wine or one shot of hard liquor per day.

Although the immediate effects of these Sickening Six can be both stimulating and pleasurable, the ultimate impact of *excessive* amounts is far more damaging; each significantly depletes life energy and impairs the capacity to thrive. To varying degrees, these substances, when consumed excessively, can either constrict arterial blood flow, diminish the transport of oxygen to every cell and tissue in the body, or weaken the immune system. We live in a society based on fast food and instant gratification. We tend to mistake the stimulants in processed foods for actual nutrients. But, though it works subtly and slowly, nature's digestive process will eventually tell you what your body needs. Use the Thriving Food Pyramid to begin to identify those foods and those amounts that are healthiest and most nutritious. They are usually foods that will naturally strengthen your energy an hour or two after you eat them. As you gradually try new foods, you will develop a greater sensitivity to the effects of those different foods on your body. This sensitivity will direct you in making healthier food choices. The Thriving Food Pyramid is just a starting point in training for optimal health. You will learn to adjust your diet to fit your particular needs.

The four criteria for identifying the most healthful foods are their nutritional content, their long-term energizing effect on the body, their cleansing properties, and their fiber content. Healthful foods provide the fuel for ATP production in the cells, which strengthens the immune system. They produce healthy red blood cells (which carry oxygen), and they enhance the function of white blood cells (which protect the body by fighting infection). The most nutritious foods are organically grown **whole foods**—raised without pesticides, artificial fertilizers, antibiotics, or hormones, and processed without added sugars or preservatives. They cost more but they are well worth the expense in their ability to strengthen immune system response, cleanse the blood, and provide fuel for energy production. Make a point of visiting your local health food store and start using it as a primary resource. The high fiber content foods consist of fruits and vegetables, and legumes

(beans). These contribute to the cleansing process by sweeping the large bowel of waste and other toxins that would otherwise accumulate on the intestinal walls and be reabsorbed into the bloodstream to slowly poison our systems.

Some of the most important food substances for energizing and cleansing the blood are **antioxidants.** These nutrients counterattack the harmful effects of highly toxic molecules called free radicals. Although free radicals can fight disease by bonding to unhealthy molecules (such as bacteria and viruses) and killing off these invaders, sometimes, due to an extra electrical charge, these free radicals will bind with healthy cells, causing cell-wall destruction, disease, and acceleration of aging. In recent years, a number of researchers have identified free radicals as causative factors in many chronic diseases, including heart disease, cancer, arthritis, and infection, and also in aging. By neutralizing free radicals, antioxidants can prevent harmful cellular destruction.

Deepak Chopra, M.D., author of *Ageless Body, Timeless Mind,* calls free radicals "the metabolic end products of environmental pollution, food toxins, carcinogens, and emotional toxins." Although the body produces its own antioxidant enzymes to protect us against free radicals, those of us living in highly industrialized, toxic environments require supplemental antioxidant nutrients to help the body offset these destructive free radicals.

Returning to the Thriving Food Pyramid, let's examine each food group more closely. Because they are highest in vitamin, mineral, and fiber content—while providing almost all of the supplemental antioxidants—**fruits and vegetables** are critical to optimal health and thus form the foundation of the Thriving pyramid. The most powerful antioxidants contained in food are **vitamin C, vitamin A** (in the form of **beta-carotene**), **vitamin E,** and the minerals **zinc, selenium, copper,** and **manganese.** However the most powerful antioxidants of all are found in grape seeds (called grape seed extract) and in the bark of European coastal pine trees (called pycnogenol). This antioxidant, called proanthocyanidins, was discovered thirty years ago by French professor Jack Masquelier, Ph.D., at the University of Bordeaux. After extensive testing, proanthocyanidin has been found to be fifty times more powerful an antioxidant than vitamin E and twenty times more powerful than vitamin C. The earliest clinical tests verified its use for improving conditions of the arteries and capillaries, in prevention of infections, as an anti-inflammatory (especially for arthritis), and for antiaging. Most European physicians consider it their first choice for hay fever, and it is also widely used in treating asthma.

Those fruits and vegetables highest in **vitamin C** in roughly descending order, are

- guavas
- oranges
- cantaloupe
- strawberries
- red chili peppers
- red sweet peppers
- green sweet peppers
- kale

- parsley
- collard greens
- turnip greens
- mustard greens
- broccoli
- brussels sprouts
- cauliflower

Remember, the vitamin content of fruits and vegetables is always higher when eaten raw. In my experience, vitamin C has been extremely effective in the treatment and prevention of both colds and sinus infections. In addition to its antioxidant properties, vitamin C is essential to the manufacture of collagen, the main supportive protein of skin, tendon, bone, cartilage, and connective tissue. It has an anti-inflammatory effect, especially in some autoimmune diseases such as lupus and rheumatoid arthritis; it facilitates the absorption of dietary iron, enhances the immune response and white blood cell activity, and in conjunction with vitamin E strengthens arterial walls. In a recent study conducted by researchers from the USDA and National Institute on Aging, vitamin C was shown to provide protection against cholesterol buildup (by raising HDL—the good cholesterol) and to reduce the risk of heart disease.

Most vitamin A comes from its precursor, **beta-carotene,** which is converted to the vitamin form in the gastrointestinal tract. Beta-carotene is found in yellow, orange, or red fruits and vegetables. Listed in descending order of beta-carotene content, these foods include

- carrots
- sweet potatoes

- yams
- kale
- spinach
- mangoes
- winter squash
- cantaloupe
- apricots
- broccoli
- romaine lettuce
- asparagus
- tomatoes
- nectarines
- peaches
- papayas

Vitamin A itself can be obtained directly from cod-liver oil, liver, kidney, eggs, and dairy products. Vitamin A helps to maintain the integrity of mucous membranes, is required for growth and repair of cells, is necessary for protein metabolism, protects night vision, and protects against cancer. Beta-carotene has been shown to be effective as an anticancer nutrient—a discovery made by Japanese researchers more than twenty years ago. Adequate beta-carotene in the diet should supply the vitamin A you need, but vitamin A deficiency in the United States is not uncommon.

Foods highest in **vitamin E** are

- unrefined soybean oil
- wheat germ oil
- fresh wheat germ
- whole grains
- raw nuts (most varieties)
- all green leafy vegetables

Vitamin E can help protect against heart attack and strokes. It is also a natural anticoagulant and powerful antioxidant.

Foods with a high **zinc** content are beef liver and the dark meat of turkey. Zinc appears to be critical to the release of vitamin A from the liver and is vital to the production of new cells and the metabolism of protein for the repair of body tissues. Zinc is also helpful in maintaining a healthy prostate gland.

Foods high in **selenium** include

- whole-wheat products
- fish
- whole grains
- mushrooms
- beans
- garlic
- liver

Although selenium is a potent antioxidant, it can be toxic to the body in large doses. Selenium reinforces the immune system and helps fight cancer. A study presented in the *Journal of the National Cancer Institute* reported that men with lower levels of selenium in their blood were most likely to develop some cancers of the lung, stomach, and pancreas. Low selenium levels have also been linked to bladder cancer and asthma.

Antioxidant value aside, the **fruits** ranked highest in nutritional value, according to the Center for Science in the Public Interest (CSPI), are in descending order

- watermelon
- papaya
- cantaloupe
- mangoes
- oranges
- grapefruit
- bananas
- cherries

- plums
- grapes

The **vegetables** with the highest nutritional value are

- fresh spinach
- fresh collard greens
- sweet potato
- fresh kale
- winter squash
- carrots
- fresh broccoli
- fresh asparagus
- cucumber

To include the healthiest fruits and vegetables in your diet, look for those that appear on both the antioxidant and nutritional-value lists. For example, cantaloupe, broccoli, and kale appear on the vitamin C and beta-carotene list, as well as on the CSPI nutritional-value list.

The second tier from the bottom on the Thriving Food Pyramid consists of **grains,** which include bread, cereal, rice, and pasta—all **carbohydrates.** As distinguished from the USDA recommendations, the *Thriving* model specifically calls for *whole* grains whenever possible. In addition to being the primary source of carbohydrates, whole grains also provide vitamins, minerals, and protein. These **whole grains** include in roughly descending nutritional value

- bulgur (cracked wheat)
- whole-wheat pita bread
- whole-wheat bread
- millet
- brown rice
- quinoa
- barley

- oats
- couscous

Finding a processed cereal without sugar in most supermarkets is like trying to find the Holy Grail. If you are concerned about sugar in your cereal—and you should be—read the list of ingredients, which by law are ranked in order of the greatest percentage of content. Sugar-free breakfasts cereals *do* exist, but you have to hunt for them in the health food aisle or at a health food store. If you still crave sweetness in your breakfast cereal, sprinkle chopped bananas or raisins on top.

Complex carbohydrates are a food category comprised of **starchy vegetables, whole grains,** and **legumes.** Complex carbohydrates digest more slowly and release their sugars into the bloodstream more gradually. Complex carbohydrates include

- starchy vegetables
  - potatoes
  - sweet potatoes
  - yams
  - winter squash (acorn & butternut)
  - pumpkins
- complex-carbohydrate whole grains
  - brown rice
  - millet
  - quinoa
  - amaranth
- legumes
  - black beans
  - garbanzo beans
  - lima beans
  - aduki beans
  - navy beans
  - kidney beans

- lentils
- black-eyed peas
- split peas

The main sources of **protein** in the *Thriving* diet are

- fish
- chicken
- turkey
- soy
- nuts and seeds (in order of nutritional value)
  - sunflower seeds
  - almonds
  - peanuts
  - cashews
  - pine nuts
  - pecans
  - walnuts
  - sesame seeds

Chicken and turkey should be antibiotic- and hormone-free. In addition to being a source of protein, nuts and seeds also provide fiber, vitamins, and minerals, as well as fat and calories. You may want to eat them more sparingly.

As for the top tier of the food pyramid— fats, **oils,** and sweets—we have already dispensed with animal fats and sugar. For cooking and salads, olive oil is the healthiest choice. Flaxseed oil is a healthy choice on salads, or as a daily nutritional supplement, because it is rich in omega-3 fatty acids, which benefit connective tissue and skin. However, flaxseed oil is not suitable for cooking. In recipes that call for sugar, substitute a half quantity of honey. Avoid all artificial sweeteners; some studies indicate they increase the incidence of cancer.

The following are a selection of nutritious meals that any thriving man should be able to prepare for himself. The total number of servings in these sample menus conforms to the daily requirements outlined in the Thriving Food Pyramid. If you can change a tire, you can learn to make these meals. Each menu offers three options ranging from light to medium to heavy caloric content. Choose according to your level of exercise and present weight. Try to eat fruits separately, between meals. During meals, try to limit your beverage intake (including water), because drinking can dilute the digestive juices and slow the process of breaking down of food. Unfortunately, there are no healthy desserts. Even fruit, which most people assume is a healthy dessert, actually impedes digestion when mixed with other food. Just remember the *Thriving* axiom: "Everything in moderation, including moderation."

Breakfast

Light

- 8-oz glass of fruit juice
- 2–3 pieces of fruit or half a cantaloupe
- 1 cup of cottage cheese
  (*4 total servings*)

Medium

- 1–2 cups of sugarless cereal with 1% milk (or soy milk) sprinkled with banana, or hot oatmeal
  (*5 servings—1 fruit, 1 milk, 3 cereal*)

Heavy

- vegetable omelet (2 eggs)
- whole-wheat toast (2 slices)
  (6 servings—1 vegetable, 2 eggs, 1 cheese, 2 bread)

Lunch

Light

- vegetable salad
- sliced chicken breast, or tuna
  (5 servings)

Medium

- turkey sandwich on whole-wheat bread with lettuce and tomato
- low-fat mayonnaise or mustard
- a bowl of soup (no cream soups) or a glass of vegetable juice (V-8, or better yet, fresh carrot juice)
  (5 or 6 servings)

Heavy

- medium pizza with vegetable toppings
  (7 servings)

Dinner

Light

- Caesar salad (see recipe)
- corn on the cob or baked potato with chopped vegetable toppings
  (9 servings)

Medium

- grilled fish or chicken
- sautéed vegetables (in olive oil, with tamari—soy sauce—and spices)
- two slices of fresh bread and brown rice
  (10 servings)

Heavy

- pasta with clam sauce or marinara (tomato sauce)
- salad or brown rice with vegetables
  (11 servings)

RECIPE FOR CAESAR SALAD

Dressing

$\frac{1}{2}$ cup olive oil
6 anchovy filets
1 clove garlic (minced)
$1\frac{1}{2}$ tsp Worcestershire sauce
$\frac{1}{2}$ tsp salt
$\frac{1}{2}$ tsp dry mustard
$\frac{1}{2}$ tsp freshly ground pepper

Combine the above ingredients and allow to sit in the refrigerator for a $\frac{1}{2}$ hour.

Wash and dry 2 large bunches of romaine lettuce. Rub the inside of a wooden bowl with $\frac{1}{2}$ clove of garlic. Add the lettuce and dressing and toss. Add $\frac{1}{4}$ cup fresh lemon juice, and toss again. Add 1 cup of seasoned croutons, $\frac{1}{4}$ cup grated Parmesan cheese, and serve.

Caloric Content of Common Foods

Apple, medium	70
Banana, medium	85
Beer, 12 oz	148
Chicken, 3 oz	115
Egg, 1 scrambled	110
Orange juice, 8 oz	110
Pasta, 8 oz.	155
Potato	90
Whole-wheat toast, 1 slice	55
Bagel	296
Beer, nonalcoholic, 12 oz	144
Cantaloupe, half of 5-inch melon	60
Corn, 1 ear	70
Fish, 3 oz	175
Orange, medium	75
Pizza, 1 section, 5½-inch dia.	185
Rice, brown, 1 cup	185

The food recommendations in this chapter will start you on your way to creating optimal health. However, due to stress, the unhealthy state of our environment, and the fact that we can't always eat pure, organically grown foods, we need help in obtaining enough vitamins, minerals, and antioxidants. **Vitamin supplements** and some **herbs** are indispensable for thriving and preventing a multitude of chronic diseases.

The daily recommended vitamin, mineral, and herb dosages in the following table will help you to maintain optimal health. Use the higher recommended dosages on days of higher stress, less sleep, increased air pollu-

tion, or other sources of high toxicity, or on days when you're not eating as well as you should be. Take at least the minimum dose every day. All vitamins should be taken with meals.

RECOMMENDED DAILY NUTRITIONAL SUPPLEMENTS

*Vitamin C (as polyascorbate or ester C)—1,000 to 2,000 mg 3x/day

*Beta-carotene—25,000 IU 1 or 2x/day

*Vitamin E—400 IU 1 or 2x/day

*B-complex—50–100 mg of each B vitamin

*Selenium—100–200 mcg/day

*Zinc picolinate—20–40 mg/day

*Calcium citrate or apatite—1,000 mg/day (to help regulate nerve and muscle function while building strong bones)

*Magnesium citrate or aspartate—500 mg/day (complements calcium in regulation of nerve and muscle function and may act as a relaxant to help promote sleep at bedtime)

*Chromium picolinate—200 mcg/day (to help stabilize blood sugar)

*Manganese—10–15 mg/day

*Copper—2 mg/day

Proanthocyanidin (grape seed extract or pycnogenol)—100 mg 1 or 2x/day

Flaxseed oil (or omega-3 fatty acids in fish oil)—2 tbsp/day (to thin the blood

These vitamins can all be found in a single megadose multivitamin or mineral preparation, or you can take them all separately.

for prevention of heart attack and as
an anti-inflammatory for arthritis)
Saw palmetto berry—160 mg 1 or 2x/day
(for men over 45 to help prevent prostatic
enlargement)

The first requirement in changing your diet is to try to obtain all of these vitamins from eating a healthy diet. Rather than trying to radically change your diet in two days, try to implement the above changes gradually over one month. The first week, start by changing your breakfast menu to conform with the recommendations in the *Thriving* pyramid and sample menus. The second week change your lunch menu. One week after that, start including the suggested dinner plan in your new diet. If you are intimidated by the prospect of swallowing a handful of vitamin pills two or three times per day, you can take just a few at a time. I apologize for all the pills, but it really doesn't take long to get used to it. If you are concerned about getting the most value for your money, consult with the health food store clerk; they are usually fairly knowledgeable and objective because they carry several brands. Most importantly, pay attention to how you feel after a meal. Try to listen to your body and to sense whether each food enhances or depletes your body's energy. That's the essence of eating for optimal health. Learn to create a highly personalized diet based on your own unique constitution, balanced with the fundamental nutritional requirements outlined in this chapter. Do the best you can. As you will soon learn in chapter 4, when it comes to holistic health, *it's not so much what you eat, but what's eating you.*

Exercising and Playing

Unhappy people, I am convinced, would increase their happiness more by walking six miles every day, than by any conceivable change in philosophy.

Bertrand Russell

For almost the entire 4 million years of evolutionary history—until this century—most men have been used to significant daily physical labor. However, in the past sixty years we have slowed our pace considerably. The majority of men today spend nearly ten times as much time watching athletes perform on TV as they do exercising themselves. But we pay a heavy price for the underuse of our bodies.

Studies have shown that sedentary people, on average, don't live as long or enjoy as good health as those who get regular aerobic exercise: brisk walking, running, swimming, cycling, or similar workouts. Some researchers now believe that getting no exercise might be a more significant risk factor for decreased life expectancy than the combined risks of cigarette smoking, high cholesterol, obesity, and high blood pressure.

Although the following chapters present a

variety of ways to enhance your ability to thrive, there may not be a better way than exercise. In my twenty-five years as a health care practitioner, I have found nothing that contributes more to optimal health than regular exercise. No single activity demonstrates a commitment to thriving more convincingly than undertaking and maintaining an exercise program. If you would like to feel thirty when you're sixty, then exercise is the key. The health benefits of exercise, according to Robert A. Anderson, M.D., in his book *Wellness Medicine,* are

1. Dissipation of tension; decreased fight/flight response, depression, anxiety, smoking, drug use; increased self-esteem, positive attitudes, joy, spontaneity, mental acuity, mental function, aerobic capacity, sense of energy; and improved quality of sleep.

2. Decreased back pain; increased muscular strength and flexibility; prevention of osteoporosis.

3. Decreased blood pressure; increased oxygen-carrying capacity (oxygen in the bloodstream).

4. Decreased LDL cholesterol (bad cholesterol), triglycerides, glucose, insulin, cortisol; increased HDL cholesterol (good cholesterol).

5. Decreased recurrence of myocardial infarcts (heart attacks), angina, ischemic heart disease, strokes.

6. Decreased incidence of cancer and improved free radical control.

7. Decreased weight; increased lean/fat ratio.

8. Increased longevity (least fit have a morality rate 3.5 times that of most fit).

From this list you can see that the rewards of exercise go well beyond the physical. In my own experience, a hike in the foothills or a bike ride never fails to invigorate my body, quiet my mind, or raise my spirit.

Although there are multiple benefits to moderate exercise, a recent Harvard study tracking over seventeen thousand middle-aged men for more than twenty years found that strenuous exercise increased their longevity. According to the study, men who reported doing at least 1,500 calories' worth of vigorous activity each week lowered their death rate by 25 percent compared to those who expended less than 150 calories a week.

To attain these results, a man would have to do the equivalent of jogging or walking briskly for fifteen miles a week. Any of the following activities would also achieve the same result:

- Walking at four to five miles per hour for forty-five minutes five times a week.
- Playing one hour of singles tennis three days a week.
- Swimming laps for three hours a week.
- Cycling four times a week for one hour.
- Jogging at six to seven miles an hour (equivalent to a ten-minute mile) for three hours a week.
- In-line skating for two and a half hours a week.

• Two to three one-hour sessions of yoga or martial arts each week.

The first step in embarking on an exercise program begins with recapturing the sense of play we enjoyed as boys: the creativity, spontaneity, and freedom, usually in an outdoor setting. The more your exercise feels like play, the greater the likelihood you'll stick with it. Most men who exercise perform a highly structured "workout" at an indoor health club or in their home gym. Although this workout could qualify as strenuous or aerobic exercise, it often can end up being little more than a physical form of work designed to achieve a health benefit, unless you stay focused within your body. The type of exercise that provides the greatest thriving benefits will be an activity that feels like fun and reconfirms our connection to life energy. These thriving *play-outs* could include competitive sports—such as tennis, basketball, racquetball, and soccer—or individual activities, such as hiking, biking, skiing, in-line skating, yoga, or martial arts. I have a good friend living in the mountains who loves to jog naked along remote national forest trails near his home. . . . Whatever turns you on! The activity you choose will depend largely on preference and previous experience as well as convenience, time constraints, and location. Your level of commitment to any exercise program and your willingness to make it a priority will be determined by the rewards it pays. We're already familiar with the physical rewards, but let's not underestimate the emotional and spiritual rewards. That feeling of well-being you experience after a workout is not merely the result of the release of endorphins, but encompasses an experience of *the zone* and a sense of power and capacity that transcends previous limits. It's a way of living in the realm of possibilities rather than in the confinement of limitations. This attitude of freedom and power can easily transfer to career and relationships.

If you haven't exercised for years and you're concerned about your poor physical condition, you might choose to see a physician for a thorough examination. Or you could take the Canadian fitness appraisal test, consisting of the following seven simple questions.

1. Has your doctor ever said you have heart trouble?
2. Do you frequently have pains in your heart and chest?
3. Do you often feel faint or have spells of severe dizziness?
4. Has a doctor ever told you your blood pressure is too high?
5. Has your doctor ever told you that you have a bone or joint problem such as arthritis that has been aggravated by exercise or might be made worse with exercise?
6. Is there a good physical reason not mentioned here why you should not follow an activity program even if you wanted to?
7. Are you over the age of sixty-five and not accustomed to vigorous exercise?

If you have answered no to all of the above questions, then it should be safe for you to get started. If you have answered yes to any of these questions, consult your physician before engaging in any type of exercise. If you are ready to start your exercise program but would like to objectively monitor your progress, then arrange an evaluation by an exercise physiologist. (Either your physician, local YMCA, or health club would be able to recommend one.) This individual can measure your baseline aerobic capacity, body composition (lean/fat ratio), muscle strength, and flexibility.

In selecting activities that will enhance your physical fitness, choose a blend that will increase *aerobic capacity, strength,* and *flexibility.* For example, weight lifting, which provides strength, usually does little by itself to build aerobic capacity and can even diminish flexibility. The answer is to balance your lifting with a stretching routine and perhaps an aerobic workout such as basketball or racquetball on alternate days. Let's look more closely at each of these aspects of exercise.

Aerobic Exercise

The word *aerobic* literally means "with oxygen" and refers to prolonged exercise that requires extra oxygen to supply energy to the muscles through the metabolizing of carbohydrates and fat. In general, aerobic activity causes moderate shortness of breath, perspiration, and the doubling of the resting pulse rate. A few words of conversation should be possible at the height of activity. This is the type of exercise that produces the greatest benefits to the cardiovascular system and provides more oxygen to every other part of the body. The long-term results include slower heart rate, greater cardiac (heart) efficiency, lower blood pressure, and greater physical fitness. If you are looking to decrease the effects of any chronic disease and attain a greater overall feeling of well-being, I recommend a regular program of aerobic exercise. If you have a chronic disease and/or have not exercised for some time, start *very* gradually. This could consist of walking fifteen to thirty minutes daily at a speed that would keep your heart rate below your fitness level (see the fitness–heart rate formula below). Over time, you'll work your way up to the minimum aerobic level at your own pace and continue progressing from there. The important factors are consistency and comfort. Don't push yourself so hard that the activity becomes painful and discouraging.

Aerobic conditioning does *not* have to entail a great deal of time. Keep in mind the *fun* factor ("What activity would I like to do?" or "What might feel good to me?") and convenience ("How can this be done in the least amount of time?" or "How can I best fit this into my schedule?"). Aerobic exercise is based on maintaining your target heart rate. To determine your **target heart rate,** use the following formula: 220 minus your age multiplied by 60 to 85 percent equals your target heart rate. Keep in mind that 60 percent is considered low intensity aerobic exercise. Seventy percent is moderate, and 85 percent is high intensity. For example, a forty-year-old's target heart rate is between 108 and 153 beats per minute. To accurately take your pulse, use your index and middle finger to feel the pulse either on the thumb side of your wrist or at your neck just below the jaw. Using a watch with a second hand, count the number of beats in fifteen seconds, and multiply that number by four to determine your heart rate in beats per minute. Remember, low to moderate aerobic exercise for forty-five minutes is just as beneficial as high intensity for twenty minutes.

A minimum program of aerobic exercise need consist of only three thirty-minute workouts weekly, maintaining your fitness heart rate two-thirds of that time. A more intensive program could call for five forty-five- to sixty-minute workouts weekly, maintaining your fitness heart rate for the entire period. If you don't have time for a thirty-minute workout, you can still derive some aerobic and weight-loss benefit from three ten-minute sessions, even if spaced as widely as several hours apart.

See the next page for a list of common exercises with their relative aerobic values.

Once you have attained your fitness heart rate (after about five to ten minutes of exercising), try to maintain it for at least twenty minutes. It is also beneficial to cool down (working out at a slower heart rate and with less intensity) for five to ten minutes following the twenty minutes at the fitness rate.

The most convenient forms of aerobic exercise involving the least wear and tear on the body are brisk walking, hiking, swimming, jumping rope, and cycling. If you have easy access to regular cross-country skiing, add that to the list. Having seen many patients with running-related complaints, usually in-

volving the knees and feet, I recommend that, if you run, stretch thoroughly before and after, use good running shoes and orthotics—if indicated—and use supplements, including calcium, vitamin C, and collagen to strengthen your bones, cartilage, muscles, and tendons. For year-round cycling, try either a good ten-speed with a turbo trainer for indoor cycling or a stationary bike. Treadmills, rowing machines, stair climbers, and cross-country ski machines also offer an opportunity for excellent indoor aerobic exercise, as do low-impact aerobics classes. Several sports also provide terrific aerobic workouts, such as racquetball, handball, badminton, tennis (singles), and basketball. Exercise outdoors if at all possible, where it is convenient and safe to do so. The combination of fresh air and sunshine provides greater health benefits than indoor exercise.

Remember that exercise may increase your intake of air by as much as ten times your level at rest. For chronic respiratory disease sufferers, and for those practicing respiratory preventive medicine, air quality is a critical factor in determining where and when to exercise. Ozone, a harmful air pollutant, is created by the combination of nitrogen oxides, hydrocarbons, and sunlight. A bright sunny day in the downtown area of most large cities would produce high concentrations of ozone. The EPA considers air unhealthy when ozone levels top 0.125 parts per million. However, in a study conducted by New York University's Morton Lippman, M.D., thirty healthy adults showed decreases in lung capacity during a half hour of exercise at

Activities That Rate High in Cardiorespiratory Benefits and Their Approximate Energy Requirements

Summarized are some of the better cardiovascular-respiratory exercises and the number of calories expended per hour of the exercise. An important concept is to select several of these activities that are enjoyable, and to use them in such a way that scheduled exercise sessions are looked forward to, not dreaded.

Caloric consumption is based on a 150-pound person. There is a 10 percent increase in caloric consumption for each fifteen pounds over this weight and a 10 percent decrease for each fifteen pounds under.

Activity	Cal per hour	Activity	Cal per hour
Aerobic dance (intense)	550	Rowing machine	840
Aerobic dance (moderate)	420	Running	
Badminton, competitive singles	480	5 mph	600
Ballroom dancing	210	6 mph	750
Basketball	360–660	7 mph	870
Bicycling	600	8 mph	1,020
10 mph	420	9 mph	1,130
11 mph	480	10 mph	1,285
12 mph	600	Sawing hardwood	600
13 mph	660	Shoveling, heavy	660
Calisthenics, heavy	600	Skating, ice or roller, rapid	700
Gardening; much lifting,		Skiing, downhill, vigorous	600
stooping, digging	500	Skiing, cross-country	
Golf	340	2.5 mph	560
Handball, competitive	660	4 mph	600
Mowing (pushing hand mower)	450	5 mph	700
Racquetball (singles)	720	8 mph	1,020
Rope skipping, vigorous	800	Snowshoeing	660

Activity	Cal per hour	Activity	Cal per hour
Squash	870	Up stairs	600–1,080
Swimming, 25–50 yards per min.	360–750	Uphill, 3.5 mph	480–900
Table tennis	280	Weight training (circuit training)	400
Tennis (singles)	450	Weight training (free weights)	350
Walking		Wood chopping	560
Level road, 4 mph (fast)	420		

Source: E.L. Wynder, The Book of Health: The American Health Foundation *(New York: Franklin Watts, 1981). Used with permission.*

ozone levels below the federal limit, compared to exercising in cleaner air.

Writing in the May/June 1989 issue of the journal *Hippocrates,* Benedict Carey suggested scheduling exercise around the rise and fall of pollution levels. In the summer, Carey noted, ozone builds up during the morning, reaches its maximum late in the afternoon, and then ebbs in the evening. In the winter, ozone isn't such a problem, but cold night air can trap a layer of carbon monoxide, nitrogen dioxide, sulfur dioxide, and particulates that can linger into the early morning. A good general practice is to do outdoor exercise in the morning during the summer and in the evening during the winter.

If you are used to walking, biking, or jogging along main roads, lung specialists recommend that you stay away from these high-traffic areas during rush hour. Avoid waiting beside stop signs or stoplights, where carbon monoxide builds up. If you're jogging in place next to cars at stoplights, you might

as well smoke a cigarette. On windy days pollution disperses quickly as you move away from the road. On calm days it can extend about sixty feet from either side of the road.

If all of these concerns pose too great an obstacle, if you live in a highly polluted city, or if you experience a wheeze, cough, or tightness in your chest during your workout, it's time to head indoors for aerobic exercise. Remember that mouth breathing during exercise bypasses the nose and sinuses, your body's natural air filter. Air pollution can therefore more easily aggravate asthma and chronic bronchitis during exercise. Ozone levels in most homes, gyms, and pools are about half that of the outdoors (in polluted cities)—even less with a good air-conditioning system.

Some allergists recommend that patients with respiratory difficulties follow regular workouts with wet steam exposure. This can improve breathing, increase mucus flow and expectoration, and reduce nasal and throat congestion. Following your twenty to thirty minutes of aerobic exercise, and after your heart rate has dropped to its pre-exercise level, give yourself five to ten minutes of exposure to wet steam. This can be done in a steam room at a health club, in the shower at home, with a Steam Inhaler®, or by standing over a boiling pot of water with a towel over your head. You should do nasal/abdominal breathing, as described earlier in the chapter. Do this as many days as you can, whether you exercise indoors or outdoors.

Low to moderate exercise is less strenuous than high intensity aerobic exercise, but is still beneficial (45 minutes of low to moderate aerobic exercises = 20 minutes of high intensity aerobic exercise). This could include rapid walking, bowling, gardening, yard work, even home repairs, dancing, and home exercise for about an hour daily. A treadmill test determined that those who engaged in this much leisure-time exercise had healthier hearts than those who got less or none, although no added benefit occurred in doing more than one hour's worth. Even a brisk walk with your dog after dinner pays dividends. Robert E. Thayer, Ph.D., a professor of psychology at California State University, Long Beach, has found that brisk walks only ten minutes long can increase people's feelings of energy (sometimes for several hours), reduce tension, and make personal problems appear less serious. Not only does it nourish mind and body, walking is also by far the easiest, safest, and least expensive form of exercise. Briskly walking two miles at 3.5 to 4 miles per hour (fifteen-minute miles) burns nearly as many calories as running at a moderate pace and confers similar fitness benefits. By swinging your arms, you'll burn 5 to 10 percent more calories and get an upper-body workout as well. To make walking part of your routine, consider parking your car farther from your office and walking ten minutes to and from work. Walk to the park-n-ride. Whenever practical, use steps instead of the elevator.

To avoid indigestion, make sure your aerobic exercise precedes meals by about a half hour or follows them by at least two and a half hours. Don't begin an aerobic activity in the heat of an emotional crisis, especially if you're very angry. Wait at least fifteen to twenty minutes. Sudden heart attacks have been reported as occurring under these circumstances.

Every type of aerobic exercise has its own distinctive rhythm. The more you practice, the more your body naturally falls into the cadence of these movements. Don't try to control your breathing; instead, let it fall into a natural rhythm in sync with the movement. Try breathing abdominally with aerobic exercise. The more you practice, the more harmonious and dancelike your workout becomes. Before you know it, your workout will feel more like play.

Building Strength

Strengthening workouts can be broken down into three categories. *Strengthening without aids* includes calisthenics such as sit-ups, push-ups, jumping jacks, and swimming. *Strengthening with aids* includes chin-ups, dips, weight lifting, or weight machines. *Strengthening with aerobics* takes in various forms of interval training, which can be done running, bicycling, circuit training with weight machines, rope jumping, or even working out on a heavy bag. The idea of interval training is to work intensively, reaching your maximum heart rate for a short interval, then to lower the level of activity to recover. By repeating this process with your heart rate remaining in its target zone, you shorten recovery time, and your cardiovascular system becomes more well-conditioned as you strengthen various muscle groups. An interval workout on a heavy bag may consist of eight two-to-three-minute rounds of punching and kicking, with a one-minute recovery in between consisting of light calisthenics.

To design a weight program to fit your specific needs, consult a personal trainer. He or she will probably advise you to work out two to three times per week. Keep in mind that you needn't lift huge stacks of weight to build and tone muscle. More repetitions with less weight will tone muscles and provide definition; fewer reps with increased weight builds mass. For each exercise, perform three sets of six to ten reps, with thirty seconds' to a minute's rest in between. Diminishing the number of reps by two for each set, use an amount of weight that will cause fatigue on the last repetition of each set. For example, when bench-pressing one hundred pounds, on the tenth repetition of the first set you reach your fatigue. On the sec-

ond set, this fatigue will occur at eight repetitions; and on the third set it will occur at six repetitions. *Remember to breathe out as you exert effort,* use a spotter for free-weight exercises, and wear a weight belt to help keep the spine properly aligned. If you feel any back or joint discomfort, use less weight. If the discomfort persists, consult your doctor. Should a personal trainer be unavailable, you can find helpful guidelines for specific weight programs in any number of books or periodicals.

Increasing Flexibility

The third component of your workout, *flexibility,* is overlooked by most men. It includes stretching and yoga. Flexibility contributes significantly to strength and function by allowing muscles to perform at maximum efficiency. Limited range of motion can severely inhibit performance, increase the potential for injury, and weaken posture. Muscles exist in a homeostasis, or state of static tension wherein antagonistic muscles exert forces of similar magnitude to create a state of balance. If an antagonistic muscle is weak or inflexible, it disrupts this balance and can cause reduced function or postural misalignment.

In addition to increasing flexibility of muscles, stretching can improve circulation and enhance the suppleness of connective tissue—tendons and ligaments. Stretching not only enhances strength and flexibility, it builds body awareness. As men age, they lose elasticity through collagen breakdown. Athletes who continue to perform well into their late thirties and early forties all engage in extensive stretching programs. Kareem Abdul Jabbar, who dominated the NBA into his forties, as well as Robert Parish and Joe Montana, all used stretching to prolong their careers. Chicago Bulls coach Phil Jackson has incorporated yoga into his team's training regimen.

You should stretch both before and after aerobic and strengthening workouts. Do five minutes of movement to warm up the muscles and body core to enhance circulation before stretching. Never stretch to the point of pain. You should feel a tension in the affected muscle or muscle group, then allow your breath and mental focus to elongate and relax the muscle group as you hold the posture for twenty to thirty seconds. In some cases this time may be shorter or longer. Repeat each stretch at least twice; your range should increase on the second and third repetitions.

In my search for effective holistic exercise and body-movement forms, the practice of hatha yoga stands out as one that integrates almost all aspects of fitness in a single routine. The benefits of this five-thousand-year-old system of mind/body training in improving flexibility and concentration are well-documented. *Yoga,* from the Sanskrit word *yuj,* means to yoke and refers to joining mind to body. During yoga exercises, meditation and physical exercise are combined to unify body, mind, and spirit in a single posture or gesture. Called *asanas,* yoga postures affect specific muscle groups and organs as they simultaneously reshape the emotional and mental body. Yoga is not just another workout technique, nor is it a religion. It can impart bodily strength and flexibility as well as peace of mind. It has been widely accepted in the West as a powerful tool for stress reduction, fitness, and mental health.

Hatha yoga postures include forward bends, back bends, spinal twists, and inverted poses such as the shoulderstand and headstand. There are thousands of postures or *asanas,* which move literally every muscle and joint in the body. These postures help to develop a healthy spine and flexible back. Yoga is considered the best form of prevention and rehabilitation for chronic low-back problems. As the core of our central nervous system, the spine remains healthy and flexible only through movement in all directions. Breathing with slow and rhythmical breaths—full and deep—throughout a yoga practice brings a mindfulness and calm to our bodies as well as a deep relaxation and oxygenation of all our tissues. Though not considered aerobic in the traditional sense, yoga promotes oxygenation of all the cells in the body through both conscious deep breathing and the sustained stretching and contraction of different muscle groups. There are also now more vigorous styles of yoga that link postures together in a flow series at a nearly "aerobic" pace.

The strengthening aspect of yoga is often overlooked for the more obvious benefits of increased flexibility and range of motion. Yoga systematically works all muscle groups, including many not normally worked by other forms of exercise (such as deep abdominal muscles, back and neck, wrists and ankles, hands and feet). By balancing a workout with full isotonic contraction and extension of each muscle or muscle group, muscle tissue is strengthened in a balanced way without shortening or limiting range of motion so common with other forms of strengthening exercise such as weight training. Yoga also increases body awareness, which can contribute to improved posture, balance, coordination, and athletic performance.

The obvious benefit of increased flexibility pays big dividends to the body and mind, as yoga enables one to live more comfortably in one's body and to resist the deteriorating effects of gravity and stiffness that old age brings with it. Many professional athletes now use yoga to increase flexibility and range of motion. Reports of increased reach or body height are common, as space is created between vertebrae and in the joints of the body. Yoga also benefits the endocrine system and internal organs of the body. Forward bends, twisting movements, and inverted poses stimulate the entire internal system, including the lymphatic system. It gives the body a boost that is not easily attained through other forms of exercise. Many forms of yoga are available. Don't attempt to teach yourself the forms out of a book. Instead, enroll in a class with a qualified instructor. After at least a few months of formal instruction, you can probably benefit from a number of yoga videotapes. The one I like is Ali MacGraw's *Yoga, Mind and Body*.

Balanced Conditioning

Martial arts are an excellent form of exercise that can provide all three aspects of conditioning: aerobic capacity, strength, and flexibility. In addition to these conditioning benefits, martial arts teach practical methods of self-defense. Furthermore, they can transform the self by using the training mat as a crucible in which the student observes the relationship between his mind and body in revealing ways. He learns to manage his habitual reactions to stress and fear and develops new strategies for responding to the challenges of life.

Martial arts can be divided into hard and soft styles. The harder styles consist of punching, kicking, sweeping, throwing, or grappling techniques that are repeated in various combinations, coordinated with the breath, until they become reflexive. Harder styles are generally more aerobic and strengthening. Some hard martial arts use weapons such as staff, sword, or short-jointed sticks called *nunchaku*. These hard arts include *karate, judo, taikwando, jujitsu,* and *kendo*. The techniques of these arts can be practiced individually, against a heavy bag, or with a training partner. The focus, clarity, and concentration that enables the practitioner to react spontaneously develops by training the body from the outside in. As the training progresses, the relationship between mind and body deepens as does the understanding of body energetics—the channeling of life force energy called *ki*.

Soft styles work from the inside out. They tend to be practiced more slowly, focusing on the coordination of precise movement with breath, sensing energy as it is directed by the mind through the limbs into the movements. The softer styles emphasize flexibility and the flow of *ki,* or body energy, first. Self-defense and conditioning are secondary. *Tai chi* and *ba gua* are two of the most popular soft styles.

Generally, younger men gravitate to the ballistic movements of the harder martial arts styles, whereas older men will appreciate the gently flowing, meditative qualities of the softer styles. Both offer tremendous conditioning benefits as well as developing body-mind awareness. They can be practiced almost anywhere and instill a centeredness and sense of calm that provides a proven method of alleviating stress.

Martial arts not only encompass all three aspects of exercise—aerobics, strength, and flexibility—they also possess a dimension that connects body and mind in the creative act of *doing.* It is why karate and judo are called martial *arts* instead of *sports.* As art forms they embody the creative elements of play and spontaneity within an established structure of movements. In fact, in the Orient, martial arts practitioners are called "players"—karate or judo players.

Ideally, every workout should have this dimension of play, because not only will your exercise be more fun, but you will also be more likely to make a greater commitment to your exercise program. If it's not martial arts, choose some activity that engages you in both body and mind to the extent you are fully absorbed in the activity and freed from thinking about everyday worries and responsibilities.

Those activities in which you would most intensively experience this level of abandon and awareness might include cross-country or downhill skiing, mountain or road biking, rock climbing, in-line skating, or running on trails. In addition to providing exhilaration, they are total sensory experiences that entail an element of risk, or performance at the edge of control, that demand your full attention in the present moment to function optimally. Any sport or activity, from swimming to golf, in which you are fully engaged can pay similar dividends.

Sleeping and Relaxation

Our diet, use of supplements, and exercise can all benefit the function of our immune system. But perhaps the most powerful and overlooked means of immune system enhancement is the simple and inexpensive elixir called sleep. Although the average person requires between eight and nine hours of uninterrupted sleep, most men average between six and eight hours, and an estimated 50 million Americans would love to claim even that much sleep. They suffer from insomnia—the inability to sleep at night, resulting in fatigue the next day.

Most men are suckers for the ubiquitous image of the tireless CEO or head of state who apparently thrives on four to five hours of sleep per night. JFK and now Bill Clinton epitomize these overachieving insomniacs. But the reality is that insufficient sleep prevents men from maintaining an optimal level of physical fitness. Bill Clinton may be shouldering the enormous responsibilities of leading a world power, but for a man who makes time to take care of himself by jogging four miles a day, he usually looks exhausted.

Lack of sleep and the resulting depression of the immune system is almost always a factor in causing colds. I routinely prescribe additional sleep as an essential component of my treatment for this most common physical malady. Sleep deprivation has been proven to lower immunity. It can also cause a decrease in productivity, creativity, and job performance. In the majority of cases, insomnia is related to a specific event or situation that induces stress. While stress-induced insomnia is often transient, it may persist well beyond the event that precipitated the condition and become a chronic problem. Overstimulation of the nervous system (produced especially by caffeine or sugar) and simply the fear of being unable to fall asleep are other common causes.

Researchers have identified two types of sleep: heavy and light. During heavier sleep, called nonrapid eye movement sleep (NREM), your body's self-repair healing mechanisms are revitalized, enabling your body to repair itself. During lighter, rapid eye movement sleep (REM), you dream more. By resolving conflicts in your dreams, you can potentially release stress and tension.

Sleeping pills have been the conventional medical treatment for insomnia, but as with almost all medications, there are unpleasant side effects to contend with, not to mention the dependence they can create. A more natural approach to treating insomnia begins with a regular bedtime every night, as you begin to attune yourself to nature's rhythms.

According to the teachings of Ayurvedic medicine—the traditional medicine of India—the circadian rhythm, caused by the earth's rotating on its axis every twenty-four hours, has a counterpart in the human body. Modern science has shown that many neurological and endocrine functions follow this twenty-four-hour circadian rhythm, including the sleep-wakefulness cycle. Ayurveda teaches that the ideal bedtime for the deepest sleep and for being in sync with the natural rhythm is 10 P.M. Unfortunately, most people with insomnia dread bedtime and end up going to bed between 10 P.M. and 2 A.M., when sleep tends to be somewhat lighter and more active. According to Ayurveda, eight hours of sleep starting at 10 P.M. is twice as restful as eight hours beginning at 2 A.M. It is also important in resetting your biological clock to get up early and at the same time every day, regardless of when you go to bed. Establishing an early wake-up time—6 or 7 A.M.—is essential for overcoming insomnia. You'll eventually begin to feel sleepy earlier in the evening. Even if you are not actually sleeping by 10 P.M., you'll benefit just by resting in bed at that hour. Other natural aids to sleep include

• vitamin B complex—50 mg 2x/day (relieves tension)
• calcium—800–1,000 mg a day (a deficiency of either or both of the above is associated with insomnia)
• melatonin—1 mg before bed (although it is usually sold in 3-mg dosages)
• chamomile, passionflower, hops, kava kava, skullcap, and valerian herbs; they

are natural sedatives that do not alter the quality of sleep the way prescription and over-the-counter drugs do; most can be taken as a tea, while valerian, passionflower, and kava kava are available in stronger dosages in a tincture (highly concentrated liquid) form

- hot bath or hot tub before bed
- breathing exercises and/or meditation to relax muscles and relieve tension

Don't overlook the benefits of naps. Even twenty to thirty minutes of sleep in the late afternoon can provide a tremendous boost in energy. If at all possible, try to substitute a brief nap for caffeine to solve the problem of a late-afternoon letdown. Hold all calls, turn off the intercom, and find a comfortable spot to stretch out.

Most importantly, don't worry about lost sleep. In most cases, anxiety caused the problem in the first place. If you can learn to relax without drugs, you will cure your insomnia and, at the same time, give your immune system a powerful boost. By the same token, if you can learn to relax without depending on television and a bottle of beer, your relaxation becomes a more conscious practice of releasing tension. Most relaxing pastimes allow you to turn off the left-brained rational, analytical mental processes and engage the more creative, nonlinear right-brained functions. This restores balance to one's mental health. However, right-brained participation does not mean total passivity or "tuning out" completely. Although sitting in front of the TV watching sitcoms or Monday-night football offers a pleasant and relaxing

diversion (humor too can strengthen immunity), three to four hours of TV can have a hypnotic effect that deadens sensibility and depletes energy, both emotionally and physically. Furthermore, studies have shown that TV and computer screens emit large doses of positive ions that adversely affect the electrostatic balance in the air and can negatively affect mood. As with everything else, moderation and balance are critical for thriving.

Relaxation (from the Latin *relaxare*—to loosen) means literally a "loosening" of the mind's focus on a given object of scrutiny or goal. It allows the mind to return to a natural state of equilibrium—a state of balance between right and left brain. Relaxation could include any activity or hobby that engages creative mental and physical faculties: reading and writing, gardening, horseback riding, singing, playing a musical instrument, painting, drawing, dance, woodworking, or crafts. While bridge, card games, chess, board games, and puzzles may be relaxing for some, the most relaxing activities are those in which the stress of winning or losing, or the quantifiable success of performance, does not overshadow the creative activity itself. Mistakes should not preclude the enjoyment of a relaxing activity; otherwise, the degree of relaxation is greatly diminished. This ability to shift gears and disengage the competitive drive that consumes the workplace is difficult for most men, but holds the key to a deeper sense of relaxation and thriving.

If you feel you are too consumed with work to allow yourself a hobby, that's all the more reason to find one. Think back to those activities other than sports that were particularly pleasurable to you as a kid. Remember to balance hobbies with your professional life. If your job is highly physical, such as construction, demanding large-motor skills, then choose an activity with small-motor requirements such as model building or choose a more cerebral hobby such as reading. By the same token, if you spend your day analyzing briefs or scrutinizing balance sheets, choose a hobby with a more physical component such as woodworking, painting, or even a martial art.

Allow yourself to be a novice, to make mistakes, and to focus on the activity itself in a nonjudgmental way. Most importantly, commit the time (two to three evening hours a week) to engage yourself with your chosen hobby. If after a month or two you've given it a fair trial and it's still not enjoyable, it's time to try another hobby.

Bioenergy

$$E = mc^2$$

Albert Einstein

———————————◆———————————

Although Einstein's paradigm-shifting equation first appeared in 1915, we in the West are just beginning to understand its biomedical applications, which physicians in the Orient have used for over five thousand years. In its simplest terms, Einstein's equation means that all matter is composed of energy in the form of subatomic particles vibrating at varying rates of speed. Dr. John Veltheim, a reiki energy therapist, explains the relationship between energy and matter:

> Science tells us that everything is energy and that matter is nothing more than energy in a different form. The chair we sit on is simply energy vibrating at a much slower rate. Our bodies are a composite of many different energy patterns and vibrations. In fact, the universe and everything in it is made up of different levels of vibration. (Daniel Reid, *The Complete Book of Chinese Health and Healing*, 156)

If all matter is energy, the human body is a form of matter consisting of different levels of vibration. In simplest terms, we humans are energy "beings" infused with what Western science now calls bioenergy. Whether we call it life force, electromagnetism, *ki, chi,* or unconditional love, **bioenergy is the essential force that sparks life itself and determines the quality of human health.** In the *Yellow Emperor's Classic of Internal Medicine,* which was written over two thousand years ago and remains one of the central texts of Chinese medicine today, the Chinese identified the fluctuations of bioenergy that occur in the relationship between the human body and its environment. The *Yellow Emperor's Classic* documents the presence of this energy within the human body and maps the pathways, called meridians, through which it circulates. Used by 30 percent of the world's population, traditional Chinese medicine is based on achieving a balance of bioenergy throughout the body, using acupuncture, Chinese herbs, moxabustion (heat), massage, diet, exercise, and meditation. All of these ways of enhancing and regulating a balanced flow of bioenergy throughout the body constitute not only the oldest but *one of the most effective systems of disease treatment and prevention, and optimal physical fitness.* And by the way, before you dismiss traditional Chinese medicine as a collection of quaint folk remedies, keep in mind that Chinese surgeons routinely perform open-heart and brain surgery without anesthetics, using only acupuncture to eliminate pain while the patient is wide-awake on the table.

Another ancient healing art from India, Ayurvedic medicine, is also based on a bioenergy system that recognizes seven major energy centers in the body called *chakras* (Sanskrit for "wheel," to describe the way energy spins from these points). Increasingly, Western doctors are seeing the relationship between the chakras and the seven endocrine glands. Some health practitioners believe these chakras, which are located from the base of the spine to the top of the skull, correspond to the seven endocrine glands in location and emotional chemistry. In fact, America's leading proponent of Ayurvedic medicine, Deepak Chopra, M.D., embraced the Ayurvedic approach after many years as a board-certified endocrinologist. This tradition attempts to enhance and to balance the flow of energy through all of the chakras, thus improving both physical and emotional health. In *curing* chronic disease, both traditional Chinese and Ayurvedic medicine have

been far more effective than conventional Western medicine, the success of which is generally limited to *mitigating* symptoms.

For contemporary American men to achieve a state of heightened bioenergy and balance, we needn't reinvent the chakra. But we can benefit from borrowing some basic precepts. If you have already begun practicing all of the physical recommendations—abdominal breathing, adequate and healthy hydration, nutritious diet, a balanced exercise regimen, and sufficient sleep and relaxation—then you are probably feeling much better. You have already significantly strengthened your health. But in order to *thrive,* you must develop a fuller experience and greater awareness of the body's bioenergy.

To see the positive effects of bioenergy, we can look to the martial artist's breaking through solid blocks of ice or consider other incomprehensible athletic achievements, such as Miguel Indurain's superhuman time-trial performances and his five consecutive Tour de France victories. (This three-week, 2,500-mile race through France is considered the world's most challenging athletic event.) These feats require the harnessing of bioenergy to raise levels of pain threshold, stamina, power, and speed far above the limits of conventional athletic training. In the field of healing, this channeling of bioenergy allowed Norman Cousins to reverse crippling ankylosing spondylitis (spinal arthritis) through the revitalizing power of laughter. The harnessing and enhancement of bioenergy has been demonstrated in numerous documented cases of patients who have dissolved solid cancerous tumors through visualization or mental imagery.

The PNI connection that Eastern medicine has routinely practiced over thousands of years, but which has been confirmed by Western science only in the last two decades, is just now being incorporated into Western holistic medical practice. The body's gateway for the transmutation of matter into energy, and vice versa, consists of the immune, nervous, and endocrine systems. At the beginning of this chapter we saw how the energy in the feeling of well-being—an expression of bioenergy—was transmuted into positive physical properties by opioids. There are numerous physical and environmental ways to increase the body's ability to receive and generate bioenergy, triggering this same opioid/endorphin response. These include

• regular exposure to sunlight
• being in nature
• body work (Rolfing, acupressure, shiatsu, craniosacral therapy, therapeutic touch, *reiki,* and reflexology)
• regular acupuncture treatments
• body movement (tai chi, karate, chi kung, yoga, and Feldenkrais)
• sound
• walking meditation
• exercise, sports, and dance
• sexual energy

By opening yourself to the regular experience of any of these sources of bioenergy, you will discover an increase of energy as a state of relaxed vitality. You may feel a "charged" peacefulness or sense of calm accompanied at times by a slight tingling or current of energy that translates into a greater sense of aliveness. Let's look more closely at each bioenergy source.

Sunshine. Diminished bioenergy can often manifest as emotional depression and fatigue. Psychotherapists have identified that seasonal affective disorder (SAD) occurs most during winter months when sunshine is scarce. The best remedy for SAD is natural sunshine. Second best is phototherapy, using special lights to simulate the color spectrum of sunshine. Sunshine triggers a chemical reaction that produces vitamin D. Try to spend at least twenty to thirty minutes a day in the sun, while taking proper precautions with the use of sunscreen as needed.

Nature. The healing power of living and working outdoors in close proximity to nature enhances longevity. Consider the large proportion of centenarians among traditional cultural groups in many remote areas of the world: the Hindu Kush mountains, the Hunza area of Pakistan along the Afghanistan-China border, the Republic of Georgia, the southern Andes, and tropical islands in the South Pacific. These centenarians all live in harmony with the planet, almost always in an agrarian lifestyle in relatively remote and beautiful areas, enjoying a level of environmental health unmatched anywhere in the United States. Rather than making plans to quit your job and move to the rain forest, set aside time on a regular basis to expose yourself to the four basic elements—earth, air, fire, and water. Spend time in nature. Hiking in pure mountain air on a sunny day and then soaking in a natural hot spring combines all four elements and feels as much like thriving as anything I have ever done. If the mountains aren't close at hand, walk in the park, along the riverfront or beaches, or through the woods. Swim in warm-water lakes or in the ocean. A hot tub or even a hot bath can replenish bioenergy. If you are pressed for time, combine conditioning and bioenergetics by filling your interlude in nature with jogging or brisk walking while the sun is out.

According to the Chinese art of *feng shui*, which seeks to balance bioenergy in the environment, bioenergy or *chi* collects in ponds, lakes, rushing streams, waterfalls, and seacoasts. It is strongest on hilltops, in valleys, and in densely wooded forests. Remember, exposing yourself to extremes of external bioenergy in the form of too much sun, heat, cold, wind, or water will unbalance your internal bioenergy. Trial and error will teach you, usually after the fact, how much is enough. With time, you will learn to identify before it's too late the body's subtle indicators that you are getting too much of a good thing.

Body work. A variety of hands-on healing techniques adjust body structure and improve the flow and awareness of bioenergy. Rolfing (sometimes described as deep-tissue massage) works primarily by using pressure to loosen the fascia, or sheath of tissue that binds muscle fibers. It can enhance the flexibility of ligaments and tendons that bind bone to bone and muscle to bone, respectively. Rolfing can be painful, especially

when the Rolfer is working on constricted areas of the body resulting from physical trauma and emotional stress. Most who experience Rolfing describe it as a good pain, which disappears on release of the pressure, and increases range of motion and flexibility. Personally, I have found Rolfing to be as powerful in improving emotional health as it has been in restructuring my physical body. By contrast, regular massage is less invasive and more of a relaxing experience, although its transformational effects are not as penetrating. A variety of "energy medicine" modalities such as therapeutic and healing touch, craniosacral therapy, and *reiki* channel the practitioner's own bioenergy to heal dysfunctional organs and dis-ease in the patient. Like acupressure, acupuncture, and reflexology, these bioenergetic forms of healing often use the meridians defined by traditional Chinese medicine to enhance the flow of *chi*—or bioenergy—thus restoring harmony to the organs and enhancing their optimal function.

Although medical science has still not conclusively proven the therapeutic value of any of these energy-medicine modalities, the National Institutes of Health (NIH) Office of Alternative Medicine is currently funding studies to document their effectiveness. Keep in mind that the Chinese, Indians, and Japanese have been using these techniques for thousands of years. For the past ten years, I have had personal experience with every one of these techniques and so have most of my holistic medical colleagues. To find competent practitioners of these therapies, contact the AHMA to obtain the *Physician Referral*

Directory (see chapter 8). This will help you locate a holistic physician in your area, who could then direct you to one of these qualified practitioners.

As in any other field, you will occasionally run into incompetence. In seeking out practitioners of these alternative therapies, be prepared to ask them several fundamental questions to see if they are well-qualified:

1. How does this therapy work?
2. Where did you receive your training?
3. Have you ever successfully treated my condition before?
4. Can you refer me to several patients with my condition that you've successfully treated?
5. How long will it take to complete this particular treatment plan?

Acupuncture. Practitioners of Chinese medicine see disease as an imbalance between the body's nutritive substances, called *yin,* and the functional activity of the body, called *yang.* This imbalance causes a disruption of the flow of vital energy that circulates through pathways in the body known as meridians. This vital energy—*chi*—keeps the blood circulating, warms the body, and fights disease. The intimate connection between the organ systems of the body and the meridians enables the practice of acupuncture to intercede and rebalance the body's energy through stimulation of specific points along the meridians with the use of needles. Acupressure uses finger pressure instead of needles on the same points.

People who have used Chinese medicine to treat particular physical symptoms frequently experience improvement in seemingly unrelated areas. This occurs because the Chinese approach tends to restore the body to a greater degree of balance, thereby enhancing its capacity for self-healing. The entire person is treated, not just the symptom, and the relationship of body, mind, emotions, spirit, and environment are all taken into account. Once I overcame my resistance to acupuncture needles, which are lightly inserted just below the outer layer of skin, I found acupuncture treatments so relaxing that I almost always fall asleep on the table.

Body movement. The two forms of traditional Chinese body movement that most increase awareness of bioenergy are *tai chi* and *chi kung* (also spelled *qi gong*). Their slow, graceful movements are designed to isolate specific meridians within the body. The movements increase the flow of energy through the meridians and improve function in their corresponding organs. Both *chi kung,* which can be used to armor the body against physical attack, and tai chi, with its blocking, warding-off, striking, and kicking motions, have martial arts applications. However, their primary focus is to enhance health and longevity. The tai chi student internalizes a series of movements or "forms" that include various combinations of parrys, kicks, and blows. These are repeated with coordination of breath and movement until the action becomes animated by *chi* instead of muscular effort. *Chi kung* uses a variety of stationary postures and movements that direct the flow of *chi* to various parts of the body. Tzu Kuo Shih is a fifth-generation doctor of traditional Chinese medicine and a master of *chi kung* and tai chi. In his book the *Chinese Art of Healing with Energy: Qi Gong Therapy,* Shih describes the benefits of *chi kung* and its practice this way:

In summary, the practice of Qi Gong is guided by three principles: regulating the body, regulating the respiration, and regulating the heart/mind. Regulating the body, respiration, and heart/mind are very important during Qi Gong practice and can directly affect the functioning of the central and autonomic nervous systems. While in a state of Inner Quiet, the body experiences physical changes that manifest mainly as a reduction of basal metabolism, oxygen consumption, and blood pressure, a slowing down of respiratory frequency, as well as a quickening of gastrointestinal peristalsis. These effects indicate that Qi Gong functions well to improve disorders of the body and the heart/mind. . . .

Qi Gong has been shown to have the function of regulating and strengthening the self-controlling capacity of the body. It is highly effective in rehabilitation and promoting rest. Qi Gong allows the body to increase its absorption of nutrients without gain in consumption. Therefore, Qi Gong acts to preserve energy. It gives the body every advantage. This is the main point of Qi Gong: that it can eliminate disease, strengthen the body, promote intelligence, prolong life, and develop the latent energy of the body.

Feldenkrais movement is one of several more contemporary forms of body movement that increase range of movement and the muscles' awareness of their own activity. Feldenkrais is used to rehabilitate injuries or simply to expand on function stunted by social, postural, and even emotional trauma. Although bioenergy is not the focus of these types of body movement, their ability to improve function allows bioenergy to circulate more freely.

Sound. Exposure to healing sounds can strengthen bioenergy while enhancing the function of diseased organs. Ayurvedic and Chinese medicine identify specific sounds for healing and strengthening the vibrational energy of various organs. Part of healing my own sinusitis included the regular practice of humming the letter *M,* which provided a nurturing resonance throughout the mucous membranes of my sinuses. Most of us are aware that listening to certain types of music can create in us a deeper sense of relaxation or compel us to get up and rock and roll. By the same token, a cacophony of noise and its stressful vibrations can weaken resistance and contribute to disease. The noise pollution in most metropolitan areas is an unconscious and unhealthy fact of life for most men, who live, work, and commute in it each day. It is clearly a significant contributor to hearing loss (the second leading health problem among men over forty-five). As far back as the late seventies and early eighties, studies by Gary Evans, a professor of design and environmental analysis at Cornell University, showed that chronic exposure to urban noise levels raised levels of epineph-rine and norepinephrine, the hormones that increase blood pressure. Evans further traced to the noise pollution of urban areas learning disabilities, hearing impairment, and lan-guage problems in children. In today's metro-politan areas, we rarely experience a level of silence that allows us to hear the sound of our own breath. Computers, televisions, refrigera-tors, and heating and air-conditioning vents provide a steady, almost subliminal noise that disturbs our peace of mind and keeps us from effectively hearing one another and the sounds of our natural environment. If we can create more opportunities to experience an aural environment of peace and quiet, we can provide a major boost to our bioenergy and op-timal health. Silence is even more golden than we think.

Meditation can take many forms. You can fix your attention on a visual image or design. You can repeat a mantra or contemplate a koan (a riddle meant to trigger a sudden ex-perience of higher consciousness, called *samadhi* in Sanskrit). Or you can simply clear your mind, loosen your attention, and follow the succession of thoughts and impres-sions as they diminish in frequency with the deceleration of breathing and heart rate until the mind is calm. You can meditate seated on a pillow with your legs crossed or seated in a chair. In either case, keep your back straight with the hands folded in your lap as you breathe abdominally. See the breathing exer-cises that begin on page 56. More important than the external model that you may choose

to emulate for your meditative posture is the internal experience of insight into the chain of sensations and attachments that fill your attention. Observing places in the body where you hold tension will help you to more dispassionately observe the flow of associa-tions that fill the mind.

The meditative posture can be either mov-ing or stationary, but the common denomina-tor is the observing of a string of thoughts or sensations until the mind is empty and fo-cused in the moment, or on the task at hand. That task could be simply observing one's breath, playing a musical instrument, doing martial arts, or climbing a rock face. Becom-ing attuned to the sensory manifestations of life force is the essence of all meditative practice; it synchronizes our experience of mind and body. In the next chapter, we will explore meditation in greater depth as it re-lates to mental and emotional health.

Visualization, or mental imagery, is al-ready a habit for many men. Picturing the re-laxed execution of a golf stroke or tennis serve before you address the ball or step up to the baseline is a familiar way of programming the body to improve performance. Similarly, picturing yourself—your organs, muscles, or joints—as vital and healthy can program pos-itive change on a cellular level as well.

Increasingly, **humor** has been identified as a powerful healer. Think of the energy of laughter as inner jogging; it increases blood flow and produces neuropeptides, which bol-ster the immune system. We'll look more closely at visualization and humor and how they strengthen bioenergy in the next chapter.

Exercise, sports, and dance certainly contribute to heightened bioenergy, which is a by-product of these activities, although not their central purpose. Nonetheless, an awareness of bioenergy or *chi* in the performance of these activities can significantly increase performance. The "zone" inhabited by all peak performers is nothing more than the synchronous awareness of energy as it informs and animates athletic movement.

Sexual energy is both a reflection of and a means of strengthening bioenergy. For many men, sexual stimulation triggers feelings of being most alive, and when they can't experience it, they feel impotent or "powerless." With practice, it's possible to strengthen sexual energy and direct it throughout the body. We will explore this further in chapter 6.

The above list includes only physical and environmental methods of strengthening bioenergy. In the following chapters, we'll examine mental, emotional, social, and spiritual sources for enhancing this energy. If "unconditional love" is synonymous with bioenergy, as described in chapter 1, then these recommendations for physical fitness are all methods of "loving" your body by nurturing it with optimal air, food, water, exercise, movement, body work, and rest.

One important way to enhance awareness of bioenergy is by identifying parts of the body, joints, muscles, even organs, where energy is "locked up." To develop an awareness of the flow of energy through the body, you need to sense where patterns of energy are

held as tension. Through the contrast between the tension, or constriction of energy, and its freely flowing circulation—felt as relaxed vitality or a sense of feeling quietly charged—we become more aware of the currents of bioenergy and the physical and even emotional blockages that can impede it. As we shall see in later chapters, these patterns of tension, or blockages, can be as powerful as they are unconscious and turn us into physical or emotional cripples.

The sources of external energy are numerous and inexhaustible, and yet most of us live in the midst of a perpetual energy crisis. Strengthening your bioenergy begins with developing an awareness of the energy residing in these external sources and learning how our body nourishes and renews itself through contact with them. To sense the subtle currents of energy that flow from our environment into our bodies, we must first let go of the rational ideals or analytical paradigms we've imposed on our bodies. Typically, these models dictate how we think the body should look and how it should function: how we should stand, sit, walk, and even how big our pecs and biceps should be. Since childhood, we have unconsciously modeled our physical, emotional, spiritual, and social bodies according to the prescriptions of higher authorities (doctors, priests, coaches, magazine editors, scientists, teachers, and other so-called experts). By conforming to their models of how we should experience our bodies, we bypass the most sensitive and accurate instrument for perceiving and meeting our most fundamental physical needs—our own senses. In our culture, we have focused a lot more attention *on* our bodies than on *actually being in* our bodies.

Much of the body work or somatic therapy that developed early in this century was pioneered by women such as Elsa Gindler, Ida Rolf, Charlotte Selver, and Judith Aston. Don Hanlon Johnson, director of the Somatics Program at the California Institute of Integral Studies in San Francisco, describes in his book *Body: Recovering Our Sensual Wisdom* the process of discovery that these women used to explore the connection between mind and body, energy and function:

The technology they employ bears curious resemblances to the old witchcraft. In contrast to the complicated diagnostic and therapeutic methods of scientific medicine, somatic therapies are based on immediate empiricism. Like modern dance, their practitioners are people who are skilled at perceiving. Diagnosis is done by looking, feeling, and listening. Healing is simple: sometimes it is accomplished by manipulating muscles and limbs; at other times, by guiding people's awareness to specific areas of their bodies or teaching them basic forms of movement and exercise.

The discoveries that led to the creation of this technology were based on a return to the obvious, an acknowledgment of the authority of perception unmediated by instruments and mathematics.

Elsa Gindler, for example, had to deal with tuberculosis, which she contracted in Berlin in 1906. Her physician told her to go to a sanatorium and predicted she would die. Refusing to accept his diagnosis, she spent six months directing her awareness to the movement of breath in her left side. Her lungs healed, and she became a pioneer in teaching others the curative powers of simple awareness, a method now commonplace throughout Europe and the United States. . . . These people had the courage to assert the forgotten obvious: that we have more immediate access to our own bodies and perceptions than any scientist or instrument; all we need do is revive our skills of paying attention.

Here are some practical recommendations for sustaining your commitment to strengthening your bioenergy:

- Choose an activity that you enjoy, or one that you have been interested in learning about. It should be convenient and not too time consuming.
- Setting is extremely important. Choose a quiet location, preferably outdoors, and one in which you are comfortable and secure.
- Try combining more than one activity. For example, a jog along a park trail on a sunny day that includes a twenty-minute stop for a *chi kung* session, combines nature, sunshine, aerobic exercise, and a form of body movement.
- If you are engaging in a new activity, or you're interested in taking a familiar pursuit to a new level, find a teacher or class.

Discovering bioenergy is ultimately a function of listening to, observing, and truly *being in* your body. Learning to listen to your body on a regular basis and acting upon that feedback can positively transform your life.

Conclusion

To become a physically fit man you advance through the same four stages outlined in chapters 1 and 2: commitment, pain, power, and harmony. Unfortunately, most men seem to need a crisis, or at least a strong warning from a physician, to begin taking better care of their bodies. You needn't wait that long. The journey to optimal health may seem like a thousand miles, but it begins with the first step toward physical fitness. In chapter 7, "Putting It All Together," you will find a detailed step-by-step program for *Thriving*, including optimal physical fitness.

The first step for improving any aspect of health consists of **commitment,** no matter how small, just so it is consistent. This could mean as little as five minutes each morning of the Quiet Five breathing exercise. The ripple effect of this one simple change in your life can be considerable. Give yourself at least two weeks of daily practice; and even if you do nothing else, the results will be noticeable.

To make these small commitments manageable, you must include the new activities within your daily schedule and assign them the same priority as a business meeting with your boss or top client. In effect, even if it is only five minutes a day, you are scheduling an appointment with yourself. Over a period of months, you will gradually increase the length of time you commit to physical fitness.

You will find that your priorities naturally change, as the health dividends of these activities become more obvious.

Eventually, a daily routine could consist of going to bed by ten and getting up around six. After awakening, possibly without an alarm clock, and even before getting out of bed, you could stretch and perform a Quiet Five or Brain Booster. If you have one, a hot tub is a good place to do your breathing exercises. You could follow this with one or two glasses of water, followed by some body movement: stretching, yoga, tai chi, or *chi kung*, followed by either aerobic or strengthening exercises. On weekends, it will be easier to do both—bioenergy and exercise. On weekdays, if time is scarce, then alternate your program: Monday, Wednesday, and Friday—bioenergy; Tuesday, Thursday—exercise. (If you have more time at the end of the workday for bioenergy and exercise, do it then and follow it with dinner.) Follow your morning exercise with breakfast. With all of your meals, begin to pay more attention to food choices and the Thriving Food Pyramid. Be conscious of not stuffing yourself; eat only enough to satisfy your hunger. You can always have fruit as a snack. It may take you several months to establish this routine, but there's no hurry. Remember that this process of creating healthy behavior will become a regular component of your life, as are a variety of environmental factors that impact your life: air, water quality, sunlight, even noise. The key to maintaining and deepening your commitment to your body's health is to make the process *enjoyable*. To see how well you are doing, periodically check the commitment column on the Thriving Self-Test for the Body.

As you deepen your commitment to physical fitness and strengthening your body, you will probably experience some degree of **pain** or discomfort. Whether it is the discomfort of muscles fatigued by exertion through an extended range of motion or by expanded lung capacity, you should expect some of this type of feedback if you are challenging yourself. As we will explore more thoroughly in chapter 4, this pain may even be in part a reflection of emotional conflict. Most men grew up with the old adage "No pain, no gain." Unfortunately, most of us took this to mean that working out was going to be nothing but pain. More accurately, this statement applies to *beginning* to work out, as you extend range of motion and load muscles in new ways. The greater your awareness of physical limits, the more you can gently push your body without injuring yourself. For example, if you start to lift weights, having never done so before, the buildup of lactic acid in the muscle fibers will cause your biceps to ache afterward when you bend your arm. As you continue to lift and your muscles become stronger and more adept at flushing out the lactic acid, the soreness diminishes. But you must be able to stay with the weight-lifting program long enough to clear that first hurdle. This period of adjustment is just as necessary for other activities as well. If you have made a commitment, you will be able to stay with your new regimen.

The goal of your physical fitness program is to learn how to become more responsible to and how to nurture your body. If you are be-

ginning an exercise regimen with some physical limitation such as arthritis, a bad back, or obesity, then you will need to progress more gradually. Over time, as you become more aware of the relationship between body and mind and their patterns of response, you will begin to address and release chronic physical disabilities.

As you commit to a consistent program of physical fitness, *within a few weeks* you will begin to reap some of the rewards. Your reservoir of both physical and life-force energy will have grown larger. You will be physically stronger, more **powerful,** and more flexible. You will develop a more positive self-image and feel better about how your body looks and performs in every realm of activity. You will feel more sexually alive and experience a greater awareness of life-force energy. And if you have been spending more time outdoors, you will feel more connected to and empowered by nature. Your most immediate benefit will be improved endurance and aerobic capacity.

After several months of training to thrive, you will work through different levels of pain. You will experience a surge of power, and you will begin to appreciate a feeling of **harmony** within your body. It may first manifest as an enhanced sense of balance and flexibility. But the underlying physical basis will be experienced as *an effortless flowing of all bodily functions and fluids.* Your breathing will become more abdominal and less restricted, providing a greater supply of oxygen to every cell as it flows through less constricted arteries. Enhanced by an increased intake of water, your circulation will in turn allow your kidneys and bowels more complete elimination of toxins and waste. Your more nutritious diet will provide better nourishment and more energy to your cells. And your more regular and effortless bowel movements will be more conducive to maximum absorption of nutrients. Your body-movement and exercise programs will even further facilitate the nourishment of all cells, tissues, and organs.

As you begin to thrive, you are sleeping more deeply and making time for relaxation. While charging your body with bioenergy, you enjoy greater sexual energy and often greater endurance and pleasure. You are not only becoming more appreciative of the miracle of your own body, and the intelligence and efficiency with which it regulates its systems, but you now have an understanding of how it exists in harmony with the environment and systems surrounding it. You can even sense how this improved harmony may enhance your longevity.

Your body is simply working better. As a result, it can provide you with some of life's simplest but greatest pleasures: deep sleep, uncongested breathing, graceful movement, unrestricted urination, easy bowel movements, and an awareness of the unimpeded flow of life energy that connects us to one another and to our environment. You have taken responsibility for your health, and you are no longer worried about being "in control" of your life. Instead, you are "in harmony." You are well on your way to thriving.

The Emotional Body:
"You Can't Heal It Till You Feel It"

Just as the health of the physical body requires a free flow of oxygen, blood, nutrients, and wastes, so the emotional body requires the unimpeded experience and expression of feelings of every type, no matter how joyful or painful.

Thriving, chapter 4

Why Most Men Are Emotionally Impotent

Have you ever walked into a room and felt another person's rage without his saying a word or moving a muscle? To what exactly were you responding? At times like these, we say the air felt charged, that the tension was so thick you could have cut it with a knife. Rage, like any emotion, consists of energy. Depending on the emotion you are feeling, this emotional energy emanates from different parts of the body, and we characterize it accordingly: "I have a gut feeling." "My heart aches." "The words caught in my throat." "She gives me a headache." "Don't be such a pain in the ass!" We use these expressions without thinking about them, but they each describe a discomfort associated with a specific emotion localized in a particular part of the body. In connecting us to our bodies, our emotions ground us in the physical world. They comprise an energetic structure of their own that I will refer to as the *emotional body,* with a strong correspondence to the physical body. They give us our bearings and balance. Together, with our genetic history, the emotions identify our uniqueness and put us in touch with what we really want and who we really are. The problem is that most men tend to keep their emotions inside, where they go unexpressed and ignored. A 1996 *Men's Health* magazine–CNN survey entitled "How Men Deal With Stress" found unsurprisingly that the most common source of stress for adult men was job-related. According to the survey of the most common ways of dealing with this stress, 74 percent of men chose to keep it inside, 50 percent got angry, and almost one-third (29 percent) used alcohol to relieve it.

Emotions such as fear or exhilaration are expressions of bioenergy that control our mind and body and affect our behavior far more than we know. Their positive, loving expressions can boost our creativity, enhance physical health, and help ensure intimate relationships. In their negative, fearful form, emotions can help us to survive an immediate crisis. They are remnants of fight-or-flight instincts that have enabled our species to evolve. However, in their protracted or habitual form, long removed from a real or present danger, these negative emotions can stunt personal growth, cause dis-ease, and poison marriages. *Ignoring, denying, or repressing emotions almost always results in destructive energy.* We all know individuals—even our own family members—who consistently embody unnecessary negative energy. These "sappers" are difficult to be around. Their emotional energy is so constricted and so debilitating that they can drain our own resources and leave us feeling exhausted and frustrated. *Just as the health of the physical body requires a free flow of oxygen, blood, nutrients, and wastes, so the emotional body requires the unimpeded experience and expression of feelings of every type, no matter how joyful or painful.*

Human experience alternates between two basic emotional poles—love and fear—both of which require our full attention for us to thrive. The energy associated with feelings of love or joy (trust, intimacy, approval, power, exhilaration, and peacefulness) is more expansive in character. The energy of fear or painful emotions tends to be more constrictive in nature; emotions such as anger, anxiety, depression, guilt, and shame are all expressions of fear. The polarity between love and fear— joy and pain—exists in a dynamic balance, and the trick to thriving is staying flexible and attentive enough to maintain that equilibrium.

At any given moment, we experience a combination of love and fear. However, for a variety of reasons men in particular are reluctant to express both emotions. In our efforts to hide or ignore these feelings, we attempt to contain our experience of all emotions. We try so hard to control our emotions that we prevent ourselves from simply experiencing them. As a result, we often fail to receive emotional messages that are trying to tell us what we *really* care about.

I can't count the number of times I have asked male patients to describe their feelings about a painful crisis or conflict, only to have them respond with an extended rational analysis of how and why the situation developed: "I think it was unfair." "She should have done it this way." "She's wreaking havoc in my life." In describing these situations, men almost always exclude their feelings. This is partly because, as boys, we were discouraged by parents, society, and especially our peers from expressing sadness, fear, and tenderness, feelings that were characterized as feminine. (On the other hand, girls were discouraged from expressing anger, aggressiveness, and curiosity because these external, outgoing emotions were considered more masculine.)

Men also use their brains to contain their feelings because no one ever gave us "permission" to have those emotions. Not only did many of us grow up feeling that we were "bad boys" if we *expressed* our fundamental feelings, such as fear or sadness, but many of us were shamed into believing that something was intrinsically wrong with us for *having* these feelings in the first place. As a result, we grew up with only a fragmentary sense of self-awareness shaped by internal statements that constantly challenged the reality of our emotions: "I shouldn't feel this way." "There's no reason to react this way." "I'm not going to let this (feeling) get to me."

The consequences of boys denying their feelings show up in some revealing statistics cited by psychotherapist Michael Gurian in his book *The Wonder of Boys:*

- Infant boys are cuddled, talked to, and breast-fed for significantly shorter periods of time than girls.
- By the age of nine, most boys have learned to repress all primary feelings except anger.
- Emotionally depressed boys outnumber girls four to one.
- Learning-disabled boys outnumber girls two to one.
- Boys are six times as likely to be diagnosed with hyperactivity.
- Male infants suffer a 25 percent higher mortality rate.
- Boys are twice as likely to be victims of physical abuse.

Nothing shapes the emotional landscape of a young boy like a parent—especially a father. Never underestimate the power of a son's identification with his father, nor that father's continuing emotional impact throughout the life of the son. Parents take their cues about gender appropriateness from their own parents and from society at large, and they tend to pass on their insecurities in the form of judgments, reprimands, and disciplines that stifle healthy childhood emotions. Mes-

sages such as "Big boys don't cry" or "There's nothing to be afraid of," especially coming from those on whom we depended most, had an overwhelming effect on how we prioritized and expressed emotion. As a consequence, we learned to reveal only those emotions that we knew were most acceptable, and we hid the rest. We were never able to benefit from what those other emotions were trying to communicate to us.

The fact was, most of us were victims of "unconscious" parenting. Our parents were not evil or malicious. Believe it or not, they probably loved us, but were unaware of our emotional needs, just as they had been of their own. Having grown up during the Depression and World War II, many of our parents were too preoccupied with survival to take time to understand their emotions. Our fathers, in particular, passed on this survivalist mind-set to us through the powerful and automatic impact of our identification with them.

In his book *Emotional Intelligence,* Daniel Goleman describes the "emotional contagion" that occurs between two individuals or groups of people by which they mirror the emotional state of the other. Goleman cites a dramatic example of emotional contagion that occurred during the Vietnam War. An American platoon and a unit of Vietcong were in a heavy firefight in the middle of a rice paddy, the two forces positioned on either side of a berm bisecting the rice paddy. According to an American soldier, David Bush, who witnessed the incident, suddenly out of nowhere a line of six monks walked across the berm, calmly poised between the two firing lines.

No one fired at them and the fighting entirely stopped. "I just didn't feel like I wanted to do this anymore, at least not that day," said Bush. In questioning how this magical transmission of emotion occurs, Goleman suggests:

[The] most likely answer is that we unconsciously imitate the emotions we see displayed by someone else, through an out-of-awareness motor mimicry of their facial expression, gestures, tone of voice, and other nonverbal markers of emotion. Through this imitation people re-create in themselves the mood of the other person—a low-key version of the Stanislavsky method, in which actors recall gestures, movements, and other expression of an emotion they have felt strongly in the past in order to evoke those feelings once again.

As infants and toddlers, this same identification occurs between child and parent hundreds of times a day and is especially magnified between parent and child of the same gender. During early childhood, we mimic every facet of that constant, powerful display of gesture and expression. Each frown or smile becomes fixed as part of a larger emotional pattern that strongly affects how we now behave as adults.

Most of us assume that we escaped the emotional influence of our parents when we moved out of their house. In fact, we did not escape as much as we might have thought. Like most men, we failed to complete this process of emotional self-determination in our late teens. Instead, we jumped into other responsibilities: education, a job, or family of our own. In transposing our emotional energy into job performance, income level, and lifestyle, we took our attention away from understanding the pressures that had shaped our emotional life in the first place. We described these new responsibilities to ourselves as essential to our "functioning in the adult world." *We committed our energy and discipline to performing as well as possible; but emotionally, we remained children, unconsciously avoiding the same old childhood insecurities.* This has been particularly true of men, who typically were not encouraged to explore their emotions as fully as women.

Our popular culture only reinforces the emotional retardation of men. Consider the emotional content of most popular movies made for men—action movies. They feature a stoic, physically powerful hero who goes about blowing up cars or buildings, and shooting villains, but expressing little, if any, emotion. Be it Gary Cooper, John Wayne, Steve McQueen, Clint Eastwood, or Bruce Willis—the American hero has always been a laconic figure who speaks more through action than words. His sense of understatement creates a dynamic inner tension that magnifies the force of his character. His pregnant pauses and long silences generate a vacuum that sucks up the audience's emotional energy. As men brought up on these models and fed a steady diet of competition and aggression, we were discouraged from showing insecurity or any weakness that might be used against us. Most of us didn't have to go to the movies to be exposed to men like this; they were living in our own homes. As a consequence, the majority of us have learned to repress feelings of pain, fear, or sadness to the extent that *we are unaware that we even have them.* With its ubiquitous ads for beer, pain relievers, and antacids, contemporary American pop culture perpetuates the promise of a pain-free existence. Its ads primarily target men and teach us to suppress our daily stress quotient. Although they may be trying to deliver important emotional messages from the unconscious, the tension headache or the pain of an ulcer are unpopular in the workplace because they threaten productivity. It is no wonder that 80 percent of serious drug addicts are men, or that men are three times more likely to become alcoholics.

Physical Symptoms of Emotional Dis-ease

If we spent less time avoiding emotional pain and made an effort to understand it instead—accepting it and relaxing into it—the pain would diminish or even disappear. However, if we continue to ignore and deny pain, it often manifests as a physical discomfort or disease. In the early 1990s, Redford Williams, M.D., the director of behavioral research at the Duke University Medical Center, published a study suggesting that chronic hostility is so damaging to the body that it ranks with, or even exceeds, cigarette smoking, obesity, and a high-fat diet as a powerful risk factor for early death from heart disease. Williams reported that people who scored high on a hostility scale as teenagers were

much more likely than their more cheerful peers to have elevated cholesterol levels as adults. Williams's finding establishes a clear link between unremitting anger and heart disease.

In light of this strong relationship between hostility and heart disease, it's no surprise that heart disease is the leading killer of men. Clearly, anger is the predominant emotion I find in my male patients—at least it is the emotion they are most conscious of. As we discuss it together, the patient usually finds that what they're aware of is only the tip of the iceberg. My experience with male patients has convinced me that we live in an epidemic of frustrated perfectionists—men in our society who were never quite good enough to earn their father's praise, let alone their affection. As adults, men internalize that paternal critic and continue to fear his harsh judgment. It's not the only source of hostility for men, but it probably does account for a large chunk of it.

Addictions such as sex, alcohol, drugs, and especially work are the primary tools for men trying to deny or suppress emotional pain. Workaholism is perhaps our most popular addiction because of the status and money that come with high performance. Men are obsessed with performance . . . in automobiles, sexual partners, athletes, and mutual funds. *Performance is the top male criterion for measuring value, and it is, therefore, the heart and soul of male self-esteem.* In its most fundamental sense, performance implies an audience. Most men act the way they do because they believe others are watching. As performance-driven creatures, we are so in the habit of filtering emotion to make sure our performance is acceptable that we can no longer identify genuine emotion. Men have lost their bearings because they are no longer grounded in genuine feeling.

Ask most men to tell you who they are, and they usually respond by telling you what they do for a living. Ask most men what they want, and they will list cars, homes, and private schools for their kids. What they really want is harder for them to identify because they don't really know who they are. Most men don't allow themselves to think about either question, because they are convinced these questions will interfere with . . . performance.

As you learn to address specific causes of chronic diseases in Part II, you will find that *most of these ailments are associated with unexpressed painful feelings.* In training to thrive, a crucial part of your commitment will require the honesty and courage to directly experience *all* of your emotions. In his insightful book *Celebrate the Temporary,* Clyde Reid, director of the Center for New Beginnings in Denver, describes this new "lifestyle":

> Leaning into life's pain . . . is far more satisfying than the avoidance style. It requires small doses of plain courage to look pain in the eye, but it prepares you for more serious pain when it comes. In the meantime, all the energy expended to avoid pain is now available for the business of living.

Pain is not a prerequisite for thriving and happiness. I am not advocating that you

needlessly seek out painful experiences, nor am I proposing that you endure prolonged or persistent pain: that is called suffering. Life is to be enjoyed, but the notion that it can be lived totally without painful feelings is an unrealistic and unhealthy belief. Pain and joy— fear and love—are intertwined, and the more you allow yourself to experience the full blend of these feelings, the greater will be your emotional and physical health.

Fortunately, it is never too late to become emotionally fit. We can start by assuming responsibility for our own emotional health and not expecting some "magic pill" to clear up the emotional confusion bred in us by the oversights or indifference of our parents, teachers, or peers. In short, we must learn to parent ourselves. We can learn to release patterns of repression that have inflicted pain and continue to cause us to turn away from experiencing and understanding our deepest emotions. The first step on the road to emotional fitness is learning to *identify* feelings and to unlock the hidden messages that they communicate to us. Once we are able to identify and experience our feelings, we can receive the powerful messages they carry that enable us to function as more conscious adult men.

The Path to Emotional Fitness: Identify, Experience, Express, and Accept

Men frequently ask one another "How are you doing?" or "How is it going?" It's a coded way of asking how we are feeling. Typically, the response might be "I'm okay" or "Fine" or "Great." We say it so automatically that we rarely ask ourselves, "What am I really feeling?" If you're honestly feeling great, why? What emotions have contributed to this state of mind? What is it that feels so good to you? Are you feeling appreciated, approved of, a sense of accomplishment or achievement, proud? By the same token, if you feel stressed or you are just "getting by," why? What emotions caused this state of mind? Are you worried, angry, sad, or feeling a sense of loss? Once you have identified the emotion, ask yourself if it was caused by an *action* or a *belief about that action.* Most of the time our reactions to stressors are determined by a belief system instead of being a response directly to the event itself.

For example, the belief "If I don't work sixty hours a week, I might lose my job" reflects a basic fear about your job and notions of success relating to it. That fear may be justified because you work in a high-pressured, competitive environment and you frequently see coworkers being replaced due to poor performance. On the other hand, it may be a belief instilled in you by your father's work ethic, which bears little relationship to the reality of your job and its responsibilities. In either case, the underlying belief causes high anxiety. Once you have identified the fear and its precipitating belief system, you can decide whether it is real and appropriate or not. Based on that understanding, you can make a conscious decision whether to stay in the job or not. In the first case, perhaps you should seek another job in a healthier environment.

In the second case, you need to address a disease in your own belief system. Painful emotions frequently stem from distorted beliefs.

Distorted thought patterns can profoundly affect our emotions by generating attitudes that skew our perception of a given event or experience. This is the foundation of *cognitive psychotherapy*. Discussed in greater depth on page 123, this type of therapy originated with psychologist Albert Ellis, Ph.D. He believes that "virtually all 'emotionally disturbed' individuals actually think crookedly, magically, dogmatically, and unrealistically."

Most of our painful emotions—anxiety, hostility, shame, inappropriate guilt, depression, etc.—are usually the result of distorted thinking, even if those thoughts seem perfectly valid at the time. By changing your perspective and eliminating distorted thinking patterns, it is possible to quickly shift your mood, without having to drink a few beers, take a tranquilizer, or even consult with a psychotherapist.

As we discussed in Chapter 2, the majority of us hear some of these negative messages on a daily basis. If you think about it the next time you feel badly, you'll probably recognize at least one of the following common thought distortions lurking in the darkness of your bad mood.

- *Black-and-white thinking.* You designate things into rigid, all-or-nothing compartments. You mistake a part for the whole, and you consider a single mistake or loss as a perpetual pattern of failure.

- *Negative "glasses."* You see only the negatives, while overlooking your achievements or positive qualities.
- *"Shoulding" on yourself.* You judge yourself and others by using the words "should, shouldn't, must, ought, have to, and supposed to."
- *Loss of perspective.* You exaggerate the significance of situations or shrink their importance.
- *Confusing emotion with logic.* You reason from how you feel. If you feel stupid, you assume you are.
- *Expecting the worst.* Without strong objective evidence, you speculate that people feel negatively toward you. Or, you expect bad outcomes.
- *Name-calling and scapegoating.* You identify with your faults. Instead of saying "I made a mistake," you tell yourself, "I'm a failure, a lousy _____ (broker, golfer, lover, etc.)." You blame yourself (or others) for something you (or they) weren't responsible for.

At different times, each of us has been guilty of employing some, if not all, of these self-limiting strategies. The recurrence of painful feelings almost always accompanies negative or critical beliefs. As the second of our stages to thriving (commitment, pain, power, and harmony), *experiencing* **pain** *has the potential of unlocking life energy and a sense of thriving.* As it relates to understanding the sources of physical and emotional disease, *pain* is an indicator that tells us when we are avoiding emotions or ignoring the reality of our lives. The body has an uncanny capacity for representing to us those painful emotions that have gone unrecognized by the mind and remain locked in the unconscious. These warnings could show up in any number of physical symptoms: chest pains, headaches, or back pain, just to name a few.

For example, suppose you were worried and angry because your boss, the executive vice president at your company, has decided to present a major deal to a group of investors that you have spent the last year working on almost single-handedly. You know you could do a much better job of selling it, but he wants to take the credit and get the recognition from the CEO. Not only are you feeling powerless, but you're also afraid he might blow the deal. Over a period of weeks these painful feelings can manifest as hyperactivity in your stomach, and eventually as an ulcer. However, if you understand how your body mirrors emotion and can express your feelings to a spouse or a close friend, then you can probably begin to relieve both the physical and emotional pain while preventing the ulcer. *Just as physical pleasure mirrors exhilaration, physical discomfort reflects emotional pain.*

There is a saying in the martial arts: "Energy follows attention." It describes the way our body and emotions follow the direction provided by the constructs of the mind. That which we fear most we tend to attract into our lives. If you are worried about losing your job—and keep expressing to yourself the belief "I know I'm going to be laid off"—this belief may hinder your performance enough to bring on your dismissal. On a psychological level, the energy of these painful emotions—loss, anger, and sadness—may manifest in the body as a constriction or tightness in the neck and shoulders, or as an empty feeling in the pit of the stomach. Over time, if these patterns of energy due to emotional disease are not discharged, they can transform into actual physical disease. *If you are experiencing physical pain, you can assume you are suffering some emotional pain that has contributed to causing it.* If we can fully understand the mind-body relationship and the way the body clearly mirrors the unconscious mind and emotions, we can begin to bring these feelings to light. To do so, try using this four-step process that helps us to **identify, experience, express,** and **accept** our emotions.

Identifying Pain

The first step to emotional fitness is learning to **identify** specifically what we're feeling. This means becoming a detached observer of your body and its held emotional energy. A simple way to identify feelings is through the following five-step **Body-Emotional Scan.**

1. Find a quiet space where you will be uninterrupted. Begin with a minute or two of abdominal breathing.
2. Spend ten to fifteen minutes doing a Body Scan (see page 60 in chapter 3). Scan your body for chronic aches, pains, or tense, constricted areas. Don't worry about attributing a specific cause to the pain. Simply experience it as fully as possible. Describe to yourself the nature of the pain. Without using medical terminology to label the discomfort (as an ulcer or arthritis), be as precise as possible in characterizing the pain. Is the pain sharp, stabbing, dull, achy, intermittent, persistent, hot, cold, numb, tingly, pulsating, viselike or constricting, pressured, migratory, stationary, superficial, or deep? Is the pain located in a joint, muscle, bone, or organ? As you explore your body for sensations of pain, you will discover your own ways of describing the pain and pinpointing its location. Try to maintain an openness to these sensations, without anticipating or directing your attention to areas where you know you have a history of problems.
3. Once you have identified a specific physical sensation (maintaining this relaxed state of abdominal breathing with your eyes closed). Try to visualize an incident or experience associated with that felt sense of pain. *The resulting image can be real or imagined.* Again, be specific, and describe the experience of that physical and emotional pain encapsulated in this event—real or imagined—as fully as possible. For example, your knees bother you and you experience an aching numbness that reminds you of playing eighth-grade football in full pads. The pain calls to mind the experience of being cross-body blocked from the blind side. You not only had your legs cut out from under

you at the knees, you never saw it coming because you were wholly focused on making a tackle across the field.

4. The next step is to relate that experience to an emotion. Ask yourself what emotion relates to this physical sense of pain: fear, humiliation, anger, betrayal, grief, etc. The emotions that accompanied the image may well be a contributing cause of your present physical pain. The previous example of stomach pain is associated with feelings of powerlessness or loss of control. I've seen several male patients in my practice whose low-back pain recurs whenever they're feeling financially insecure. Sinus pain almost always accompanies repressed anger.

To go back to the example of our cross-body block, the sudden sense of surprise, rage, humiliation, and loss of control and stability, at being suddenly upended and knocked off course, is an emotional trauma that is still strongly associated with a current experience of knee pain. A highly charged situation in the present that elicits feelings reminiscent of an old real or imagined trauma can actually trigger the same physiologic sense of pain. Try to identify the situation that triggers the physical and emotional pain. Ask yourself what, where, when, or who triggers this pain. For example: "When do I notice this pain?" "Am I at work, at home?" "Is it only on weekends?" "Does it only occur after talking to or thinking about my parents or ex-wife?"

5. The final step is to ask yourself how these powerful emotions trigger a belief or a set of beliefs that strongly affect your behavior. Ask yourself, "How does this pain limit me?" or "How does this pain benefit me?" The answer may be as surprisingly simple as "It prevents me from going to work at a job that I now realize I detest." Or, "It benefits me by making my wife give me more attention." I even had one AIDS patient who responded by saying, "I've always been afraid of intimacy. Now that I'm HIV-positive, it keeps people at a distance." Another AIDS patient said that once he was diagnosed as HIV-positive, his family, who had been estranged from him for years, were suddenly supportive. The point is that physical pain, in the way it reflects underlying emotional pain, may exist to achieve objectives we're often not consciously aware of. This is far from an easy concept to accept. But to truly take responsibility for your physical and emotional health, assume temporarily that in some way we do unconsciously contribute to creating our own disease. If you prefer, think of this perspective on illness as an exercise, and see where it leads you. What can you learn from it? You may find that it changes your entire understanding of *dis-ease* and its role in your life.

BODY-EMOTIONAL SCAN

1. Find a quiet spot; breathe abdominally.
2. Do a Body Scan; find areas of pain.

3. Identify an event or situation connected to this sensation of pain.

4. Identify an emotion related to this experience.

5. Ask how this physical and emotional pain affects your behavior: What does it prevent? What does it gain?

Most men live their lives with a limited emotional palette. How many of the emotions in the diagram on page 120 can you identify in your own life? How many of these feelings do you experience in a day? The six basic emotions expressed by the adjectives in the center of the circle—scared, mad, sad, peaceful, powerful, and joyful—are the sources from which the other feelings emanate. If you identify with any word on the outer circles, you can trace it back to the fundamental emotion in the inner circle. For example, feeling "embarrassed" is an aspect of being "scared" (fear).

To change the current pattern of behavior resulting from the specific emotions we have just identified, it is essential that we go back and actually *reexperience* those feelings in a safe context. In avoiding the emotional experience, we only magnify its control over us. However, by bringing those hidden emotions into consciousness, we are able to discharge their energy and release them from their entrapment in the body.

Having identified what it is we are feeling, we need to reexperience that emotion more truthfully, in a way that gives it a human scale and sense of reality, as distinguished from the overwhelming magnification we confer on it

through a lifetime of avoidance. To reexperience these feelings, we should place ourselves in a safe and secure environment, where we can shout or cry, without drawing attention to ourselves. By going back and safely reexperiencing a traumatic event and actually feeling the emotions relating to it, we realize its impact is often not as overpowering as we had thought.

I learned about the power of buried childhood emotion and its impact on adult behavior by reexperiencing a deep sadness that had occurred as the result of my family's moving when I was ten years old. My experience felt traumatic because I had been living in a comfortable neighborhood where I had plenty of friends and a strong sense of belonging and self-esteem. When I was suddenly moved into a setting in which I was the first new kid in the class in four years, I felt like an outsider. As the first Jewish student in the school, I also experienced my first taste of anti-Semitism. I had abruptly dropped from the top of the world to the depths of feeling like an outcast. As a result of not being able to express my intense rage and deep sense of loss, I became severely depressed.

Many of us as children have had emotionally traumatic experiences, but few of us have made the effort to understand how we carry these emotional scars from childhood into our adult psychic life. When I began my thriving training program, I made a conscious effort to reexperience my feelings relating to this trauma, and I was gradually able to fully express these emotions for the first time. At first, like most men, I was self-conscious

The Feeling Wheel

about crying and allowed tears for only a few seconds at a time. However, over a period of years I was able to experience a powerful physical release of these emotions and was able to cry more freely. The practice gained from directly reexperiencing this sadness helped tremendously during this same period, when I had to deal with the chronic sense of grief surrounding my father's progressive physical and mental deterioration due to Parkinson's disease. Having allowed myself to finally experience the sadness and a sense of loss relating to my "new school" experience, I was better able to identify and experience these same emotions as they related to the ongoing "loss" of my father.

In recognizing this traumatic pattern as it related to my family's move and starting a new school, I clearly saw a pattern of resistance to encountering other major changes in my life. I realized how frightened I had been of change. But since I began training to thrive, I have practiced making major changes, and the fear has lessened with each undertaking. Bringing hidden emotion into consciousness helps with other painful feelings as well. The experience of expressing sadness through tears, and rage through punching a heavy bag, helped me to diminish my fear of other painful emotions and rewarded me with an almost immediate sense of well-being.

Expressing Painful Emotions

Even though current emotional pain is often a "reflection" of past trauma, the benefit of fully experiencing both is to perceive their true dimensions and to discharge their locked energy from the body. This can occur not only through feeling emotion, but by **expressing** it as well. Because most men are new to this emotional arena and have had little practice expressing their feelings, it is important to find safe, reliable techniques and therapies that you can do alone, with your spouse, partner, or with a mental health professional. These include keeping a journal, recording dreams, expressing feelings to your spouse, psychotherapy, and anger release and body work.

If you are looking for a simple way to start tracking your emotional life and to express feelings, consider keeping a journal. This practice, also called **journaling,** means making a written record of your feelings, thoughts, and any other information you would like to clarify for yourself. If journaling is done regularly, it can increase self-knowledge and prove highly enlightening. In a sense, you become your own therapist or your own best friend; instead of trying to convey what you are feeling to another person, you "write" it to yourself. For some, journaling allows greater clarity and ease than expressing feelings to another, probably because there is much less concern about judgment—you are the only one who will be reading what you write, and you don't have to worry about spelling or grammar. *Opening Up,* by James W. Pennebaker, Ph.D., documents in detail the benefits to one's physical health that can be gained by writing about upsetting or traumatic experiences. It is an excellent resource for learning to journal, as is Kathleen Adams's *Mightier Than the Sword: The*

Journal as a Path to Man's Self-Discovery. If you write on a regular basis, your journal becomes an instructive emotional "diary," instead of merely a record of events.

Dreams are always symbolic expressions of your inner emotional life. **Recording dreams** is another technique for developing a greater understanding of these feelings. "Expression" of these dreams, and even writing down dream fragments, can trigger a direct "experience" and understanding of hidden emotions. "Dreams are extraordinarily reliable commentaries on the life you really live—the people you care about, the events you anticipate, the problems you are trying to solve," says Robert Langs, M.D., a psychoanalyst and chief of the Center for Communicative Research at Beth Israel Hospital in New York City. "Every dream reflects an unconscious response to an emotionally charged situation in waking reality. [Dreams] consistently point out aspects of your feelings that you have overlooked, ignored, or tried to keep at bay. My own studies have indicated that the very process of remembering a dream promotes emotional stability. Analyzing dreams is an extremely helpful way of maintaining your equilibrium and your emotional balance."

At least two obstacles prevent us from using our dreams as tools for better emotional health. First, most dreams are quickly forgotten. Second, the few that we do remember are filled with symbolism and imagery that do not lend themselves to simple interpretation. Dr. Langs believes that it is more natural to forget a dream than to remember it, because of our

unconscious efforts to protect ourselves from mental and emotional pain. Langs urges us to trust our unconscious intuition. "When the conscious mind is ready to cope with the meanings embedded in a dream," he says, "in most instances you will dream some other version of it later—and remember it."

If you are able to recall dreams and would like to use them in self-healing, keep a pad and pencil or a tape recorder by your bed. By writing dreams down or verbally recording them immediately after you awaken, you will retain more of the details. The more often you do this, the better you may be able to understand the symbolism of your dreams. Some psychotherapists, usually with a Jungian orientation, are skilled in dream interpretation and can help you. Three books I recommend are *Do You Dream?* by Tony Crisp, which offers many alternative interpretations of symbols; *The Dictionary of Symbols* by J. E. Cirlot; and *What Your Dreams Teach You* by Alex Lukeman. A dream, however, is highly personal, and ultimately, the dreamer is the only one who can appreciate its deepest meanings.

Talking to your spouse or partner about your feelings can be one of the most therapeutic methods for creating emotional health as well as intimacy. We will examine how to develop these communication skills between partners in chapter 6. As you will discover, marriage can potentially be the most therapeutic relationship in your life.

If you don't feel comfortable doing this emotional work by yourself or with a spouse or partner, you might consider **psychotherapy.**

Classical psychotherapy is based on Freudian principles of intellectual understanding of past emotional trauma buried in the unconscious. Like traditional medicine, this conventional approach to the treatment of mental and emotional disorders offers a disease-oriented approach in which patients come to be "fixed." Nonetheless, psychiatrists, psychoanalysts, and psychotherapists might have distinctly different ways of treating the same problem. Other popular types of psychotherapy include

Jungian: A disciple of Freud's, Jung used a more spiritual orientation in working with the unconscious. Jungian psychotherapy emphasizes work on archetypes (personality types), *animus* and *anima* (male and female aspects of an individual psyche), and dreamwork.

Family Therapy: Based on systemic thinking that views the family as interconnected. Problems occur as a result of the way a family is structured or relates, not due to a flaw in any one person.

Cognitive/Behavioral Therapy: Based on the understanding that our beliefs affect our emotions and behavior (discussed more fully in the following pages).

Brief/Solution-Focused Therapy: More frequently used today especially in conjunction with managed care. Short term (one to eight sessions), present-focused, and goal-focused. Objective: to break larger problems into smaller, manageable parts and solve them in brief episodes.

Humanistic/Existential Therapy: Develops awareness of each individual's uniqueness, emphasizes strengths and positive attributes, and has faith in a person's innate ability to solve problems through his own choices.

Today, the majority of patients who see psychiatrists are labeled with a psychiatric diagnosis and treated with psychotherapeutic drugs. As researchers explore the physiology of the human brain, the arsenal of these drugs is constantly expanding. In fact, Prozac, an antidepressant, has quickly risen almost to the top of the list of the most prescribed drugs in this country. Psychiatry is definitely moving in the direction of less counseling and more drug therapy, although every one of these drugs has potentially unpleasant side effects. The emphasis is on treating the symptom with drugs rather than encouraging the patient to change attitudes or behavior, or even simply to understand his pain and learn from it.

A new wrinkle in psychotherapy, which appears to be one of the most effective, is the rapidly expanding field of cognitive therapy. Therapist and theorist Albert Ellis, Ph.D., has pioneered a psychotherapy that stresses the importance of cognition—ideas, beliefs, assumptions, interpretations, and thinking processes—in the origins and treatment of emotional disturbance. There are many different types of cognitive therapies, all of which teach people how to evaluate critically their own thought processes and to trust in their own reasoning ability, rather than adhere to the standards and norms of others. These theories are based on the power of people to transform their current beliefs, similar to the technique of using affirmations discussed in chapter 2. Unlike the Freudian approach, the focus of cognitive therapy is not on the past but on the present: *If you can change what you think, you'll change the way you feel.* This brief form of psychotherapy usually takes under a year, much less time than the traditional psychotherapeutic approach.

The thought distortions enumerated by David Burns earlier in this chapter typify the lack of awareness of self-talk and beliefs that can be reversed through cognitive therapy. Mark Sisti, Ph.D., associate director of the Center for Cognitive Therapy in New York City, agrees that antidepressants can help people with severe depression, but says that "in mild to moderate depression, cognitive therapy works as well or better." In addition, it costs less and has no side effects. For other mood problems—anxiety, stress, guilt, or phobias—cognitive therapy is more helpful than medication. A recent study by researchers at the University of British Columbia in Vancouver analyzed twenty-eight separate studies comparing how patients responded to various kinds of mental health therapy. Patients using cognitive therapy fared almost 70 percent better than those who took antidepressant drugs, those who tried a variety of talk psychotherapies, or those using behavioral therapy.

Dr. Sisti formulated seven effective steps to overcome anxiety and depression. Don't think of these measures as a onetime panacea. Instead, use them over time to create the habit of identifying limiting beliefs and their subsequent emotions that negatively affect your behavior.

1. Write everything down. "Jotting things down provides perspective and helps people detect distorted thinking more easily," says Dr. Sisti.
2. Identify the upsetting event. Ask yourself what is really bothering you.
3. Identify your painful emotions connected to this upsetting event.
4. Identify the self-critical or limiting thoughts or beliefs that accompany your painful emotions.
5. Identify thought distortions (see page 115) and substitute more reasonable and realistic responses.
6. Reconsider your upset.
7. Plan corrective action.

Increasingly, the work of psychotherapy is being done by health care professionals other than psychiatrists: psychologists, social workers, pastoral counselors, and anyone else with a counseling degree. Although this book is intended to be a self-help guide, and holistic medicine focuses on self-healing, I strongly advocate cognitive psychotherapy as an important means of improving your health. Almost any form of psychotherapy is preferable to none at all. In addition to the obvious mental and emotional benefits, physical effects have now also been documented. Norman Cousins conducted a study at the UCLA School of Medicine that involved two groups of cancer patients. The group that had psychotherapy for one and a half hours a week for six weeks showed profound positive changes in their immune systems. The group that received no counseling had no change in immune function.

More and more therapists are becoming aware of the connection between psychotherapy and spiritual growth and have incorporated spirituality into their therapeutic program. In addition to cognitive therapists, I would also suggest the option of seeking a therapist who has made this transition and who understands and appreciates the importance of spirituality in healing. Most of these therapists have a Jungian orientation. Whether it is a cognitive or spiritual psychotherapist, he or she should be someone with whom you feel comfortable. It would be prudent to interview several before selecting one.

Goals are extremely important. Try to clarify what it is you want from psychotherapy. Be as specific as possible. The clearer your goal, the shorter your therapy will be. However, you might be in such emotional pain, or so deeply depressed, that drug therapy may be appropriate. In this case, the emphasis is on a pharmacological "solution" (treatment of a symptom), instead of a cognitive understanding. Remember, only a psychiatrist can prescribe drugs. If you go this route, find a psychiatrist who can clearly outline the choices for you. This psychiatrist should be someone with whom you can talk easily. You also have the option of seeing a holistic physician, who typically includes psychotherapy as part of his or her treatment program.

Some therapists have found that the combination of sound and body movement is far more effective in releasing the highly charged emotional energy of anger than is just sitting and talking about it. In recent years some psychotherapists have begun teaching their clients effective methods of **anger release** using sound and body movement. Not surprisingly, the most common of these techniques is screaming. It certainly worked well when we were kids. The most difficult problem with screaming is finding a place where you won't attract attention or be considered crazy. Doing it in the basement of your home, in a closet, or in the car with the windows rolled up (not while you're driving!) are all possibilities. If you want to make less noise, you can hold your hands over your mouth when you scream. Take a deep abdominal breath just before screaming, and try to bring up the sound from your diaphragm or from deep in your chest, and not from your throat, in order to protect your vocal cords. Slowly move your upper body or trunk from side to side and up and down while you're screaming (this will be a real challenge if you're sitting in a car). Two or three screams in succession are enough.

Although it doesn't involve sound and body movement, I know a holistic physician who recommends the following technique to almost all of her patients to help them release anger. She tells them to write a list of all the reasons they're angry at their spouse, boss, or usually parents. Then, after reading it, they're instructed to tear it into small pieces or burn it.

Punching (a bag, not another person) is another effective method for venting anger. I have a heavy punching bag and boxing gloves, and I make daily visits to the basement for just a couple of minutes of punching. I do this preventively rather than waiting until I'm in a rage. However, when I do feel a lot of anger, punching is a great way to release it. Instead of punching a bag, you can also hit or punch pillows or your sofa, using your fists or a baseball bat or broomstick.

As an adolescent, tennis was my favorite sport. I loved to hit the ball hard, and my cannonball serve and powerful forehand were often accompanied by a slight grunt. Now, in retrospect, after learning that repressed anger is the primary fuel for depression, I'm realizing another reason why I may have felt so good after playing tennis. I was unconsciously releasing a lot of anger on the tennis court—not quite at the same level as John McEnroe, who seemed to be enraged a good bit of the time that he was playing, but it was still quite helpful. Any strenuous exercise accompanied by audible exhaling can serve as a release for anger or stress and return the physical and emotional body to equilibrium. Evidence indicates that strenuous exercise immediately following intense emotional upset can precipitate a heart attack. It's advisable to wait at least one-half hour before exercising.

If you have young children, an inflatable pop-up punching bag may help you teach them that it's okay to give expression to their anger. A gift of this toy shows that you accept and approve of your children's anger. You can encourage them to use the punching bag as a means of venting anger, instead of punching you or their siblings. A friend of mine has done this with his children and it works quite well. What a gift of emotional health to give your kids—to let them know that it's okay to express anger and to provide them with an acceptable means of doing so.

As you will see throughout this book, repressed anger and hostility contribute significantly to causing many of men's most common chronic diseases. Therefore, the expression of anger is an essential component of thriving. Find some way to *safely* express anger daily. It may take only a couple of minutes, but it can add years to your life.

When we try to deny, judge, or even justify our emotions, we restrict the flow of emotional energy and create a corresponding constriction in the physical body. Over a lifetime these constrictions can manifest as postural abnormalities, musculoskeletal dysfunction, organ impairment, and chronic disease. Deep tissue **body work** such as Rolfing can be extremely effective in releasing the bound emotional energy in the fascia, tendons, ligaments, and muscles. Regular (monthly) sessions with a highly skilled practitioner over the last nine years have done as much or more for my emotional fitness as any other single technique or therapy.

Accepting Your Emotions

The lesson of **acceptance** is one that, unfortunately, most of us never learned as boys. Whether it was displaying anger, fear, or sadness, most of us grew up in a society that frowned on expressions of painful emotions. As more men learn to identify, experience, and express their feelings, our society as a whole will become more accepting of the health benefits derived from emotional fitness. We will all become more fluent in the language of emotional health. *Self-acceptance is the art of loving your emotional body.* Its skills consist of identification, experience, and expression of feelings, the process that we have considered in depth earlier in this chapter. Acceptance allows the emotions to flow freely. The more we practice these techniques of emotional fitness, the greater will be our level of acceptance and the more easily life-force energy will fill both our physical and emotional bodies.

Nothing quite epitomizes this free flow of energy so well as **laughter.** The ability to laugh at ourselves—at our weaknesses, flaws, and shortcomings—represents the essence of self-acceptance. In this regard, laughter is a powerful preventive medicine and the perfect antidote for most men, who take themselves far too seriously. In the words of Paul Case, the twentieth-century esoteric scholar, "[Humor] pacifies the subconscious and dissolves mental complexes and conflicts." Similarly, in a hymn to the sun god Ra, we read, "Thy priests go forth at dawn, they wash their hearts with laughter."

Although men's unwillingness to express painful emotions is a primary cause of our dis-ease, our inability to fully experience positive emotions has also handicapped us in our efforts to thrive. We have little problem identifying positive feelings—such as love,

trust, innocence, approval, peacefulness, and exhilaration—but we often don't give ourselves permission to fully savor these emotions. Why? We might consider it too self-indulgent. Our sense of duty keeps us focused on the job at hand. Sometimes we simply feel awkward with emotions that we've experienced all too infrequently. To thrive, we need to start engaging feelings of pain *and* joy more fully. Part I is all about teaching yourself how to do just that in body, mind, and spirit. Just as we identified, (re)experienced, expressed, and accepted *painful* emotions, we should do the same with *joyful* feelings.

"I Sing the Body Electric": Tapping Into Healing Energy

In chapter 3 we discussed the concept of bioenergy. Feelings are one form of bioenergy, part of the energy system that unites our bodies and minds. Feelings exist on a subconscious level as forms of energy that communicate with us through a coded logic of sensation and imagery. The underlying structure to this energetic system has been identified by both traditional Chinese medicine and Ayurvedic medicine, disciplines that are thousands of years old. Each of these Eastern healing arts is based on balancing the flow of *chi* or *prana*—the Chinese and Indian names for life-force energy.

To understand the relationship between energetic and emotional bodies as defined by Eastern medicine, let's focus on the Ayurvedic system of chakras. (The Ayurvedic system is not necessarily preferable to the Chinese system; it is merely simpler.) Ayurvedic medicine identifies seven major energy centers—chakras—located along the midline of the body. *Chakra,* meaning "wheel," describes the spinning vortices of life-force energy that flow into and emanate from each chakra center. Each chakra has its own "frequency" characterized by a specific color, sound, and range of emotions. For several thousand years Ayurvedic medicine has used chakras to treat specific physical and emotional conditions. By balancing the energy in a given chakra, the Ayurvedic practitioner can heal an organ located in the corresponding area. For instance, the thyroid gland and the larynx located at the base of the neck are associated with the throat or fifth chakra. Hypo (underactive) or hyper (overactive) thyroid, voice problems, neck pain, or dental problems can be treated by strengthening and balancing the energy of this chakra. One of the ways in which this is done is by addressing the emotions associated with the chakra. In the throat chakra, these are predominantly emotional issues relating to support and self-expression. As part of a treatment program for such problems, the patient might address issues related to feeling criticized, a loss of faith, and inability to express those feelings. In much the same way, each of the other chakras has a specific emotion embodied in the energy of that chakra.

The electromagnetic energy of the chakras can project as far as a foot from the surface of the body and sometimes more. When there is an imbalance, as there is when you walk into a room and feel another person's rage, this energy radiates strongly enough to be felt across the room. Emanating from the root chakra, this energy in the form of rage can be emitted when someone feels that their survival is at stake. That we can sense this emotion without any visual or auditory clues indicates just how strong this energy can be. Conversely, if we try to hide or repress these basic energy states, or feelings, we can deplete enormous stores of life energy and subsequently weaken the immune system. Just as we learned to identify and safely express emotion, we should be equally aware of how we store and produce these same emotions through our energy centers. The chakras not only hold energy in the form of emotion, they transmit that energy to the other centers and can profoundly affect our mental and physical states of being. The chakras can tip us off to hidden emotional responses that we need to consciously address. Think of how your body feels the next time your boss criticizes you and you have to sit there and take it. Ask yourself, "Where am I storing this energy?"

The first or **root chakra** is located between the anus and scrotum. It is associated with feelings of security, survival, and vitality. Root chakra energy connects us to the earth and to our "tribe," which might consist of other men, our country of origin, ethnic background, or religion. Sexual energy is also a component of the root chakra and can overlap with the lower belly chakra. Physical dysfunction relating to an imbalance in this chakra might include impotence, prostate, rectum (including constipation), and immune system problems. The color associated with the root chakra is ruby red.

The second chakra—sometimes called the lower belly or **sex chakra**—is located four finger-widths below the navel. As the body's natural center of balance and movement, the second chakra provides a focus of concentration and energy for martial artists, dancers, and athletes. It is the center of power and control (money), sex and relationships, creative energy, and feelings of mental, emotional, and spiritual pleasure. Recent research has identified the lower abdomen as a second brain directing vital, unconscious bodily functions, particularly those relating to the parasympathetic nervous system, which quiets and calms the body. It has also been suggested that this concentration of nerve endings is the source of many emotions. An obstruction of the free flow of energy through this chakra might result in a lack of creativity, as well as in problems with the large intestine, bladder, hips, and lower back. The color associated with the second chakra is orange.

The **solar plexus chakra** is located in the central hollow just below the breastbone or sternum. Its emotional energy is associated with feelings of personal power, charisma, and self-confidence. This chakra influences the adrenal glands, which produce the hormone adrenaline to fire up the sympathetic nervous system and activate our fight-or-flight response. Physical problems associated with this chakra, other than adrenal dysfunction, include those of the stomach, liver, kidney, pancreas, small bowel, and middle back.

The color associated with the solar plexus chakra is yellow. If this chakra is open and balanced, you will have a greater sense of self-esteem. You will experience feelings of wholeness and expansiveness and have a better sense of who you are in the universe.

Although it lies close to the anatomical position of the heart, the **heart chakra** is located at the center of the chest, about one inch above the base of the sternum where the ribs come together. The emotions associated with this chakra are the same as those we usually relate to the anatomical heart: compassion, unconditional love, and harmony, as well as grief, anger, and self-centeredness. Heart, lung, and circulatory problems, in addition to dysfunction of the thymus gland (causing reduced immune function), typify an imbalance in the heart chakra. The color associated with the heart chakra is green.

As we have already mentioned, the **throat chakra** relates to feelings of self-expression, addiction, judgment, criticism, and faith. Located at the base of the neck, the chakra's predominant color is blue.

The sixth chakra is called **the third eye.** It is located in the center of the forehead, between and behind the eyebrows. When this chakra is clear, you experience a heightened sense of intellect, intuition, imagination, and awareness. You encounter a level of reality that transcends the ego. Physical dysfunction related to this chakra include eye problems, hearing impairment, nose and sinus problems, sleep disorders, and limited or "stuck" thinking (which can contribute to any chronic disease), and brain and nervous system problems. Hormonal imbalance related to the pineal gland is a dysfunction of the third eye. Melatonin is the primary hormone secreted by the pineal gland. Synthetic melatonin is now widely used to treat insomnia and jet lag, while enhancing immunity. Balanced third-eye energy can contribute significantly to the creative process and imaginative vision needed to fulfill professional and financial success. The Brain Booster breathing exercise in chapter 3 (see page 59) is an effective exercise for stimulating the third eye. The color associated with the third eye chakra is indigo.

The seventh or **crown chakra** is located above the center of the top of the head. Through the crown chakra you experience mystical feelings of spiritual power, unlimited potential, ability to trust life, selflessness, and a profound connection to God. Through this center you can experience the expansiveness of the soul—realms of peace, silence, and wonder. Many hormonal disorders associated with the pituitary gland are related to an imbalance or obstruction of life energy through the crown chakra. Skin and musculoskeletal problems are also related to this chakra. The color most associated with the crown chakra is violet.

Chakra-Charging Visualization

Because the chakras function interdependently, if one is out of balance or obstructed, it can potentially affect all of the others depending on the degree of the imbalance. Clearing or balancing the chakras is a powerful technique for creating both physical and emotional fitness and can be done in just a few minutes in conjunction with the Quiet Five exercise or abdominal breathing. I call the following method of balancing the chakra energy **chakra-charging,** because it will energize you with a feeling of clarity and power. Although I often do this exercise while jogging, walking, or hiking, it is important to maintain a sense of being grounded and focused on the exercise. It may be even more effective to do this sitting comfortably with your eyes closed. Chakra-charging is a visualization exercise in which you will picture energy flowing up from the earth beneath your feet, spiraling through your body and into each of the seven chakras.

Begin by visualizing a bright white light rising up through your feet and into your legs. Continuing through the legs, the light converges at the root chakra between your scrotum and anus. As you visualize this light (which may assume different colors as it ascends through each chakra), you will begin to experience a sense of relaxation in your pelvis. This can elicit feelings of safety, security, and stability, along with a strong connection to the earth. This sensation of energy or comfort signals a balanced charge in the root chakra. Once you have expressed this feeling, allow the light to spiral up to the next chakra.

When the light enters the sex chakra in the lower belly, four fingers below the navel, you will begin to experience a sense of relaxation in this area and possibly feelings of sexual energy and pleasure. This again indicates a charge of balanced energy in the second chakra.

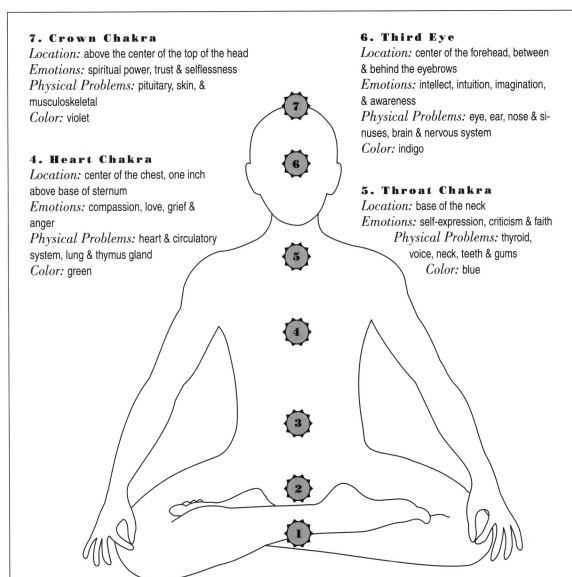

7. Crown Chakra
Location: above the center of the top of the head
Emotions: spiritual power, trust & selflessness
Physical Problems: pituitary, skin, & musculoskeletal
Color: violet

4. Heart Chakra
Location: center of the chest, one inch above base of sternum
Emotions: compassion, love, grief & anger
Physical Problems: heart & circulatory system, lung & thymus gland
Color: green

6. Third Eye
Location: center of the forehead, between & behind the eyebrows
Emotions: intellect, intuition, imagination, & awareness
Physical Problems: eye, ear, nose & sinuses, brain & nervous system
Color: indigo

5. Throat Chakra
Location: base of the neck
Emotions: self-expression, criticism & faith
Physical Problems: thyroid, voice, neck, teeth & gums
Color: blue

3. Solar Plexus Chakra
Location: central hollow below the breastbone
Emotions: self-confidence & charisma
Physical Problems: adrenals, stomach, liver, pancreas & small bowel
Color: yellow

2. Sex (Lower Belly) Chakra
Location: four inches below navel
Emotions: power, sex & relationships
Physical Problems: large intestine, bladder, hip & lower back
Color: orange

1. Root Chakra
Location: between the anus & scrotum
Emotions: security, survival & vitality
Physical Problems: impotence, prostate, rectum & immune system
Color: ruby red

Repeat this process of directing energy as light to the solar plexus, heart, throat, third eye, and crown. As you visualize each concentration of light and its corresponding chakra, you will experience those nurturing or positive emotions characteristic of each center: power and self-confidence from the solar plexus; compassion and love from the heart; faith and self-expression from the throat; imagination and intuition from the third eye; and spiritual power or selflessness from the crown.

The whole chakra-charging visualization can take up to fifteen minutes, depending on distractions in your environment and your degree of concentration. Do not move from one chakra to the next until you have fully experienced the energy and nurturing emotion related to that chakra. Always end this visualization by returning your focus and energy to the second chakra in order to leave the body in a balanced state. Because this visualization demands full concentration, don't attempt it while driving or while operating heavy equipment. If performed with attention and focused awareness, chakra-charging will almost always result in a feeling of heightened energy and vitality. It will build awareness and an experience of nurturing feelings and enhanced emotional fitness. There are numerous variations on this basic visualization. There is no one right way to do this.

Conclusion

The biggest obstacle for most men along the path to thriving is our largely unconscious denial and repression of emotional pain. We deny emotional pain primarily through our addictions. These enable us to (1) divert emotional energy from actual pain to pleasurable substitutes and (2) to engage in a known experience or routine that alleviates the fear of an uncertain or uncontrollable outcome. The most common addictions among men are workaholism, alcoholism, sex, drug addiction, and overeating. A man who anticipates the birth of his first child, and all the responsibility and limitation that might entail, may start drinking three or four beers each night instead of his usual one or two. Without his being aware of it, the comforting buzz anesthetizes him from experiencing or expressing his fear. I had one patient whose marriage was troubled; he used work as an excuse to avoid coming home. He became a workaholic and purposely overcommitted to the routines, responsibilities, and performance at the office, instead of facing up to the uncertainty and pain awaiting him at home.

Pain is the second and perhaps most challenging of our four stages—commitment, pain, power, and harmony. It is somewhat ironic that men are far more willing to endure physical pain than emotional pain, yet most of us fail to realize that *one of the greatest contributors to physical discomfort is unexpressed emotional pain.* The more we practice emotional fitness, the less our behavior will be controlled by these painful emotions. Think of these emotions as configurations of energy with their own distinctive shape and drama. When we are traumatized or have a strong emotional reaction and don't allow ourselves to feel that emotion, we lock that pattern of energy deep inside our physical body. Every time a similar emotional experience arises, we become reflexively engaged in this dramatic fragment—an unwilling player locked in a painfully familiar scene, unable to move the plot along to its denouement. And yet the script is ours to write. When we can first *identify* this pain and we learn to *experience, express,* and *accept* it, only then will the drama be allowed to unfold and the energy can assume its flow through the emotional body. Almost every physical disease results in large part from this stifling of emotional pain and our subsequent self-imprisonment within this avoidance behavior.

As you practice emotional fitness, you commit to an awareness of your pain and pleasure that enables you to determine who you really are. By letting go of your fear of experiencing life more fully, you allow yourself to "embrace" all of your emotions. You will be liberated from their unconscious tyranny. *It's only when the emotional energy of fear and love go unexpressed that we succumb to the unconscious tyranny and paralysis of a life unlived.* Only through fully experiencing *both pain and joy* can you attain the realization of those unique talents, gifts, and purpose in life that constitute your personal power and lead you on your way to thriving. Like any other skill, it gets easier with practice.

Chapter 5

Power:
Connecting to Spirit

To study the way
is to study the self.

To study the self
is to forget the self.

To forget the self
is to be enlightened by all things.

To be enlightened by all things
is to remove the barrier
between self and other.

Dogen Zenji

———————◆———————

What Is Spirit?

Suppose your parents told you as a kid there was a reason why you were here and that your main focus in life was to find out for yourself what that purpose was. They explained that you have a special gift that no one else has, and that you have a singular way of expressing that talent. All that they asked of you was to discover for yourself what that unique talent was and to use it to best serve humanity. Even if you were never so fortunate to have had such parents (who was?), it's never too

late to find your purpose and free yourself to take risks instead of fearing the consequences of every choice you make.

Exploring who you are and discovering what you are here to do requires a measure of faith—personal responsibility and a sense of adventure—that most American men never allow themselves to experience. Instead, we tend to limit ourselves, playing by the rules and conforming to institutional norms that limit awareness and narrow our options. Typically these restrictions are self-imposed. They play on our greatest fears—professional failure, loss of control, rejection, and poverty. Collectively these fears imprison us in a cell of our own making. By unconsciously accepting limiting beliefs and their attendant fears, we inhabit a jail without walls, wistfully looking out at views of majestic yet unattainable grandeur. Yet each of us has the capability of escaping from this bondage. Each and every one of us holds the key. It is called **spirit**. It consists simply of identifying our greatest gifts, realizing our purpose, and releasing past fears *by experiencing fully the power of the present moment*. The trick is to keep your eye on this empowering ball.

Spirit is the power released through the

selfless experience of the present. It is an experience you never had in Sunday school, because it is nothing that you can write on a chalkboard or memorize from a workbook. (The fact is you probably didn't want to be there to hear about it in the first place.) The first requirement for an experience of spirit is the willingness to face reality without making judgments. Thoughts, judgments, and comparisons belong to the discriminating mind—that egotistical little know-it-all voice inside your head that is constantly telling you what to watch out for and what a failure you are. These messages are based on past experience and divert our attention from knowing the reality that exists in the present moment—a reality that is knowable only by putting aside the ego. (Remember Dogen Zenji's advice: "To forget the self is to be enlightened by all things.") Selflessness is easier said than done and one of the hardest things for men to do. Asking most men to set aside their ego is like asking the Great Dane to ignore the poodle in heat.

Spirit is neither mind nor body, but animates both. Although usually referred to as God, spirit may be called many things: the creator, Jesus, Allah, Yahweh, and Buddha. It has also been called intuition, higher self, and inner healer, teacher, guide, or child. In earlier chapters we referred to spirit as life-force energy or *chi*. Spirit is located neither in the brain nor in any single organ, but the closest thing to its true reservoir is probably the heart, with its untapped supply of unconditional love.

An experience of ourselves in touch with, and part of, a larger awareness in which we all participate constitutes the power of spirit. Spirit is present in any moment in which we suddenly realize our connection with life-force energy or *chi, when we feel profoundly alive.* It occurs in the experience of watching your child's birth, of being present at the death of a loved one, but also in listening to a running stream, a favorite song, or in smelling the fragrance at the nape of a woman's neck. Most often these moments of joy surprise us, because they present us with a perception of reality suddenly freed from the usual judgments and concerns of the ego. They offer instances in which time seems to slow to a standstill as we lose ourselves in *pure awareness.* Although these moments often occur as accidental encounters, to thrive we want to encourage these experiences of spirit, to make them a more conscious and frequent part of our lives. Eventually, we will be able to access spirit and awareness at will, and to make it the basis for all our actions, relationships, triumphs, and even failures.

By generating the emotions associated with transcendent experience, using techniques described in each of the earlier chapters, we can put ourselves in touch with spirit. If you feel that you are immune to an experience of God, just think back to the last time you were in the zone, to the first time you made out with a girl you really liked, or to whenever you just felt exhilarated. What you felt was more than just endorphins kicking in: it was an experience of spirit. Like subatomic particles that can be identified without being directly observed, that sense of spirit is identifiable mostly through the traces left behind from its creative presence in our lives. It's hard to talk about because it never seems to last for more than the instant it takes us to recognize it. This chapter will try to show how to do that; it presents a series of methods for more purposefully engaging spirit, allowing it to direct our lives and to reveal a far greater dimension of power than any you have ever known.

Think of a time when you stopped to help someone—a friend or total stranger. That selfless act of giving goes to the essence of spirit. By *sharing* with others your special gifts and talents in a way that benefits them, you engage in perhaps the most powerful means of expressing spirit. The ability to *receive* from others is the other side of the spiritual coin. Most men are reluctant to receive the attention, time, or love of others, because of our insatiable appetite for control. We insist on seeing ourselves as givers and providers, but the ability to receive is a fundamental step in understanding the flow of spirit that streams both into and out of our lives. Spirit is nothing we own, but it resides in us as much as we reside within it, conscious of its presence and living it moment to moment. You don't need a Jim Bakker, Pat Robertson, or even a Maharishi Mahesh Yogi, or any other guru for that matter, to intercede on your behalf and direct your spiritual growth. There are no "carriers" or "networks" where spirit is concerned. You can get your own direct line whenever you want.

One way to make choices informed by spirit consists simply of asking, "How does this decision make me feel?" If it makes you feel bad, you're on the wrong track. Normal sweaty palms about risk-taking aside, if your decision is not in harmony with spirit, you will probably experience some form of acute discomfort: an injury, disabling muscle tension, severe headache, and/or nausea, among others. Over time these stresses add up to chronic dis-ease: prostate, heart, and substance abuse problems being perennial favorites with American men. The good news is that if you're on the right track, you will also know it: "Joy is the most infallible sign of the presence of God," wrote Teilhard de Chardin. (A twentieth-century French priest, paleontologist, and philosopher, Teilhard de Chardin also maintained that the universe and humankind are evolving toward a state of perfection.)

If the first step in accessing the unlimited source of power and awareness called spirit is setting aside judgment and seeking joy, the next requirement is making a commitment to give yourself the *time* to do so. There are specific techniques for slowing down our physical and mental activity. They allow us to disengage the body and mind from their attachment to endless rounds of thoughts and judgments, and these methods form the basis of meditation and prayer. When we plug into these techniques, we experience ourselves as expressions of spirit instead of as reflections of thought patterns and fears—the ego. They take us to that "great good place" that Deepak Chopra calls the "gap between thoughts."

Men in particular have a difficult time of

"letting go" long enough to allow themselves an experience of spirit. We're anxiety junkies and have been conditioned to believe that unless we are on top of our games, troubleshooting every detail of our jobs and our lives, we will fail. Most men derive their self-esteem from *doing*—actively using their bodies and minds for purposes of high achievement and recognition. To "let go" and give ourselves over to a process that is nonactive, receptive, and fraught with uncertainty can seem terrifying; most men would rather opt for a vasectomy. But this act of surrender is exactly what spiritual health demands. If we insist on basing self-esteem on the peak performance of body and mind alone, as manifested by external accomplishments and ephemeral successes, we are sure to be disappointed. *After all, we are at heart spiritual beings, and true self-esteem comes from a recognition of our life experience as a unique expression of spirit, rather than from the size of our bank accounts or the number of our sexual conquests.* Undiminished by age and unbounded by time, spirit is far more than a consolation for the aging of body and mind. As we discover who we truly are by connecting with spirit, we start to live more fully and become more in touch with life itself.

Accessing Spirit

Letting go of the ego entails a surrender of mind and body that most men equate with death—a thought that can be overpoweringly frightful. But just what exactly are we afraid of? What is the experience of death? Typically we think of it as the extinguishing of mind and body—the death of the self, or ego. However, as we've seen, exhilarating and transcendent experiences of spirit can also include the absence of ego, and yet we don't consider these to be frightening. If death is the freeing of spirit from the physical plane, perhaps it is not as frightening a prospect as we might imagine. Perhaps it might even be exhilarating.

It's not exactly what you might have chosen for your major, but in the last few decades a scientific field of study dedicated to death and dying has emerged. Elisabeth Kübler-Ross, M.D., who pioneered this investigation, is recognized as the leading medical expert on death and dying. She has concluded from her many years of scientific research that "death does not exist . . . that all that dies is a physical shell housing an immortal spirit." Kübler-Ross describes the time spent in our bodies on earth as but a brief part of our total span of existence. She urges that to "live well" while we are here means to learn to love—which is the active recognition, engagement, and appreciation of spirit in ourselves and in others.

Kübler-Ross is no longer alone in her belief that death is merely the shedding of a physical shell instead of an absolute ending. Her view that death, like life, is a transformational stage in our evolution as spiritual beings is one shared by a growing number of physicians and researchers who have studied the increasing number of reported "near death experiences." These episodes, called NDEs, involve people who are considered clinically dead in emergency or operating rooms, or at the scenes of accidents, and are subsequently resuscitated. These people report strikingly similar experiences, consisting in almost every case of the following elements:

- Leaving their traumatized bodies, but maintaining complete visual and auditory awareness. This may have consisted of seeing and hearing from an elevated vantage point above their traumatized bodies the emergency room staff working on them.
- The sense of traveling through a tunnel and being enveloped in a bright white light.
- A feeling of profound peace and unconditional love.
- A sense of restored physical wholeness. If they were blind, they could see. If they were amputees, they sensed their severed limb functioning again.
- A comforting greeting by loved ones or close relatives (known and unknown) who had preceded them in death.
- A panoramic review of the events in their life.
- A reluctance to leave the dimension of spirit and return to the body.
- A consequently greater appreciation for life and life's purpose, resulting in an enhanced ability to take risks, and to reduce stress and the fear of death.

The consistency of these NDE reports confirms Kübler-Ross's observation that the soul (the individual expression of spirit) remains intact beyond the death of the body. This belief forms the basis for the concept of reincar-

nation asserted by several of the world's major religions: Buddhism and Hinduism most notably, but even the mystical teachings of Judaism and Christianity. Reincarnation is the belief that souls take on a number of lives on the physical plane for the purpose of spiritual learning, until the spirit has sufficiently developed to break the cycle of birth and death. In his groundbreaking study of past lives, *Many Lives, Many Masters*, psychiatrist Brian Weiss, M.D., describes his therapeutic use of hypnotherapy to document the belief that not only has each of us reincarnated many times, but that we can recall those past lives. Weiss cites numerous cases of patients under hypnosis speaking in foreign languages, or recounting in detail past events and situations they could not otherwise have known, given their present life experience.

Whether you choose to believe this evidence or not, two facts remain: (1) our physical bodies are going to die, and (2) we continue to amass evidence that proves the existence of spirit beyond the dimensions of mind and body. The understanding and acceptance of this ultimate release into spirit has the ability to greatly heighten creativity, to enhance our healing capacity, and to free us to realize our true purpose. What this means is that you're still going to have to pay off your credit cards, but at least you'll be able to take more risks and experience more freedom while you're doing it. Even if you reject the belief in reincarnation and the world of spirit beyond death, merely accepting your mortality and living as if you knew you had only a year left to live would fill your life with a rejuvenating sense of spirit. Maybe this explains the popularity of extreme activities such as bungee-jumping, rock climbing, and skydiving. Increasingly, people are living closer to the edge, risking death, to more fully experience life. But you don't have to jump out of an airplane to connect with spirit. Randall Hassell is a martial artist who has collected numerous traditional stories about Zen and the martial arts. One of these reveals the secret to "mastery" as the willingness to accept one's own death:

Yagyu Tajima no kami Munenori was a famous swordsman who was retained as a teacher by the Shogun, Tokugawa Iyemitsu.

One day, one of the Shogun's guards approached Yagyu and asked to be accepted as a student of the sword.

"I would be happy to teach you," Yagyu said, "but it is obvious to my trained eye that you are already a master. To which ryu [school] do you belong?"

"Sensei," replied the guard, "it shames me to tell you that I know nothing of swordsmanship. I have never studied the art."

"Don't try to make a fool of me!" roared Yagyu. "I know a master when I see one, and you have obviously studied long and hard."

"Sir," said the guard. "I am sorry to upset you, but I swear that I know nothing."

"All right," Yagyu conceded, "but the way you move tells me that you are a great master of something, and you must tell me what it is."

"Well," replied the guard, "since I was born a samurai, I knew that eventually I would have to be trained for warfare, and at a very early age I determined to practice Zen to overcome my fear of death. After many years of practice and meditation, I can honestly say that I have solved the problem, and death holds no meaning for me. Perhaps this is what you are sensing."

"That's it!" cried Yagyu. "I was right. Of all the hundreds of students I have trained in the way of the sword, not one of them has yet received a certificate of mastery from me, because they are all still afraid of dying. You, however, have practiced Zen until you have completely transcended matters of life and death.

"You need no technical training. You are already a great master." (*Zen, Pen, and Sword*, 40)

The expanding body of evidence asserting our true nature as spiritual beings can help us immensely to release our fear of death and our fixation on past, painful experience, and to find our purpose in the present. One intriguing, yet unproved and controversial, idea coming out of this research is the belief that we consciously and carefully select the time, place, and parentage for each of our incarnations as directed by our spirit's purpose. If you think of this idea as more than a Star Trek premise and consider it uncritically for a while, it starts to make more sense than you'd care to admit. Face it, the next time you feel resentment for your parents because they scolded you for watching your sister in the shower or shaving the cat, consider that you chose your mother, your father, and even the city you were born in. If your family's a depressing negative for you, then start asking, "How do I take this lemon and turn it into lemonade? How do I turn a negative circumstance into a positive?" The answer is, you embrace it and say, "I chose it!" Then you can ask, "Why?" Acting with spirit means you become a cocreator of your life. It means you accept that *the ultimate responsibility for this life is your own.* Like it or not, every detail and action of your life is of your own making and imbued with a purpose, albeit on an unconscious level.

If we were lucky enough to have had a good teacher or mentor early in life, we were encouraged to believe that our natural talents and gifts would provide us with a strong sense of what that purpose is. But how we put those gifts to use and share them with others shows our full understanding of that purpose. Understanding who we are and what we are here to do may take years to realize: many people never get there. However, if you make a conscious commitment to finding your purpose, it accelerates this process. Begin by considering those life lessons that have been the most challenging and probably the most painful. They are the ones that can teach you the most. Just as we were held back in school if we failed to learn our lessons, so life provides us with the same opportunity for defining our purpose through repeated "lessons." It's no wonder these episodes seem to have the same character or feeling. Not only are our most important life experiences the most painful, we're doomed to repeat them until we understand them. Take the example of those of us who are divorced and remarry. We may

choose an apparently very different spouse, only to realize the same conflicts and crises have arisen with our new partner. Six months after the honeymoon, you have a new wife and a new job in a new city, but the same buttons are being pushed. To get at the lessons in these relationships, it may be useful to ask "What do I have to learn from these people?" or "Why have I chosen them to be in my life?" Believe it or not, you may even reach a point of understanding, where you can thank apparent enemies who have helped to enlighten you.

What we are most afraid of often relates to our purpose in life. For example, if you fear most the loss of control, it may mean that you need to understand that fear more deeply in order to loosen your viselike grip over your spouse, your children, or your employees. Identifying, experiencing, expressing, and accepting these fears can eliminate the obstacles that stand in the way of understanding and achieving our life's purpose. In this way, our fears, which can appear to us as obstacles, actually provide important guideposts. Like our greatest joys and pleasures, they can show the way to realizing and enjoying our uniqueness. Spirit is the inner teacher that inspires us to learn these lessons.

Prayer

The most familiar method of connecting with spirit—prayer—is both a spiritual exercise and the standard Western format of meditation. A Gallup poll in 1988 found that 88 percent of Americans pray. Most of those who pray have a greater sense of well-being than those who don't. A majority said that they experience a sense of peace when they pray, have received answers to their prayers, and have felt divinely inspired or "led by God" to perform some specific action. Those who said they felt an experience of the divine during prayer are the people who have the highest rating in general well-being or satisfaction with their lives. More than 70 percent of Americans believe prayer can lead to physical, emotional, or spiritual healing.

Dale Matthews, M.D., an associate professor of medicine at Georgetown University, reviewed 212 medical studies examining the relationship between religious beliefs and health. Seventy-five percent of the studies showed health benefits for those patients with "religious commitments." For patients with hypertension, the habit of prayer reduced blood pressure in 50 percent of the cases.

A 1994 National Institute of Mental Health (NIMH) study of almost three thousand North Carolinians showed that those who attended church weekly had 29 percent less risk of alcoholism than those who attended less frequently. Those who prayed and read the Bible regularly had 42 percent less risk of alcoholism than those who did neither. Another 1994 NIMH study of more than twenty-five hundred patients found that frequent churchgoers had lower rates of depression and other mental problems.

Herbert Benson, M.D., a Harvard cardiologist, has been conducting research that has conclusively demonstrated that prayer benefits health. He began his research in 1968, using subjects who practiced transcendental meditation. These subjects meditated with a mantra, a single word with no apparent meaning to its user, such as *om*. Dr. Benson found that repetition of the mantra replaced the arousing thoughts that otherwise kept his subjects tense during waking hours. This resulted in a lower metabolic rate, slower heart rate, lower blood pressure, and slower breathing.

Dr. Benson then studied Christians and Jews who prayed rather than meditated. He asked Roman Catholic subjects to repeat "Hail Mary, full of grace" or "Lord Jesus Christ, have mercy upon me." Jews used "Shalom," the peace greeting, or "Echad," meaning "one." Protestants used the first line of the Lord's Prayer, "Our Father, who art in heaven," or the opening of Psalm 23, "The Lord is my shepherd." The phrases all had the same physiological effect as the meditation. Dr. Benson has found that all major religious traditions use simple repetitive prayers. Such repetitions, his research suggests, create what he calls the *relaxation response* (RR). By calming the body, RR is the opposite of the stress reaction widely known as the fight-or-flight response—in human beings, the physical reaction to perceived danger.

As he continued his studies, Dr. Benson found that faith affects the physiological benefits of RR and that prayer initiates the relaxation response. He also found a connection between RR and exercise: when runners meditated or prayed as they ran, their bodies were more efficient. Instead of listening to a

Walkman to stimulate their heart rates, they were able to achieve even greater efficiency by matching the cadence of their short prayers to the rhythms of their strides.

Since 1988, Dr. Benson and psychologist Jared Kass have been conducting a series of programs at the Mind/Body Medical Institute at Boston's New England Deaconess Hospital. They have invited priests, ministers, and rabbis to investigate the spiritual and health implications of prayer. They found that people who feel themselves in touch with God are less likely to get sick—and better able to cope when they do. Drs. Benson and Kass developed a psychological scale for measuring spirituality both before and after prayer. Those high in spirituality, which Benson defines as the feeling that "there is more than just you" and as not necessarily religious, scored high in psychological health. They also had fewer stress-related symptoms. Next, he found that people high in spirituality gained the most from meditation training; they showed the greatest rise on a life-purpose index as well as the sharpest drop in pain. The nearly three-quarters of the American population who already believe that prayer can be therapeutic now have additional confirmation: science has shown that as prayer strengthens the spirit, it can also heal the body.

"To put it simply, we're wired for God," says Dr. Benson. "We have a tremendous healing capacity if we can tap into what I call the 'faith factor.'" For men who would like to begin the practice of prayer, I suggest you start with any prayer with which you might be comfortable or can remember from your religious training. The Lord's Prayer is familiar to most Christians, and the majority of Jews know the Shema and Viahavta. Try to establish a regular routine and repeat the prayer morning and night. Regular intervals of prayer combined with the rhythm, movement, and sound of the litany or chant can take the supplicant out of his everyday consciousness and into a state of heightened awareness. You might have a favorite psalm or a passage from the Bible or a prayer book that is especially meaningful. Add it to your daily regimen. I have found three psalms in particular to be especially protective, fortifying, and healing: 121, which I repeat every morning; 91, which I say in late afternoons or after work; and 23, which I say before bed. As originally written in Hebrew, the sound and corresponding energy of each word were carefully chosen to maximize the psalm's spiritual power; however, the psalms' messages are still potent in English.

PSALM 121

I will lift up mine eyes unto the hills, from whence cometh my help.
My help cometh from the Lord, who made heaven and earth.
He will not suffer thy foot to be moved; he that keepeth thee will not slumber.
Behold, he that keepeth Israel shall neither slumber nor sleep.
The Lord is thy keeper: the Lord is thy shade upon thy right hand.
The sun shall not smite thee by day, nor the moon by night.

The Lord shall preserve thee from all evil: he shall preserve thy soul.

The Lord shall preserve thy going out and thy coming in from this time forth, and even for evermore. Amen.

PSALM 91

He that dwelleth in the secret place of the most High shall abide under the shadow of the Almighty.

I will say of the Lord, He is my refuge and my fortress: my God; in him will I trust.

Surely he shall deliver thee from the snare of the fowler, and from the noisome pestilence.

He shall cover thee with his feathers, and under his wings shalt thou trust: his truth shall be thy shield and buckler.

Thou shalt not be afraid for the terror by night; nor for the arrow that flieth by day;

Nor for the pestilence that walketh in darkness; nor for the destruction that wasteth at noonday.

A thousand shall fall at thy side, and ten thousand at thy right hand; but it shall not come nigh thee.

Only with thine eyes shalt thou behold and see the reward of the wicked.

Because thou hast made the Lord, which is my refuge, even the most High, thy habitation;

There shall no evil befall thee, neither shall any plague come nigh thy dwelling.

For he shall give his angels charge over thee, to keep thee in all thy ways.

They shall bear thee up in their hands, lest thou dash thy foot against a stone.

Thou shalt tread upon the lion and adder: the young lion and the dragon shalt thou trample under feet.

Because he hath set his love upon me, therefore will I deliver him: I will set him on high, because he hath known my name.

He shall call upon me, and I will answer him: I will be with him in trouble; I will deliver him, and honor him.

With long life will I satisfy him, and show him my salvation. Amen.

PSALM 23

The Lord is my shepherd: I shall not want.

He maketh me to lie down in green pastures: he leadeth me beside the still waters.

He restoreth my soul: he leadeth me in the paths of righteousness for his name's sake.

Yea, though I walk through the valley of the shadow of death, I will fear no evil; for thou art with me; thy rod and staff they comfort me.

Thou preparest a table before me in the presence of mine enemies: thou anointest my head with oil; my cup runneth over.

Surely goodness and mercy shall follow me all the days of my life: and I will dwell in the house of the Lord forever. Amen.

In addition to the prayers, psalms, and scriptures of various religions, you can also engage in more personal prayer. To do this, talk to God as if you are speaking to your best friend. Just be honest. For example: "I'm having a problem and I really need some help." It is fine to want material things or health for yourself or loved ones, but first ask yourself what feeling would result from having those things you're asking for. It is more effective to pray for that feeling rather than for specific things.

An experiment performed by the Spindrift Organization of Lansdale, Pennsylvania, tested the effectiveness of directed and nondirected prayer. Those practicing directed prayer had a specific goal, image, or outcome in mind, while those using nondirected prayer had an open-ended approach in which no specific outcome was projected. (The practitioner of nondirected prayer does not attempt "to tell the universe what to do.") The results proved conclusively that chances are much greater for attaining the desired outcome when one prays only for what is best (nondirected): "Thy will be done."

Larry Dossey, M.D., former cochairman of the Panel on Mind/Body Interventions, Office of Alternative Medicine at the National Institutes of Health, has written several excellent books on the subject of prayer and healing: *Healing Words; Meaning and Medicine;* and *Recovering the Soul.* Dossey documents the value of group prayer and long-distance prayer. He cites a study by Randolph Byrd, M.D., at the San Francisco General Medical Center, where Christians were asked to pray for half of a group of 393 hospitalized heart-disease patients; no one was assigned to pray

for the other half. The patients were unaware of which group they were in. The results showed that a majority of those who were prayed for needed less medical intervention during their hospital stay and went home sooner than those in the control group.

Shaping the Imagery of Faith

How do you picture yourself getting in touch with spirit? Perhaps you picture yourself on an isolated tropical island, lying on a white sandy beach, listening to the waves lap the shore. You feel the sunlight on your body, the warm sand and gentle breeze. You feel embraced by Mother Earth. If your picture includes a pair of bare-breasted native girls giving you a full-body massage, you're still on the right track. Perhaps in another visualization, you picture a vortex of energy descending from a starry sky and connecting to your crown chakra. It's not a question of which one is holier or more spiritual. The point is, in your own ineffable way you feel at one with the universe. Take a moment and try to recapture one of your own experiences of spirit. Complete this mental picture with detailed images that may or may not have existed in the actual experience, yet contribute strongly to your sense of spirit. It doesn't matter if it is a scene of absolute fantasy; try to imbue it with an unmistakable reality. Perhaps you experience this vivid sense of spirit surrounded by white light, your body charged as energy radiates from every pore. Refine this image and keep it with you so that you can not only recall it, but reinhabit it. Situate yourself in that imagery and animate it with your breathing, bringing yourself fully into that experience. Perhaps this visualization re-creates a moment of peak performance when you were in the zone—on the golf course or delivering a key presentation. Instead of concentrating your focus on the surface memory, re-create that intense feeling of spirit in the present moment. As you sense your awareness expanding, bring that energy into your immediate environment. Let it sanctify the light in the room, the color of the furniture, the scents and sounds that fill the space around you. Use this visualization technique to soothe yourself after a busy day, or to inspire you in advance of any performance. *The resulting experience of spirit will infuse you with an energy that fills your entire being and helps you to realize your full potential.*

Rabbi Mordecai Twerski, the spiritual leader of Denver's Hassidic community, offers a variation on this technique of creating spiritual imagery. He teaches the following visualization to be practiced each morning before getting out of bed. Picture a person, a scene, or situation that you have experienced that fills you with exhilaration or happiness just at the thought of it. Create the habit of visualizing this person or scene each morning upon awakening and you will enjoy a terrific spiritual jump start to your day.

If you think back to our four stages of thriving—commitment, pain, power, and harmony—spirit is the energetic component of power. It is a part of every conscious transformational process, whether you are attempting to train for a new job, to heal a part of your body, or to resolve a long-standing conflict in a committed relationship. Think of your spiritual imagery as a personal covenant, an inner temple that you can carry with you through the desert or onto the freeway for your morning commute. These images create the spiritual connection—not through the image itself—but through the release of energy triggered by the unconscious imaginative interaction with that image. Spiritual visualization can be used in conjunction with prayer as part of an established religious orthodoxy, or as part of your own personal communion with spirit. Remember that whatever method you choose, there is no right or wrong. Religious establishment, with its dogma, trappings, and rituals, has no greater claim to spirit than the individual who prays on a park bench or mountaintop: faith in this transcendental power is the only requirement for experiencing spirit.

Denver spiritual psychotherapist Myron McClellan teaches that *faith* both begins and ends a three-stage cyclical process of spiritual growth that includes *manifestation* and *surrender*. A former teacher of theology at Princeton University, McClellan believes self-realization and finding one's purpose, begin by firmly positing the belief that your desire will be met. The strength of your faith will determine how quickly you manifest that desire. Once your desire is made manifest, surrender your attachment to its material accomplishment and let go of your ego to develop greater faith at a higher level of manifestation. This, in turn, allows you to continue connecting to a higher level of spirit. If this feels too esoteric for you, give it some time and effort. And remember Assagioli's law (from chapter 2): "All action proceeds from thought."

Meditation

If prayer is the act of using words and images to animate the spirit, meditation does the same through a focusing of breath and attention (remember: "Energy follows attention"). As with prayer, there are an infinite number of techniques, and there is no right or wrong way to proceed. Meditation can be done while stationary in a seated or supine position. It can be done moving: walking, jogging, or even while rock climbing. The martial arts are often described as a "moving meditation." All of these applications have in common a focusing on the breath and an emptying of the mind of thought.

Lawrence LeShan, Ph.D., psychologist and author of *How to Meditate,* describes the goal of meditation as working toward "our fullest 'humanhood,' the fullest use of what it means to be human." "In meditation," writes LeShan, "we find ourselves more at home in the universe, more at ease with ourselves, more able to work effectively at our tasks and toward our goal, closer to our fellow man, less anxious and less hostile." LeShan claims the physical benefits of meditation can be measured, and numerous studies have documented increased alpha waves (brain waves associated with deep relaxation), greater oxygenation (more oxygen to every cell in the body), and decreased pain (especially headache), blood pressure, and heart rate. Meditation can be used in treating heart disease and many other physical ailments. A former Harvard researcher, Charles Alexander, Ph.D., taught transcendental meditation to a group of nursing-home patients. In 1990, he reported that over three years all the meditators survived, compared with only 62.6 percent of the nonmeditators.

To get a sense of what meditation feels like, think of it as a neutral emotional state, opposite to the intense feelings of anger, hostility, or even happiness. Meditation is simply a state of heightened attention and pure awareness. For men, who are typically "gear heads," reveling in high performance and the precision of complex interacting systems, meditation technique will seem surprisingly simple. Don't underestimate its power. With a little commitment and consistency, you will reap astonishing rewards. The only recommended equipment is a cushion or a straight-backed chair. If you are seated on the floor, cross your legs comfortably while sitting on a cushion or folded blanket, so your hips are elevated above your knees. If you are sitting in a chair, it is preferable that your back is unsupported: sit forward on the chair with your feet flat on the floor. The more vertically aligned your head, neck, and spine are, the less muscle tension develops in trying to maintain your balance. Imagine that a hook is attached to the crown of your head pulling gently upward; the head then is resting directly over the sit bones. If you are seated in a chair, rest your hands on your thighs or fold them in your lap. If you are seated on the floor, you can rest your hands on your knees or rest one on top of the other in your lap. The breathing is similar to the abdominal breathing described in chapter 3 (see page 58). If possible, breathe in and out through the nose.

The simplest method of meditation is to focus on your breathing, fully sensing each inhalation and exhalation. It may help to silently say the word *in* with each inhalation and *out* with each exhalation. Allow your thoughts to come and go without attaching to them. After a few minutes, you may notice longer periods of silence between thoughts. It may take months to quiet the mind to this extent, but with consistent practice, your meditation *will* become deeper and easier. Try to sit for at least ten minutes once or twice per day, working up to two thirty-minute sessions per day. The most important part of this practice is consistency. However, don't force your meditation: if you are too distracted or pressed for time, end your session after five minutes instead of forcing yourself to sit restlessly for twenty minutes. To assure yourself enough time, budget twenty minutes at the same time each day, even if it means waking up earlier.

Some meditators silently repeat a word or phrase (sometimes with no meaning) called a mantra: *love, peace, om.* They find that the rhythm of breath and inner sound frees the mind from its relentless cycle of thoughts. Chanting uses this same principle with a voiced recitation. Hinduism and Buddhism abound with chanting meditations, and their rhythmic drone fills their temples with a contagious energy and peace. The effect of chanting is similar to that of ritual prayer in which the rhythm of breath and sound create a powerful psychophysical release.

Through prayer, and meditation especially, you can more easily put yourself in touch with your intuition, which some people describe as a quiet, inner voice: "God speaking to us." Although we have experience of intuitive moments every day, as men we are not always trusting of these messages unless we find a rational corroboration. The more we open ourselves to this process and quiet our internal "static," the clearer the signal becomes. Think of learning to tap your intuition as similar to Myron McClellan's cyclical process of *faith, manifestation,* and *surrender.* We listen for the message and act upon that message (which often entails risk-taking); this requires *faith.* We confirm the message through its physical *manifestation;* and as a result we gain greater trust in the intuitive process. This, in turn, leads to enhanced receptivity, the equivalent of *surrender:* we must empty the glass, surrendering its contents, to receive more. As we become more adept at "listening," we can learn to quiet ourselves with a few abdominal breaths and tap into the spirit wherever we are. The bottom line on spirit is that the process works, if we only allow ourselves to be receptive to it.

Spiritual Counselors

If you haven't been in the habit of listening or need help tuning in, you may consider working with a spiritual counselor. Just as you would visit a doctor to heal your physical body, or a psychotherapist to heal your emotional body, spiritual counselors can help connect you to your spiritual core. In addition to priests, rabbis, and other clergy, these may include spiritual psychotherapists, medical intuitives, astrologers, clairvoyants, and spiritual healers or shamans. (Don't knock them until you've tried a good one. Some can be astonishingly accurate and provide information that might have taken you a lifetime to acquire.) These healers have in common an ability to see beyond the boundaries of the five senses. Their services may include seeing into past lives, identifying purpose, seeing into the body for medical diagnostic purposes, communicating with "guides" and "angels," and recognizing opportunities for your spiritual growth. Most of all, they can assist you in learning the lessons of this lifetime. Because of the lack of certification in these areas, you will need to rely upon word of mouth and trial and error. Keep an open mind and see how you respond to the information provided. Some of these counselors can be truly gifted and provide you with information that can be a catalyst for transforming your life.

Finding Spirit in Nature

Many of us find our greatest connection to spirit through nature. In nature we most directly experience the four elemental forms of energy: earth, water, fire, and air. Earth energy consists of matter in its densest form. Water is the receptive, yielding principle. Fire is the transformational energy that changes the form of matter. Air is the resulting blend of the other three forces into a subtler vibration of life-force energy. For human beings, these elements comprise the building blocks of our organism: earth is cellular matter; water is blood and circulation; fire is metabolism and energy production; air is oxygen, our most critical nutrient for life. These elements also correspond to the energy of the four lower chakras. The lower three connect us to our material existence: the root chakra corresponds to earth energy; the sex chakra to water energy; the solar plexus to fire energy. As an energetic link between matter and spirit, air resonates with the energy of the heart chakra. The Chinese character for life-force energy—*chi*—symbolizes this interaction between the four basic elements: it depicts an earthenware vessel filled with water, heating over a fire to produce the vapor or steam of life-force energy. Nowhere is this creative power of spirit made more visible than in nature. By having more regular daily exposure to the four elements of nature, we can enhance the unlimited creativity within us.

As you spend time in nature, you will expand your awareness of the ways in which you embody each of the elements and their unique energy. Here are a few suggestions for connecting with each.

Earth. Spend as much time as possible outdoors in close contact with the earth, or at least in natural settings—parks, woods, beaches, or mountains. A daily walk is great, or playing an outdoor sport, riding your bike in a park, gardening, or just finding a quiet, scenic spot to appreciate the surrounding beauty. As you spend more time in nature, you will become more sensitized to powers residing in landscapes and the ways the earth retains and radiates energy. The Chinese art of *feng shui* specializes in identifying ways to harmonize with the landscape (see chapter 3, page 100) and to benefit from its energetic properties. What the American Indian often called sacred ground was land highly charged with life-force energy. Like *feng shui*, the science of geomancy studies the effects of energy found in specific landscapes and its cultural and spiritual influences on the people who live there. These "magical" places exist all over the planet. Some are said to be positive energy vortices with powerful healing properties. Sedona, Arizona, and Waimea Canyon on the island of Kauai in Hawaii are considered two such locations. Sites of positive energy were often sacred to native peoples, who lived close to the earth and built their societies around a heightened awareness of its energy. Native American tribes freely roamed our national landscape and identified many such sacred lands long before we arrived. On the other hand, many large cities and highly industrialized areas concentrate negative energy. Near urban areas, many sacred sites have been covered with concrete and asphalt. If you know of a special natural setting in which the positive energy is still vibrant, it can provide a heightened experience of prayer and meditation.

It is commonplace to say that our urban society has robbed us of our contact with nature.

What this means on an energetic level is that we have lost touch with the life-force energy emanating from the earth, causing a depletion of the root chakra. This is in part responsible for the dramatic increase of prostate cancer. In 1981, Roger Ulrich, Ph.D., a professor of urban and regional planning at Texas A&M, performed a study with the help of Swedish scientists. He showed eighteen students slides of trees, plants, water, and cities. The students reported that the nature scenes, especially those of water, made them feel more elated and relaxed; in contrast, the urban scenes tended to elicit sadness and fear. Electroencephalograph (EEG) readings of the students' brainwave activity showed significantly stronger alpha waves when viewing the nature scenes—scientific evidence of feelings of relaxed wakefulness. In 1984, Dr. Ulrich found that exposure to nature speeds recovery from the stress of surgery. When he examined the hospital records of forty-six men and women who had undergone gallbladder operations, those with a window or view of a small grove of trees were hospitalized about a day less than patients with a view of a brick wall. They also required less pain medication and were less upset.

Water. We have already emphasized the importance of drinking plenty of water. Now I am suggesting that you immerse yourself in it. Nothing is quite so relaxing as bathing in warm water, at least once a day, morning or night. Hot tubs and spas are two of technology's greatest inventions, but if you don't have either, a bathtub will suffice. If you have ever soaked in a natural outdoor hot spring, congratulations—you have experienced one of life's ultimate pleasures. Mineral hot springs can be therapeutic for a variety of ailments. In some that are still in their natural state (without a cement foundation), you can at times feel so close to nature that it is almost as if you are floating in the womb of Mother Earth.

One of the most visible forms of *chi* in nature is the flow of water as it follows the contours of the earth and interacts with other forces. As receptive energy, water is affected by the forces acting upon it. A river, of course, flows due to the gravitational forces at work in the gradient of the landscape. Hydroelectric energy is an offshoot of this flow. However, the action of water tumbling over rocks also releases a more subtle energy in the form of negative ions, which can contribute to a feeling of well-being. Think of the sensation of standing next to a powerful waterfall or the crashing surf. Swimming in an ocean, lake, or river provides invaluable exposure to this special energy of water. The forces of wind and lunar gravitation also profoundly affect water, as evidenced in the fluctuation of tides and waves. Those of us who live near the ocean have a profound appreciation for this type of energy.

Fire. Throughout the Bible, the dominant symbol for the divine essence in man is fire or light, and candlelight provides a spiritual focus to almost every one of the world's religions. Anyone who enjoys camping can attest to the pleasure of an open campfire. A fireplace at home offers similar satisfaction, but because burning wood contributes to air pollution, I recommend a gas fireplace or simply lighting candles.

As our ultimate source of "fire," the sun provides a healing and creative energy that animates directly or indirectly every living organism. We should try to expose ourselves to the energy of the sun daily, remembering of course to use appropriate precautions: sunscreen, hats, and long sleeves and pants where indicated.

Air. Air is the breath of the planet. The Greeks equated spirit *(pneuma)* with the wind. It is the vehicle that carries and dispenses life-force energy: moisture, warmth, seeds in the form of pollen, and most of all . . . oxygen. Conversely, air can spread pollutants hundreds of miles or it can smother a city in its own carbon monoxide. It has the power to move oceans and turn fertile land into desert and vice versa, simply by altering its currents. Most importantly, as the earth's lung and diaphragm, it activates the exchange of carbon dioxide and oxygen that allows the planet to breathe. When the farmer in the Amazon burns his acreage of rain forest to create grazing land for cattle, he affects the amount of oxygen available to the fisherman in Iceland. When the earth breathes deeply and freely of pure, vital air, every plant, animal, and human thrives.

Spiritual Practices

Here are a number of simple habits and rituals that will enable you to connect with spirit on a routine basis. Like anything else, the more you do these, the more accessible spirit becomes.

Sabbath. "Remember the Sabbath day and keep it holy." Although more than three thousand years old, the Ten Commandments remain a worthy set of ethics. To the Jewish people, the Sabbath is still the holiest day on the calendar, even though it occurs every week. A Sabbath day is observed in many of the world's religions. It is meant to be a day completely devoted to love—of God, self, family, and friends. I am not suggesting that you observe any particular day of the week, or even a full day if you can't afford the time. For your spiritual health, however, I recommend setting aside the same time each week to indulge yourself in this celebration of life. Try to abstain from anything even remotely resembling work.

Fasting. The ancient ritual of purification by abstaining from food can have a cleansing effect upon the body. According to the Bible, Moses and Jesus were both able to sustain fasts for forty days. Unless you have attained their level of spiritual mastery, please don't attempt a fast of that duration. I recommend one day, during which you abstain from both food and water. Doing this can definitely elicit a heightened spiritual feeling, as your focus shifts away from physical concerns. Select a day when work and family responsibilities are limited and you won't be too active. Plan for some quiet time alone, and during the final two hours of the fast drink six to eight glasses of water. This helps to cleanse

your body of toxins. See how it feels after you have fasted once or twice, and if you think it has been beneficial, try fasting on a regular basis, perhaps monthly. You will be surprised at how much easier it is with each subsequent fast. If you are interested in attempting longer fasts, consult first with a naturopathic physician. (NDs are specialists in natural medicine who treat both acute and chronic disease primarily through the use of clinical nutrition and herbal medicine. Their practice is based on the concept that the body is a self-healing organism.)

Eye contact. Looking at yourself, especially your eyes, in a mirror for five minutes every day can be a powerful exercise. It works best to look into your left eye, which is connected to the more "receptive" right side of your brain. Doing this practice daily can help you to love what you see. Louise Hay recommends that while doing this mirror work you add a positive affirmation expressing approval or self-love. Hokey though it may sound, this technique can be quite powerful. Remember, the eyes are the windows to the soul.

Touch. Several topics don't fit easily into one single component of holistic health but offer several healing benefits simultaneously. Touch is one of them. I have included it here because not only is it one of the most effective healers, it might well be the most powerful and direct means of conveying love.

According to Saul Schanberg, M.D., Ph.D., a professor of pharmacology and biological psychiatry at Duke University, "Humans need to touch and be touched, just as we need food and water." His research and that of other experts on touch were cited in *Hands-on Healing*, edited by John Feltman.

- In a study involving forty premature infants, half of them were gently stroked for forty-five minutes a day; the other twenty were not. Although all were fed the same amount of calories, after ten days the touched babies weighed in 47 percent heavier than the unstimulated group. The stroked babies were also more active, more alert, and more responsive to social stimulation.

- When a person's wrist is gently held by someone else, the heartbeat slows and blood pressure declines.

- Children and adolescents hospitalized for psychiatric problems show remarkable reductions in anxiety levels and positive changes in attitude when they receive a brief daily back rub.

- The arteries of rabbits fed a high-cholesterol diet and petted regularly had 60 percent less blockage than did the arteries of unpetted but similarly fed rabbits.

- Rats that were handled for fifteen minutes a day during the first three weeks of their lives showed dramatically less cell deterioration and memory loss as they grew old, compared with nonhandled rats.

In spite of the many health reasons to touch and be touched by other human beings, Americans indulge very little in this simple pleasure. One study in the 1960s noted the number of touches exchanged by pairs of people sitting in coffee shops around the world. In San Juan, Puerto Rico, people touched 180 times an hour; in Paris, France, 110 times an hour; in Gainesville, Florida, twice an hour; and in London, England, the pairs never touched. The implications and possible causes of this phenomenon would entail a lengthy discussion, although I am sure the puritanical legacy of associating touch with sex has had a profound effect on American attitudes. This is probably especially true of men. William E. Whitehead, Ph.D., an associate professor of medical psychology at the Johns Hopkins University School of Medicine, believes that a significant part of the blame lies with the father of modern psychology, Sigmund Freud. "Freud encouraged austerity in dealing with children. And parents bought into that behavior," says Dr. Whitehead. "People who aren't cuddled a lot as kids," he adds, "tend to develop into nontouching adults. The cycle then repeats itself, generation after generation."

As an osteopathic physician, I learned early in my medical training about the therapeutic value of the "laying on of hands." Although almost all of our courses and textbooks were the same as those used to train allopathic medical doctors (M.D.'s), we were also taught a holistic approach to health care that included osteopathic manipulative therapy. Soft-tissue stretching (somewhat similar to massage) and adjustments or corrections in the position of the spine and other body parts (similar to chiropractic adjustments) are part of this therapy. It has taken me a while to realize that patients responded well to this treatment not only because of the prescribed techniques, but also because of the healing potential of touch itself. Touch is a primary healing ingredient in a number of other therapies, including acupressure, the Alexander technique, applied kinesiology, Aston-patterning, the Berry method, chiropractic, craniosacral therapy, the Feldenkrais method, Hellerwork, hydrotherapy, myotherapy, oriental massage, physiatry, physical therapy, polarity therapy, reflexology, Reichian therapy, Rolfing, Swedish massage, therapeutic touch, and the Trager approach. I will not discuss the relative merits of these methods other than to say that all of them deserve to be recognized as legitimate disciplines in the full spectrum of the healing arts.

I have always viewed the practice of medicine as the business of caring. As our health care system continues to change radically, the most insidious shift has been the erosion of the doctor-patient relationship. As it becomes more impersonal, there is less mutual trust and intimacy. Within the conventional medical community there is a greater fear of closeness due to the increase in malpractice suits. Touching of patients is limited to that which is strictly necessary in the course of a diagnostic evaluation. In fact, sick people need the comfort of human touch more than healthy people—a reassuring pat on the shoulder, hand-holding, or even a hug.

If caregivers are to do their best job, this powerful method of healing must be learned. Touch has to become a larger component of every physician's therapeutic black bag. If you are interested in experiencing hands-on healing techniques, I suggest trying a practitioner of one of the many therapies previously mentioned. See how it feels and give it a fair trial. If it works for you, that's great. If it doesn't, try something else.

Touch is a gift you can give to yourself every day. It requires allowing yourself to receive and to feel deserving. If you are meditating, praying, or just lying in the bathtub, try touching your chest over your heart in as gentle and compassionate a way as you know how. A loving touch is healing, no matter who gives it.

Animals are perfectly fine sources of tactile comfort, says Alan M. Beck, Sc.D., director of the Center for the Interaction of Animals and Society at the University of Pennsylvania. Numerous studies, he adds, "definitely show that petting an animal can lower one's blood pressure." If you don't have a pet, my prescription for maintaining your spiritual health is to get several hugs daily!

There is no question that we have become too distant from one another. There is clearly a movement in this country to compensate for that deficiency and restore our sense of wholeness and balance. The trend toward more touching is a return to some of the more positive norms and values of preindustrialized societies. Most of these cultures are very touch oriented. I have lived with one such native group in Fiji, for whom touch is their primary method of healing. These people believe that their healers have a gift bestowed by God, and that the healing energy that flows through the healer to the patient is God's love. Whatever its source, the healer's touch works extremely well for a variety of ailments. By our standards these people might be considered primitive or underdeveloped, but they are clearly much healthier than most Americans in body, mind, and spirit.

Gratitude. Most religious traditions provide for specific prayers or grace before meals as a means of thanking God for the food and for our physical sustenance. As with other spiritual practices, there is something to be gained from these rituals, or they wouldn't have survived for thousands of years. The more you can appreciate the spirit of the practice rather than merely following its form, the greater its value will be. Science is just beginning to appreciate the multifaceted benefits of spirituality.

Feelings of gratitude can elicit similar life-enhancing benefits. Rabbi Twerski's "wake-up" visualization (see page 145) elicits the feeling that you would never have had that experience if you weren't living. It prepares you to expect that something equally wonderful can happen again. What a great way to instill an attitude of anticipation and appreciation for being alive and to begin the new day.

Most of us tend to take life for granted. Suppose you choose instead to see your life as a gift, to be thankful for all that it has provided you—both the pleasure and the pain. As we've seen, adversity can give you the opportunity for tremendous growth. You might not be too happy about it at the time, but in retrospect you can be grateful for the lessons you've learned.

Gratitude can produce powerful feelings of joy and self-acceptance. It is an attitude that anyone can choose to have, just as you can choose to be positive or negative, to be forgiving or unforgiving, to see the cup half full or half empty. It has been my experience that when people choose to look at the up side of life, more positive things start to happen. *It seems that we attract whatever feeling we radiate.* When you focus on gratitude, wonderful things happen. When you focus on what you do have, not on what you don't have, you feel a sense of abundance, which enables you to let go of negative thoughts and attitudes.

This isn't easy to do. If you are feeling a great deal of fear and anger, it is especially difficult to superimpose gratitude, but if you can release some of those feelings through forgiveness and acceptance and put your heart into practicing gratitude, it will work for you. As long as you are alive, blessings will come your way. I rarely go through a day without thanking God for something, and every time I do, there is an accompanying feeling of joy.

Conclusion

As we learn to diminish fear in our lives, we are able to relax more into the present moment and to embrace the power of spirit. By living each day as if it were our last, our inner resources guide us to realizing a purpose greater than material success or financial security alone. As men, we are driven by images of accomplishment or achievement because they hold out to us the promise of control and power. By moving beyond these limiting goals and exploring within, we can tap that unlimited source of power that enables us to create the reality of our choosing. Spirit can take us by the hand and guide us to the threshold of unlimited possibility. This path into the unknown is fraught with risk and fear as long as we cling to the brittle trappings of our ego. Once we embrace the spiritual identity that ties us to every living creature, we experience a freedom that empowers us to explore every facet of our being. Only in this spiritual realm can we fully embrace the reality that death does not exist and experience heaven on earth, in which we live fully while we are alive. Once again, this understanding that "death does not exist" is the basis for Elisabeth Kübler-Ross's "Key to Life":

> There is no need to be afraid of death. It is not the end of the physical body that should worry us. Rather, our concern must be to live while we're alive—to release our inner selves from the spiritual death that comes with living behind a facade designed to conform to external definitions of who and what we are. Every individual human being born on this earth has the capacity to become a unique and special person unlike any who has ever existed before or will ever exist again. But to the extent that we become captives of culturally defined role expectations and behaviors—stereotypes, not ourselves—we block our capacity for self-actualization. We interfere with our becoming all that we can be. . . .

It is the denial of death that is partially responsible for people living empty, purposeless lives; for when you live as if you'll live forever, it becomes too easy to postpone the things you know that you must do. You live your life in preparation for tomorrow or in remembrance of yesterday, and meanwhile, each today is lost. In contrast, when you fully understand that each day you awaken could be the last you have, you take the time that day to grow, to become more of who you really are, to reach out to other human beings.

Chapter 6

Happiness Is a Harmonic Relationship

Better to shower the people you love with love,
show them the way you feel.
Things are gonna be much better if you only
will.

Lyrics from "Shower the People"
James Taylor, 1975

In April of 1996, ABC television aired an hour-long special on happiness. In preparing the show, the producers conducted an extensive survey of a cross-section of Americans to find out the most important factors contributing to the feeling of happiness. At the top of the list by a large margin was *close relationships*. Surprisingly, *money* did not even make the top six, except in cases of poverty or extreme financial hardship. Rounding out the top six were *control over one's life, challenging and fulfilling work, a sense of optimism, faith in God,* and *a sense of purpose.*

All of these ingredients for happiness ap-

peared in previous chapters discussing how to create optimal health: clearly, happiness is synonymous with holistic health. Happiness also corresponds to our fourth and final stage—**harmony:** that feeling of confidence and peace with ourselves, others, and our environment. In the first five chapters we explored the journey of self-awareness in body, mind, and spirit, learning how to nurture ourselves and how to cultivate an *internal* sense of harmony.

In chapter 3, we learned how the feeling of harmony in the **body** requires a free flow of oxygen, blood, and nutrients as well as aerobic capacity, flexibility, balance, coordination, and strength. We also saw how a nurturing environment—a living and working space that is relatively free of toxins and stressful noise while providing plentiful exposure to the life-force energy found in sunlight and nature—contributes to the body's internal sense of harmony.

Peace of **mind** comes from making a commitment to nurture yourself with beliefs and attitudes that endow the psyche with feelings of well-being. In chapter 4, we saw how this mental harmony manifests as high self-esteem, acceptance of one's feelings, and a sense of tranquil exhilaration. Typically, as boys, we experienced this sense of well-being through the abandon of play. Training to thrive can reawaken this feeling of freedom and take us to an even higher level of awareness.

Spiritual harmony is the empowering experience of your body and mind's unique configuration of energy (soul) in relationship to the universal energy that permeates all matter (spirit). Chapter 5 identified the essence of spiritual harmony as unconditional love. In chapter 6, we will learn how to directly experience unconditional love with others through committed relationships. *This chapter marks the transition from concentrating solely on the self and its internal experience of harmony to a sense of harmony that we share externally with others through thriving relationships.*

So far, training to thrive has depended on your commitment to yourself to do this work. Now you are about to enlist the aid of a partner. In so doing, you will face one of the toughest challenges in your training, but one that potentially offers the greatest rewards: a committed relationship. Although it won't require six weeks of boot camp, a committed relationship will demand a systematic effort to learn new ways of communicating. You have already acquired some of these skills: you have learned to listen more attentively to your body, you have learned to identify critical self-talk and feelings, and you have learned to articulate new goals and visions by creating and using affirmations. Each of these skills can pay big dividends in enhancing your relationships at home or at work. While close friendships are important to thriving, a committed, intimate partnership or marriage can be invaluable. It offers the most fundamental spiritual practice, the potential for the greatest experience of unconditional love, and a lens through which you can focus your awareness of relationships with all family and close friends. Think of harmonic relationships as *a balance between the autonomy of the self and the interdependence of intimacy with others.*

Community: The Importance of Social Connection

With people we love, men are capable of expressing great warmth, nurturing, and selflessness. We can be great friends, lovers, husbands, fathers, brothers, and sons. Like women, men profoundly enjoy a sense of belonging. However, unlike women, men are quick to exile themselves from a group or relationship from which they feel disapproval or criticism. Men are sensitive to feelings of rejection. It is often easier for us to withdraw behind the defenses of our ego and fight than it is to communicate our feelings and negotiate.

Social health depends on connection to other human beings: "No man is an island." Whether we view ourselves as warriors, pioneers, or power brokers, our fear of loss of control and rejection compels us to create a self-sufficiency that often keeps us at arm's length from those with whom we need to be closest. Social health requires a balance of autonomy with intimacy. Not surprisingly, our relationships are the most difficult area for us to improve and one that can have a drastic effect on our health and survival. A 1990 study at the University of California, San Francisco, found that single men between the ages of fifty-five and sixty-four were twice as likely to die within a ten-year period as married men their same age. Another similar study showed that unmarried people end up in the hospital with mental disorders five to ten times as frequently as those who are married.

Some of the reasons for this pervasive sense of isolation among men were explored in chapter 1. Through our fathers many of us experienced the results of a fear-based mentality caused by economic depression and world war. It forced them to focus their energy on the goals and competition of their jobs, often to the exclusion of their sons, as well as their wives and daughters. As role models, our fathers unknowingly conditioned us to value professional accomplishment and material goals over close relationships. We reacted by alternating between solipsistic self-examination and blind ambition. We embraced both the excessive self-involvement of the late sixties and seventies and the material obsession of the eighties encapsulated in the bumper sticker "He who dies with the most toys wins."

Our self-absorption has created a profound sense of alienation and isolation. It has separated adults from one another, children from their parents and families, and it contributes to both our social and physical *dis-ease.* The importance of social relationships has been documented in studies showing a high incidence of illness and death after the loss of a loved one. Dean Ornish, M.D., a professor at the University of California School of Medicine at San Francisco, found that a common denominator among heart disease patients was their feeling of hostility and a sense of isolation. In a study of terminal cancer patients with long-term survival rates, conducted by Kenneth Pelletier, Ph.D., a professor of medicine and psychiatry at the University of California School of Medicine at San Francisco, one of the strongest factors contributing to longevity was their relatively high degree of social involvement. University of Michigan sociologist James House and his group of researchers concluded that *social isolation is statistically just as dangerous as smoking, high blood pressure, high cholesterol, obesity, or lack of exercise.*

Two other studies powerfully demonstrate the health benefits of close relationships and a strong sense of community. In the small town of Roseto, Pennsylvania, the citizens consumed what would today be considered a dangerously high-fat diet. They had been eating this way for several decades, into the mid-1960s, when Stewart Wolf, M.D., began studying the health histories of Roseto's inhabitants, most of whom were Italian immigrants. As a result of Dr. Wolf's findings, the town has become famous because of its surprisingly low death rates. According to researchers, there is only one clear-cut explanation for the finding: the extraordinarily close-knit family and community ties among Roseto's residents.

Another convincing study was conducted by federal researchers, and the findings were published in November 1993 in the *Journal of the American Medical Association.* It showed that despite poverty, poor access to medical care, and a lack of health insurance, Hispanics are surprisingly less likely than whites to die of major chronic diseases, including all forms of cancer, heart disease, and respiratory ailments. It found that with certain notable exceptions, including diabetes, liver disease, and homicide, the overall health outlook for Hispanics is significantly better than for whites. Most researchers cannot explain these findings and believe the reason for this health disparity between whites and Hispanics is still a mystery. Some health experts, however, including former Surgeon General Coello Novello, a Latina who was the first woman to serve in that post, theorize that Hispanic culture—which frowns on drinking and smoking and promotes strong family values—helps keep that population healthy in spite of socioeconomic disadvantages. These and a growing number of other studies reinforce our understanding of the life-enhancing power of social connection.

We are beginning to see a movement in America toward a greater sense of community. Support groups for those sharing common values, experiences, and goals are becoming much more commonplace. Men's groups, women's groups, AA groups, and couples' groups, perhaps affiliated with a church or synagogue, are gathering all over the country, some for the purpose of enhancing spiritual growth, but all benefiting from the social connection. This trend is a positive and healthy response to a widespread deterioration of the family that has caused an unspoken yet almost epidemic sense of isolation among Americans.

As a society we are plagued by a divorce rate that tops 50 percent, a general sentiment of feeling overworked, dual-career marriages, and a generation of children more adrift and alone than any that has preceded them. According to *Turning Points,* the 1989 report of the Carnegie Council of Adolescent Development, almost half of all adolescents are at significant risk of reaching adulthood unable to meet the requirements of the workplace, to make the commitments to family and friends, and to accept the responsibilities inherent in a democratic society. The study finds them susceptible to "a vortex of new risks . . . almost unknown to their parents and grandparents."

In her study of ways to rebuild the family, *The Shelter of Each Other,* Mary Pipher, Ph.D., a Nebraska psychotherapist, attributes the breakdown of the family to a new set of realities and pressures that drive families apart. These include (1) *longer working hours* that overextend parents and keep them away from home; (2) *excessive television* and inappropriate programming that oversexualize children or subject them to far too much violence; and (3) *computer games* that further isolate children and engage them in *a virtual reality that excludes them from contacts and relationships in the real world.*

Television contributes significantly to this sense of virtual reality that has distanced us from natural relationships, responsibilities, and communities. It has turned us into a nation of self-centered media surfers, who increasingly embrace the synthetic relationships of television and the Internet at the expense of the commitments and realities of actual human connection. The average American watches about thirty hours of television a week, and it is both a distraction from and a frequent guest at dinner tables across the country. A recent Gallup poll revealed that among those who dine at home with family, nearly four out of ten watch TV, study, work, or read while eating.

As a start to reuniting you and your family, I suggest trying to share at least the evening meal without television. Find other ways to escape the virtual-reality trap by spending more time together as a family, playing, working, providing community service, worshiping, or simply reading together. Designate a regularly scheduled time during the weekend for family activities. Setting aside time together allows your family the opportunity to *re-create* your relationships and yourselves individually. Rotate the leader, so that each family member has a chance to choose the activity. Don't underestimate the value of play. Having fun together can sometimes accomplish what many sessions of family therapy are unable to do.

Just as we reflect the world of our fathers, our children reflect the world we have shaped for them. They may interpret that world in ways quite different from what we had intended. As a result, what may seem dysfunctional in your child's (or particularly in your teenager's) behavior might actually be a functional way of dealing with the environment of limited or superficial relationships that we have created for them. For example, the Internet, with its vast array of information and services, has proven an enormously valuable tool. However, its often addictive exposure to "virtual" communities can replace real human contact with digital relationships. As a result, our children have lost the ability "to look others in the eye." Maybe the ABC poll identifying close relationships as the key to happiness actually reflects an underlying desire to renew our sense of community.

In the last decade, the excesses of competition, consumption, and self-interest have changed the character of our society. Built on fairness, equality, and cooperation, our nation has become increasingly divided by the ethos of getting ahead at all costs. The nobler truths of independence, trust, and honor have been replaced by selfishness, money, and cynicism. Look at any major metropolitan newspaper and you'll find that the economic news, which used to be confined to business pages, has spilled over into other sections, even superseding performance as the lead story in sports, entertainment, and the arts.

Typically men have grown up fed on a steady diet of competition. When it was enlisted in the service of a community, country, or even corporation, competition was frequently tempered by virtues such as patriotism, loyalty, and honor. But now that the bottom line has affected the way we measure individual worth in our society, the perennial virtues are being tossed aside. Add in the factors of a shrinking job market, rapidly changing technologies, corporate downsizing, increased competition from international markets, and the entry of women into the job market, and it's not hard to see why men have never been more competitive and less trusting of one another. As a consequence, we are more isolated from each other than ever before. *We are like gladiators thrown into an arena, so consumed in a fight for our own survival that we fail to see how we are destroying ourselves and our families in the process.* This crisis of competition among men has spawned a number of organizations that have tried to remedy our social ills. Former football coach Bill McCartney's Promise Keepers fills stadia around the country, asking Christian men to pray together and recommit themselves to their responsibilities as husbands and fathers. Black Muslim leader Louis Farrakhan's Million Man March asked for a similar commitment from Afro-American men as a way of raising self-esteem and regenerating their communities. These rallies are outgrowths of a burgeoning men's move-

ment started by Robert Bly, Michael Meade, James Hillman, and others, who urged men to seek a deeper emotional connection with one another by healing psychic wounds together. From early boyhood on, men have always spent time together at work or play, but in ways that excluded expression of their inner emotional life. As a consequence, most of us suffer in silence without ever knowing the inner joy and pain felt by many of our closest friends. Whether you are drawn to large rallies, a small circle of friends, one or two coworkers, or a single male friend, the need to find other men with whom you can forge lasting bonds based on emotional integrity and openness has never been greater. Our need for close fraternal relationships goes to the very heart of what it means to be a man.

Marriage and Committed Relationships: Discovering Intimacy

The model for all committed relationships is marriage. However we may feel about our own marriage(s), present or past, the fact remains that marriage promotes physical health. Statistics show that men who are single, divorced, or widowed are twice as likely to die prematurely than those who are married. Committed relationships can promote physical, emotional, and especially spiritual well-being, by bringing us into close contact with that positive energy in another. In this way, our relationships can make us more aware of that energy in ourselves.

It doesn't matter whether your partner is

female or male, whether your marriage is recognized legally by the state, whether you're in a thirty-day or thirty-year relationship; the most important ingredient to any committed relationship is **intimacy.** Just as the first five chapters of this book provided a systematic program for you to become more intimate with *yourself*—to create a greater sense of self-awareness—this chapter will give you exercises for becoming more intimate with your *partner* in a committed relationship. Think of intimacy as *into-me-see.* Having developed the skills for seeing into yourself, and having learned to appreciate what you see, you can now apply these skills to "seeing into" your partner and allowing your partner to see into you.

One of the biggest stumbling blocks for men in establishing committed relationships is the fear of exposing their true feelings to the scrutiny and potential judgment of another person. In both business and personal relationships, men typically avoid this situation at all costs by relating to others in a superficial way. Although most of us may not be aware of it, as men we now *probably fear criticism, embarrassment, and rejection as much as—if not more than—we feared physical intimidation as boys.* For men, this fear of rejection lies at the heart of their avoidance of intimacy and its accompanying sense of exposure. Growing up in a world of competition, men are hypersensitive to exposing their deepest feelings to criticism or ridicule that may result in rejection. Let's face it, if you have been conditioned to reject or hide your feelings (as most of us have since boyhood),

you will no doubt be wary of exposing those feelings to the scrutiny of others, even if it is a spouse or loved one. As we saw in chapter 4, thriving on an emotional level begins with complete acceptance of your own feelings. The same exercises from chapter 4 that helped you to become more *accepting* of yourself can also show you how to bring unconditional love into a committed relationship. Use these exercises to communicate your feelings more freely to one another and build a truly harmonic resonance within your partnership.

The key to a successful marriage is a commitment to each other and to the growth of each partner. Once that pact is made, the relationship becomes an entity greater than the sum of its parts. In her book *Intimate Partners,* Maggie Scarf describes the creative possibilities of such unions this way: "When space is provided within the system—space for changing, growing, being different over the course of time—marriage can be the most therapeutic of relationships, the fertile terrain which permits both partners to expand, flourish, and attain their full potentials." The positive change that can take place in a committed marriage entails letting go of conditional responses and behavior, and as you do so, realizing that in giving more to the relationship you are ultimately giving to yourself.

After almost twenty-nine years of marriage, my wife, Harriet, and I share with other couples what we have learned together through our respective practices. The recommendations that follow are distilled from the counseling the two of us have received; from the couples classes we teach; from Harriet's marriage and family-therapy practice; from two insightful books, *Getting the Love You Want* by Harville Hendrix, Ph.D., and Maggie Scarf's *Intimate Partners;* and from our many years of working to make our own relationship a more conscious one. The following is a brief discussion of the methods and exercises we find helpful. They will improve any committed relationship: marriage, partnership, gay relationship, or close friendship. If you are interested in making a deeper commitment to your relationship, I suggest you begin with couples counseling. As with any new course of study, it doesn't hurt to find yourselves a good teacher.

Creating a Shared Vision

A vision is really a way of defining your mutual goals and focusing your energy on their attainment. Without a vision, your relationship can become aimless, and your problem-solving behavior will reflect a crisis orientation. You have given thought to your individual list of goals and affirmations as suggested in chapter 2. Now you and your partner should create a list of affirmations describing how you see your relationship. The "relationship" affirmations should be in the present tense. They should be *positive*, short, descriptive, specific, and begin with *we*. For example, "We trust each other," "We can safely express all of our feelings to one another," or "We are very affectionate and touch each other daily." Your list of affirmations might include statements about the way you feel about each other, where you live, how

you play together, how you resolve conflicts, what your sex life is like, and anything else that applies to your situation. Before sharing your vision with your partner and creating a mutual vision list, prioritize in numerical order the items on your own list. The next step is to begin combining lists by starting with the affirmations having the highest value and alternating between the two lists to form a composite vision. As you proceed, you should try to combine similar sentences from both lists while capturing their essence. When you have completed this "mutual relationship vision," schedule a time every day to read it to each other, or record it on cassette and listen to it together. Do this exercise daily for at least sixty days. This is just one of sixteen exercises described in Dr. Hendrix's book.

A Listening Exercise

Most men are poor listeners. We're usually convinced we can do more than one thing at a time. It's not unusual for us to be watching a game on TV and assuring our wives or partners that they have our undivided attention. The fact is we *hear* but we don't *listen*. The difference is that hearing can be unconscious while listening requires conscious effort. Since communication is the foundation of any relationship, and listening is a critical aspect of effective communication, this exercise can go a long way toward creating greater intimacy and autonomy. It can also be good for your health. At the University of Maryland, James Lynch, Ph.D., found that people who do not listen well, who jump at the first chance to answer back, tend to have higher blood pressure.

Schedule an uninterrupted forty-minute block of time with your partner once a week in a comfortable, relaxed, quiet setting. One person speaks for twenty minutes while the other listens without responding. Then the roles are reversed. The object is to be able to talk freely about whatever you're thinking or feeling without worrying about judgment or criticism. Under the usual circumstances, if you express something that makes your partner uncomfortable, you get a negative reaction right away. With this exercise the listener will still react to the words or ideas that trigger discomfort, but will not be allowed to respond. The more the listener focuses on his or her own reaction, the less he or she is actually listening. The more you practice listening, the better you become at letting go of your own thoughts and feelings and at focusing on those of your partner. Some people have described this exercise as almost meditative, because it requires you to empty your mind of your own thoughts as you listen.

As the speaker, try not to dwell on the relating of current events, but concentrate more on the feelings these situations have elicited in you. If you're the second speaker, avoid a critique of what your partner just said. It is best not to comment on anything that was said during the exercise for up to three days following it. Creating a safe environment for expressing your feelings and allowing yourself to be vulnerable with your spouse or partner is an extremely valuable tool for building trust, understanding, and, at times, exhilarating feelings of intimacy. The wife of a couple to whom we recommended this exercise said, "It felt wonderful to have my husband's total attention." Her husband added that he "really liked the fact that she was just listening without giving me any advice." Other couples have remarked that the skills learned in this listening exercise also adapt well to the workplace. This exercise is described in more detail in Maggie Scarf's book *Intimate Partners.*

Another helpful communication exercise, one that is highly effective for resolving conflict, is called **mirroring** or **reflective listening.** This skill helps couples in the midst of an argument to slow down their reactions and reduce the intensity of their interactions. It assures them that what is being communicated is accurately interpreted and validated. In this exercise, it is essential to let go of the need to resolve the conflict, and instead to thoroughly focus on understanding each other's perspective. Without blame or criticism, one partner paraphrases short segments of the other partner's conversation in a neutral tone of voice. They reverse roles and continue the process. In a way, mirroring is echoing your partner's expression, as if you were a reporter accurately recording what your partner just said and reading it back to her. Practically speaking, this exercise confirms that the message has been received and that each of you has been heard. *A couple's ability to manage conflict is the best indicator of a successful marriage.* In the book *Getting the Love You Want* by Harville Hendrix, you can find an in-depth description of this technique.

A heightened level of communication helps to create not only greater intimacy but better health as well. That's the finding of Ohio State University researcher Janice Keicolt-Glaser, who studied ninety newlywed couples as they discussed difficult issues—from money to in-laws—during videotaped sessions. By comparing before-and-after blood samples, researchers found that partners who resorted to hostile tactics showed measurably greater drops in immune function than did those who took a more supportive, less adversarial position.

Requests

When you commit to each other, you enter into a relationship in which you have promised to give and receive love. Since each of us is different, what feels like love to one person might not even be noticed by another. Most of us attempt to love our partners in ways that feel like love to *us,* and we are surprised when they do not react as we would. A good method of eliminating this problem is simply to tell each other what feels good. To insure that you both receive more of what you want, write three requests of one another. These should consist of actions or behaviors that you, the requester, perceive as most loving. Like affirmations, requests should contain only positive directions and should be as specific as possible. Requests may include statements such as "I would like you to give me two hugs daily," "I would like us to spend one night out each week," "I would like you to buy me flowers once a week," or "I would like you to cook din-

ner once a week." It can be quite a revelation when someone you have lived with for many years, a person whom you thought you knew well, tells you what they really need from you. This exercise helps explain your own feelings of betrayal when your loving actions were not reciprocated. We often expect our partners to be mind readers: "He should have known what I wanted"; "She ought to have been able to tell how I felt." We really can't know exactly what our partners want unless we are told. Be specific, make requests, and get what you need. It is extremely important to thank your partner for complying with any request. The requested task might not have been an easy or natural thing for him or her to do—otherwise you wouldn't have had to ask in the first place. Acknowledge the effort and even greater compliance will follow.

Re-creation: Having Fun Together

The pressures and responsibilities of daily life make it difficult to remember to have fun. Recreation is an important way to renew spontaneity in a relationship. It enables you to *re-create* the joy in one another that you experienced during your courtship and early years together. Think of it as a glue that reinforces relationships. (Another common glue of relationships is shared suffering, but recreation is much more fun.) To rekindle some of that excitement and sweep away the cobwebs of routine boredom, it helps to schedule fun activities together regularly. Plan a day or half-day each week to spend together away from home in an activity one of you has chosen. Alternate the responsibility for the choice of activity. Being out of the house, unaccompanied by friends or other family members, can help you focus attention on each other. Although it is more difficult, it is also possible, even with young children, to plan an enjoyable and perhaps an exciting evening at home, after the kids are in bed. Choosing something neither of you has ever tried before can add a sense of adventure to your play. If you can manage it, plan one weekend a month out of town. You might be surprised at how refreshing and invigorating regularly scheduled short trips can be for your relationship. These two-day excursions might be just what you need, especially if a real vacation isn't feasible.

Sex

Implicit, of course, in the two-day getaway, is sex and plenty of it . . . away from the house, the kids, the phone, and preferably set in a novel location with plenty of romantic atmosphere. The local Motel 6 won't do. Let's admit it up front: although *Thriving* is filled with pleasurable activities and exercises, most men find that nothing feels quite so good as having their primal unit enveloped by the warm throb of their lover's perfectly fitting yoni.

Not that we ever stop to think about it, but here is what goes on physiologically. At the point of maximum pleasure—ejaculation— the penis is engorged with blood, testosterone is off the charts, the heart is pounding, blood

pressure is peaking, and the senses are gridlocked in your crotch like Times Square on New Year's Eve waiting for the ball to drop. Does God love us or what . . . ? The fact is, most guys in their youth can reach orgasm in nothing flat. Show an eighteen-year-old male a *Penthouse* centerfold, and it's zero to sixty in ten seconds. Talk about instant gratification. . . . Biologists will tell you that men are quick on the draw because of their Neanderthal cousins, who did everything with self-preservation in mind, including sex. Yes, it's true that women live longer than men (an average of seven years), but they need every minute because it takes them that much longer to reach orgasm.

If we males have been so blessed as love machines with our rapid-fire physiology and instant hard-ons, why are so many of us impotent? According to some estimates, more than 20 million men are unable to have an erection when they want one. The word itself (*im-potent:* without power) gives us a clue as to the reasons for this epidemic of sexual dysfunction. Next to air, food, and water, men subsist on confidence. They need a sense of authority, recognition, or confirmation of their performance at work, and among friends and family, to "perform" in the bedroom. Sex is often a metaphor for what goes on in other areas of your life, and if those other areas are fraught with failure or insecurity, you are not likely to perform up to your usual standards in bed. If these problems outside the bedroom are compounded by a critical spouse who makes it abundantly clear how dissatisfied she is sexually, it can obliterate sexual confidence. The crux of our sexual problem as men is our belief that sex is a performance and that we are being graded on our ability to provide pleasure to our partners.

In the interest of providing greater pleasure, some of us are more frequently feeling the need to enlarge our equipment. Penile implant surgery that lengthens and enlarges girth has become an advertising staple in men's magazines and on sports pages across the country and a booming business for a growing number of urologists. If men knew the truth about average penis size, almost all of these surgeries would be unnecessary. Tom Lue, M.D., a urologist at the University of California, San Francisco, has conducted an extensive survey of a cross-section of men without surgical enhancement to determine average penis size. His study, measuring circumference and length in both limp and erect conditions, showed that what men frequently assume is small size and in need of surgical enhancement is, in fact, quite normal: *surgery is unnecessary.* Lue found that the average limp penile length was 3.5 inches (8.8 cm). The average erect length was 5.1 inches (12.8 cm). Limp circumference averaged 3.9 inches (9.8 cm). Average erect circumference measured 4.9 inches (12.2 cm). Of the sixty men included in the study, only one came even close to what would be considered subnormal in size (less than 2.8 inches in limp length and less than 3.5 inches in erect circumference).

Before you take out your tape measure, keep in mind that a variety of independent studies based on interviews with women have shown that size is much less a factor in determining their sexual pleasure than tenderness and attention. Unfortunately, the myth of performance is so compelling, it can lead men to self-mutilating extremes or irreparable marital conflicts. Sexual pleasure should be based not on myth or false expectation, but on the reality of shared experience, one in which both partners are open to both giving and receiving sexual pleasure. If both partners meet the criterion of a basic openness to sexual intimacy, then each will assume a natural responsibility for having his or her sexual needs met. The burden of performance is then lifted, and men can enjoy both a loving and ecstatic sexual experience. There's nothing wrong with a man's inclination to feel a sense of power or self-confidence, but let that feeling derive from participating in the moment. Where good sex is concerned, all you need is to show up and be ready to play ball. Leave behind your power tools: the bank balance, Mercedes coupe, and other money-drenched trappings. These accessories may make for a great one-night stand, but it isn't making love, and it's a far cry from thriving sex.

If men require a sense of power and confidence to feel good enough to perform sexually, what then do women need? Therein lies the problem with sexual relationships, because women, as most of us have found out the hard way, have very different needs. *Men need sex to feel intimate, and women need intimacy to feel sexy.* Most women are far more interested in feeling loved and cared for during sex than they do about being shot to the moon. It's not that women don't enjoy their orgasms as much as we do, but they need to experience more intimacy in getting off the launchpad.

One factor that accounts for this difference is purely chemical. Testosterone, the male hormone, produces a highly self-individualizing response that produces feelings of autonomy and power. Females have a corresponding sexual hormone called oxytocin, which predisposes them to connect with others and establish intimacy. For sexual compatibility in a relationship, both partners' needs must be met. This means that men need to learn patience, especially since women need extra time to make the transition from work and mothering responsibilities to becoming a lover. Although men can do this with great ease, women, as we've seen, are wired differently. Women express and receive love through nurturing.

Touching can be the most powerful way of conveying love and allowing your partner to feel nurtured. Most men zero in only on selected targets: breasts, vulva, and clitoris. Women actually prefer that you hold off on those areas until after caressing, stroking, and massaging the *whole* body. By letting her gradually reach a state of sexual arousal, you can both share in the passion of sexual intimacy.

Not every sexual encounter will be this ideal. When "making love" is called "fucking," it tends to be a little more than a quickie, or a shot in the dark, an opportunity to come without expending much effort toward your partner. Occasionally, this is fine for stress management, as long as both partners agree to it. Since men also commonly perceive themselves as initiators of sexual encounters, try occasionally to hold off and allow your partner to direct more of your sexual activity.

Perhaps the key ingredient in allowing both partners to have their sexual needs met is *time*. If you were to devote at least a few minutes of your lovemaking to include sexual exercises, you would enhance your pleasure while prolonging and intensifying orgasm. The foundation of these sexual exercises is the contraction of the pubococcygeus (pc) muscle (sometimes called the Kegel exercise), which normally contracts on ejaculation. By learning to contract this muscle at will, you can hold off orgasm and/or intensify it. Located on the pelvic floor between the anus and scrotum, the pc muscle can be identified by stopping your flow of urine in midstream. Once you know this feeling of contraction, you can practice it as often as you want. This exercise not only enhances sexual pleasure, but it can aid in reducing an enlarged prostate. To get in the habit of using the pc exercise, incorporate it into your daily routine: remind yourself to do it every time the phone rings when you are seated at your desk at work, or each time you stop at a traffic light. You can even coordinate pc exercises with your abdominal breathing by contracting the pc muscle with every inhalation. It is recommended that you start with ten to fifteen pc contractions daily. Try to do them consecutively and gradually work your way up to thirty or more. Contraction and relaxation should be about the same length of time—two to four seconds. You can gradually increase the length of each contraction beyond four seconds as your pc muscle becomes stronger. As for its sexual application, a prolonged pc contraction can be used just prior to ejaculation to avoid orgasm and maintain erection by arresting the pumping action of multiple contractions that accompany ejaculation.

As you become more skilled in the use of pc contractions, you can use them to move sexual energy from the pelvis through the rest of your body. To do so involves extensive practice in coordinating breath and visualization with your contractions. This combination is also a highly effective method for treating premature ejaculation. For further guidance on these supersex techniques called *tantra* (from the Sanskrit *tantram:* doctrine or loom), see Margo Anand's book *The Art of Sexual Ecstasy.* Tantra is an ancient system of sexual and sensual techniques designed to use the body as an instrument for consciously controlling the mind, increasing the reservoir of life-force energy and tapping the spirit. Tantra's erotic practices include the use of position, breath, and visualization to heighten sexual energy and channel that energy to each of the seven major chakras, thus expanding consciousness. The ancient civilizations of India, China, Nepal, Tibet, and Japan all developed variations of tantric practice. Taulere Appel, Ph.D., founder and teacher of Tantric Intimacy® in Boulder, Colorado, has developed a diagram to illustrate the tantric sexual cycles. To this diagram

(page 170), I have overlaid a corresponding diagram of the conventional male sexual cycle (dotted line) based on Masters and Johnson's model. As you can see, conventional male response, relegated to the root chakra (i.e., the genitals), runs its course before the second of eight tantric stages of excitement has even begun.

A word of caution: Just because at eighteen we had the ability to go from arousal to orgasm faster than a funny car devouring a quarter-mile drag strip, don't expect this same speed at age fifty. This mind-set is so ingrained by the headiness of youth that we are reluctant to let it go, even when we are older and slower. Many men interpret slower sexual performance as a symptom of failing or defective equipment. Instead of accepting inevitable physiological change, they adopt a defeatist attitude and limit themselves, gradually curtailing sexual activity because they no longer see themselves as vital sexual beings. Instead of exploring what can potentially become a period in their lives of enhanced sexual pleasure, many middle-aged men drop out of the game entirely. In what ways can sex get better on life's back nine? (1) You have an increased ability to sustain prolonged lovemaking. (2) You have better control over ejaculation. (3) You enjoy an expanded sense of orgasm that transcends genital pleasure alone and can infuse your entire body. Like getting to Carnegie Hall, enhancing sexual response as you age takes practice, practice, practice . . . and a supportive partner. But if you're willing to spend an hour each week at the driving range

TANTRIC INTIMACY® CYCLE
(ONE TO THREE HOURS)

TANTRIC AROUSAL	KUNDALINI AWAKENED	ECSTASY	ECSTASY	ECSTASY	ECSTATIC BLISS	BLISS WAVES	ENLIGHTENMENT
(two to eight minutes) ORGASM ✳			Delay and Meditate	Orgasm Directed or Relaxed Into	Conjoined Climax of Body and Soul	Float in Exquisite Sensations	Relationship with All of Life Maintains "Ecstatic Glow"
Harmonization and Bonding	Delay and Meditate	Delay and Meditate	Edge of Orgasm	Edge of Orgasm			
PLATEAU	Edge of Orgasm	Edge of Orgasm	Excitation		United with the Cosmos	Continuous Flow of Energy	
Erotic Relaxation	Excitation	Excitation				Refreshed and Revitalized	Seventh Heaven (Endless Orgasm)
EXCITEMENT	First Pleasure (Electro-Magnetic Warming)	Second Pleasure (Yearning)	Third Pleasure (Passion of the Heart)	Fourth Pleasure (Transcendence)	Fifth Pleasure (Deepest Communion)	Sixth Pleasure (Afterglow)	
	Sexual Energy (Shakti) Begins to Rise up Spine	Sexual Energy Rises to Navel and Solar Plexus Chakras	Sexual Energy Rises to Heart Chakra	Sexual Energy Rises to Throat and Head Chakra	Physical Orgasm Is Accompanied by Spiritual Bliss	Gratitude for Your Beloved as an Expression of the Divine	Sacred Sensual Intimacy Transforms Daily Life
Practice to Modulate, Prolong, Expand and Contain Pleasure to Reach Higher States of Consciousness, to Develop New Circuitry and Transmute Sexual Energy							

working on your backswing, this should be a piece of cake. If you still don't think aging and sexuality are a match that works, consider what Masters and Johnson, authors of the groundbreaking *Human Sexual Response,* had to say on the subject. They documented that men who had never stopped sexual activity continued to enjoy their sexuality—its function and response—well into their eighties. So you choose: Are you going to be a happy Hunza or a withered prune?

Fathering

If you think that a committed relationship consists only of meeting the physical and emotional needs of you and your partner like dragonflies in an endless mating idyll on a summer afternoon, you'd better think again. An unavoidable consequence of healthy sexual practice is the subject of children. . . . Which brings us to the art of fathering: not the procreative function whose pleasures can extend to several hours, but the often consequent parental responsibility replete with its array of challenges, frustrations, and rewards that can carry on for several decades.

Prior to becoming a father, a man should be able to answer two important questions in no uncertain terms: (1) *Am I consciously choosing to have kids?* (2) *Am I prepared to commit to the responsibility of parenting those kids?* Which also means: *Am I prepared to stay with their mother for better or worse?* The first question will test your motivation for having kids: Do you really know why you want them? A sixteen-year-old inner-city

gangbanger may want a child to symbolize his manhood; in some gangs impregnating young girls is required for initiation. For the thirty-two-year-old suburban yuppie, a child might offer a different brand of male self-confirmation: a way of carrying on the family name that confers a sense of immortality. As shallow as these reasons may sound, they relate to some fundamental male urges. Spreading one's seed satisfies an essential male need to participate in the dance of life as it unfolds from one generation to the next. This sense of immortality derives from a real urge to participate in something larger than oneself. We can dress up these reasons and make them sound as profound and noble as we want. Other reasons might include loving the innocence, creativity, and vitality of children; wanting to nurture and fill a parental role; wanting to re-create the good feelings of your own childhood or to redress the injuries that you suffered. Understanding your reasons for wanting to make babies will help you to commit to the long-term process that follows. Whatever your reason, you'd better understand the reality of what you're getting yourself into.

The second question—Are you ready to commit to parenting and staying with the mom?—is tougher. After all, kids are *not* low-maintenance propositions. To do a good job as a father is like any other job in which 90 percent of performance is practice: showing up and putting in the time. That's why the second part of this question is asking yourself if you are committed to staying with the mother of these children. Thirty-seven percent of the children in this country today do not live with their natural father, and the epidemic of low self-esteem and teenage crime probably bears a relationship to this abandonment by fathers. So far, the effects of "present" fathering hasn't been quantified in terms of enhanced test scores, athletic ability, or language facility; but the structure, sense of security, and especially the self-esteem that present fathers can provide their children build a critical foundation for creating a fulfilling adulthood. Know your responsibility to everyone involved and commit to accepting it. *Be a man!*

Although there are no simple approaches to what many see as life's most challenging job, it's not all work and no play. Fathering can also be one of life's most enriching experiences: a chance to play, to feel more in touch with our own "inner child," and to let go of ourselves and experience selflessness. In dealing with teenagers, in particular, we face a wonderful opportunity for practicing forgiveness, trust, self-awareness, and most of all, patience.

A useful guideline to the art of effective fathering might be to ask yourself regularly, "Will this action (response, activity, or demand) of mine help my child's self-esteem?" The same principle holds true in fathering as it does in marriage: *To love another is to help that person better love himself or herself.* Obviously, as human beings, we are not always able to meet this ideal and not impose our own selfish interests. Children are constantly trying to expand their limits (as they should), and at the same time they are testing ours.

While they seek greater independence, our job is to balance our own degree of comfort—which includes our values and levels of fear and trust—with what will most benefit these young explorers. This task requires a great deal of awareness to appreciate who these unique persons are and to best provide them the structure and sense of security they need to develop independence and discover their hidden talents. Most men take great pride in their children's achievements and strengths and disavow any connection with their weaknesses or flaws. Still, our children are a blend of genetic inheritance, environmental influence, and their own unique spirit. As parents we must respect that individuality and trust our children to "find" themselves. As they grow up, our job of fathering becomes more challenging. We must learn to do less and spectate more, showing an endless reserve of support while constantly biting our tongue.

In the field of family therapy, the family is usually seen from the systems approach. This view holds that if a member's behavior is harmful to himself or others, the problem and the solution lie not solely within that individual but in the entire family system. This perspective encourages parents to look at their roles and the partial responsibility they share for the problem. A child's crisis can reflect an imbalance in that child's individual system as well as in the larger family system. In much the same way that holistic medicine insists on treating physical symptoms within the context of the whole person, the systems approach in family therapy recognizes the need for treating the suffering individual within the larger context of the family. One of the significant advantages of family therapy is that change can occur more rapidly than in individual psychotherapy. If someone in your family is struggling emotionally, I strongly recommend family counseling.

In examining the emotional body, we saw how anger can be a cause of physical disease. Within the family, the focus of that anger is going to be yourself, your spouse, or your children. Now that you know several ways to release that anger, there is another way to use it beneficially, particularly with regard to your children. I have found consistently that those aspects of a child's behavior that most upset a parent are those that the parent either has denied or likes least about himself or herself. Perhaps it is easier to be angry with our kids than with ourselves. These disturbing behavior patterns become most apparent during adolescence and merely add to the challenge of parenting teenagers. For instance, suppose you believe your child has innate ability in a certain sport, with a musical instrument, or in a creative art, but the child refuses to pursue it for fear of making mistakes or looking awkward or silly as a beginner, or perhaps for no reason at all. You react strongly, become furious, and find yourself insisting that the youngster at least try this new endeavor. Why did you react so strongly? When you do so, it's time to stop, reflect, and use the situation as a mirror. Perhaps this particular incident is reminiscent of your own fear of trying new things. It might be bringing

up feelings of frustration and anger with yourself for the many times you failed to realize your own potential. Out of your anger with the child can arise an opportunity for you to observe yourself more clearly and to forgive and accept both yourself and your child. Opportunities for loving often present themselves in unusual ways.

Good fathering requires two essentials: **consistency** and **time.** In a June 1994 edition of *Men's Confidential* magazine, psychologists Ronald Levant, Ed.D., and Jerrold Shapiro, Ph.D., outlined four simple steps for fine-tuning the art of fathering and becoming more consistently aware of your child's needs.

1. *Learn what your child is feeling.*
   It is critical to develop the ability to read your child's emotions by tuning into what he or she is saying and learning to read nonverbal behavior. Try to be more observant of body language, tone of voice, and facial expression. A mirroring technique similar to the one described earlier in this chapter for use with your wife or partner might also work well with your child. It should consist of using a neutral tone of voice to repeat the precise content of what your child has said when you sit down to talk. Don't interrupt or try to micromanage through advice or judgment, which only serve to dismiss the child's emotions. Like your partner, when a child wants to talk, he's asking you to listen, not to fix his life. Try empathizing with his emotion and

remember that your child grows stronger and bonds more closely with you the more he feels understood. Trust him to solve his own problems.

2. *Build an emotional vocabulary.* The majority of men know lots of words for anger and aggression, because as boys those were the emotions we were most often permitted to experience. What we don't know as well are the words for the vulnerable emotions—fear, sadness, shame, hurt, and disappointment. And we are not as comfortable with the words for the tender emotions, like care, affection, and compassion. To develop a broader emotional vocabulary, I recommend using words that have fallen out of use in your vocabulary: *hurt, afraid, sad,* and *ashamed* for painful emotions, and *loving, tender,* or *compassionate* for gentler emotions. To expand this vocabulary, please refer to the "Feeling Wheel" on page 120.

3. *Establish a strong sense of identity as a parent.* List those assets that you bring to parenting as distinguished from those of your wife. If you can explain to your kids how an internal combustion engine works, recite the infield-fly rule, cook a perfect steak, or show your kid how to cast a fly rod, these are all qualities that your wife may not have been able to provide on her own. Add other qualities that you would like to offer.

4. *Share your time and wisdom equally with sons and daughters, encouraging self-sufficiency in both.* Many men teach their sons to change a tire, but not their daughters. Yet it is the daughter who is more vulnerable out on the road if the tire should blow.

In a nutshell, these four steps to effective fathering add up to a willingness on our parts as fathers to build our children's self-esteem and to let them know they are loved. But beyond the need for these expressions of love and understanding is the basic prerequisite of *time:* you must make time to be with your kids. Although you can't spend every waking hour with them, no nanny, teacher, baby-sitter, or housemaid can take your place. Time is the most essential ingredient to first-rate fathering. Unfortunately, time is the ingredient most lacking in today's society. Most men of our generation learned from their fathers that time at work takes priority over time with children. It was a painful lesson to learn and has been a difficult one to unlearn. Most of us appear to be making a greater effort to be better fathers. According to a 1996 *Newsweek* poll, 55 percent of today's fathers say being a parent is more important to them than it was to their own fathers. Sixty-one percent say they understand their children better. Forty-nine percent rate themselves better parents than their fathers. And 70 percent say they spend more time with their children than their fathers spent with them. But in spite of all this self-congratulation, the divorce rate still runs at 50 percent.

For as little time as our fathers spent with us, most of them were still available to us physically each day. They were in our lives at the dinner table, during drives in the country, at church or synagogue, family get-togethers, or sporting events. The irony of our generation's growing sensitivity and enthusiasm for good fathering is that although we make the attempt to be more emotionally present for our children, almost half of us are physically absent a good bit of the time due to divorce. The crux of the problem with divorce is the damaging message it sends to our children, telling them that commitments are merely temporary conveniences that cannot withstand the stresses of fundamental human relationship. Although our fathers rarely, if ever, told us they loved us, we could usually depend on them to come home each night and provide a sense of security. When our children watch us throw away a committed relationship with our spouse or partner, it unavoidably makes them wonder if they were somehow responsible and if we might do the same to them. Not only can this fear translate into feelings of insecurity and low self-esteem, it erodes the foundations of trust between father and child. Furthermore, since parents are the first place children learn about committed relationships, the example of divorce can easily create the expectation of failure in their own relationships. This sense of failure can surface later in their lives as a self-fulfilling prophecy that either dooms their own marriage or makes them gunshy about entering into a committed relationship in the first place.

Its impact on self-esteem and a child's view of relationships aside, divorce takes a father out of the house and robs his children of the second most important thing he can provide them—time. Whether you are a divorced single parent or married with children and find for a variety of reasons that you don't see your kids as often as you'd like, make a point of *regularly scheduling* time together. To a child encountering the world and attempting to make sense of it, you are still one of the most important contacts and filters for helping them to pattern that reality and give it meaning. If you are indifferent or impatient in relating to them and answering their questions about the world, they will assume the world is also that way. It may take them a lifetime to disabuse themselves of these limiting notions, providing they are lucky enough to meet a friend, mentor, therapist, or spouse who can help them to expand their awareness. This should give you a sense of the enormity of your responsibility as a father. Even if you cannot see your child daily, your level of participation will condition how they choose to experience the world and live their lives.

The goal of good fathering is to provide your child the security, confidence, and caring that come from being loved. This is true whether you spend time together once a week or once a day. Like any other aspect of thriving, effective fathering begins with *commitment*. It will unavoidably include doses of *pain*, as well as the joy of seeing your child *empowered*. The result: your child's ability to form *harmonic* relationships with you and others, built on intimacy and trust.

Father and Son: The Crucible of Forgiveness

Just as we learned about committed relationships from observing our parents, so we learned how to (or how not to) parent from observing our fathers. So much of our adult behavior as men has come from (or, in many cases, in reaction to) the example set by our father. The way we relate to other men derives from the way our fathers related to us. If Dad was inexpressive and never showed fear, anger, or sadness, chances are good you don't express these emotions either. Our work ethic, ambition, and need for recognition are closely related to the praise and acknowledgment that, as kids, we hungered for from our fathers.

Unfortunately, most of us didn't grow up in idyllic nineteenth-century farming communities where father and son worked together and shared the joys, hardships, and responsibilities of their lives. Instead, we inhabited artificial communities, called suburbs, purposely distanced from work and, in many cases, from extended families as well. Not only were our suburban fathers more detached from their own roots, they never had a book like this to read. If they had, we probably wouldn't need it now, which we do, because it has taken two generations to identify the kinds of social upheaval that affluence, technology, and mass culture can breed. In any case, most of us now realize intellectually—if not emotionally—that our fathers were doing the best they knew how. It is up to us to acknowledge that healing the father-son relationship is primary to restoring a man's

holistic health. Your father's love is the tie that binds you to our male "tribe," to your masculinity, and it may be the most significant factor in the development of your self-esteem. To a great extent, this relationship will determine how you relate to your own son. Father-son is a bond that for most of us needs strengthening. There are positive steps to take to heal the wounds that have created a distance between you and your father, and perhaps between you and your son.

In my own work with men, I've heard bitterness, anger, and hostility when I initially questioned them about their feelings toward their father: "That SOB was never there for me!" Although sons of alcoholics probably have the greatest animosity, most of our fathers were physically or emotionally absent due to some type of addiction. Workaholism was far more prevalent than alcoholism. As a result, almost all of us were, to some extent, wounded by unmet needs. Yet as hardened as many men seem to be by this experience, there is obviously a soft spot in our hearts for our fathers, and not too far below the surface. In my patients, I have observed a deep desire that never dies to love and be loved by their father, regardless of their age or whether or not their father is still alive.

No doubt, our fathers were probably parenting in much the same way that they had been programmed to do so by their fathers; nonetheless, the distance between father and son and its emotional pain persists. Although we intellectually acknowledge that many social factors account for this rift, and we try to be grown-ups about understanding them, at some level we're still hurt and pissed off, as any child would be. More often than not, this anger is reinforced by our present interaction with our fathers, because most of them haven't changed one bit and probably never will. If we're ever going to close the abyss between father and son, *we* are the ones who are going to have to change. This may be the single most important and challenging responsibility of our generation of men. If we are going to close the numerous gaps in understanding between races, cultures, economic classes, and nations, we must start with the rift between generations embodied in the relationship between father and son.

Before this father and son *re-union* can occur, there must be forgiveness. Just as we used the four stages of thriving to overcome our fear of intimacy in committed relationships with spouses, partners, and children, we can use them once again to close the distance between us and our fathers. Between father and son, many obstacles are in the way of forgiveness—competition, the need to be right and to win, the need to control, and the fear of intimacy with another man. Prior to forgiveness, it is important to fully acknowledge the pain one's father has caused. What did it feel like when he never made time for you—to play, to go to your games, performances, or award ceremonies, or to simply sit and talk together? Most men are disappointed that they never really knew who their fathers were—their hopes and dreams, their fears and regrets—and that they have been unable to share the same information about themselves with their fathers.

For those men who have the opportunity to be with their fathers day to day, it can be easier to bridge that gap: they have time together to form an intimate relationship. But for most of us, the demands of jobs and general busyness keep us apart from our fathers from week to week, month to month, and even year to year. As adults, we even seem to push our fathers away in the same fashion they kept us at arm's length when we were children. To thrive, we must break this self-perpetuating pattern of behavior. Try spending more time visiting, calling, or corresponding with your father. As in any important relationship, making a *commitment* to set aside time for that relationship to unfold is probably the most important requirement. Plan an activity that you would both enjoy. Create more opportunity for your father to communicate with you. The result can bring both joy and pain. Be realistic and don't set your sights too high. Understand that healing this relationship may not mean it will change; however, giving it your best shot will heal something inside of you that will enable you to feel a greater sense of wholeness. Remember: "It's better to have loved and lost than to have never loved at all." From this *pain* emerges an understanding and acceptance that *empowers* you to discover a new sense of *harmony* in that relationship. Although the relationship may appear unchanged on the surface, it doesn't mean that healing hasn't taken place.

The most challenging part of healing between father and son is the ability to *forgive* your father. The essence of forgiveness lies in the awareness that our fathers did the best they could. Now that they're older, many with chronic disease and disability, it is time for us to let go of the past and be there for our fathers. It's our turn to give and theirs to receive. There are times, no doubt, when they fear their approaching death, as we will too at their age. As they begin to lose their physical and mental capabilities, this fear escalates in inverse proportion to their self-esteem. They need us more than ever. Hopefully, we can learn to teach them that their self-worth doesn't depend upon the optimal functioning of their mind and body (if that were true, then ultimately we'd all be "losers"), but from their capacity to experience love. While we're at it, maybe we can learn the same lesson ourselves.

Why bother? Because every new offense, slight, or insult committed by them or us merely piles on top of the old ones and keeps dragging our energy into the past. Without realizing it, we reignite the same angry response, which may take new form as irritability, or even rage directed at our wife, kids, or coworkers. Forgiveness is the only way to heal this relationship with our fathers and to finally dry up our wellspring of anger. Only by truly forgiving the *person*, instead of holding fast to his hurtful *behavior*, can we let go of the past and bring that relationship into the healing present. Forgiveness is a *very gradual* opening of your heart and allowing yourself to feel compassion for your father, whether he is still alive or dead.

One effective way that I have found for practicing forgiveness is the following meditation adapted from Stephen Levine. Author of *Who Dies?*, *Healing into Life and Death*, and *A Year to Live*, Levine worked for many years with the terminally ill and found that almost uniformly their greatest regret was that they either hadn't forgiven a family member or conveyed how much they loved him or her. The meditation below may be read either silently or aloud to oneself. It can be used to close the distance between you and your father, even if he is estranged or no longer living. It will also work with your spouse, partner, child, or any other committed relationship.

A FORGIVENESS MEDITATION

Begin to reflect for a moment on what the word forgiveness might mean. What is forgiveness? What might it be to bring forgiveness into one's life, into one's mind?

Begin by slowly bringing into your mind, into your heart, the image of your father (your spouse, partner, child, sibling, friend), someone for whom you have resentment. Gently now invite him into your heart just for this moment.

Notice whatever fear or anger may rise to limit or deny his entrance and soften gently all about it. Use no force. Just create an experiment in truth which allows this person in.

And silently in your heart, say to him, "I forgive you. Whatever pain you may have caused me in the past, intentionally or unintentionally, through your words, your thoughts, your actions and inactions. However you may have caused me pain in the past, I forgive you."

Feel for even a moment a sense of spaciousness or release relating to that person and the possibility of forgiveness.

Let go of those walls, those curtains of resentment, so that your heart may be free. So that your life may be lighter.

Say to yourself, "I forgive you for whatever you may have done that caused me pain, intentionally or unintentionally, through your actions, through your words, even through your thoughts, through whatever you did and through whatever you didn't do. However the pain came to me through you, I forgive you. I forgive you."

It is so painful to put someone out of your heart. Let go of that pain. Let them be touched for this moment at least with the warmth of your forgiveness.

"I forgive you. I forgive you . . ."

Allow that person to just be there in the stillness, in the warmth and patience of your heart. Let them be forgiven. Let the distance between you dissolve in mercy and compassion.

Let it be so.

Now, having finished so much business, dissolved in forgiveness, allow that being to go on their way. Not pushing or pulling them from the heart, but simply letting them be on their own way, touched by the blessing and the possibility of your forgiveness.

And now gently bring into your mind, into your heart, the image, the sense, of someone who has resentment for you. Someone whose heart is closed to you.

Notice whatever limits your entrance into

their heart and soften that obstruction. Let it float.

Mercifully invite them into your heart and say to them, "I ask your forgiveness.

"I ask your forgiveness.

"I ask to be let back into your heart. That you forgive me for whatever I may have done in the past that caused you pain, intentionally or unintentionally, through my words, my actions, even through my thoughts.

"However I may have hurt or injured you, whatever confusion, whatever fear of mine may have caused you pain, I ask your forgiveness."

And allow yourself to be forgiven. Allow yourself back into their heart.

Feel their forgiveness touch you. Receive it. Draw it into your heart.

"I ask your forgiveness for however I may have caused you pain in the past. Through my anger, through my lust, through my fear, my ignorance, my blindness, my doubt, my confusion. However I may have caused you pain, I ask that you let me back into your heart. I ask forgiveness."

Let it be. Allow yourself to be forgiven.

If the mind attempts to block forgiveness with merciless indictments, recriminations, judgments, just see the nature of the unkind mind. See how merciless we are with ourselves. And let this unkind mind be touched by the warmth and patience of forgiveness.

Let your heart touch this other heart so that it may receive forgiveness. So that it may feel whole again.

Let it be so.

Feel their forgiveness now as it touches you.

If the mind pulls back, thinks it deserves to suffer, see this merciless mind. Let it sink into the heart. Allow yourself to be touched by the possibility of forgiveness.

Receive the forgiveness.

Let it be.

And now gently bid that person adieu and with a blessing let them be on their way, having even for a millisecond shared the one heart beyond the confusion of seemingly separate minds.

And now gently turn to yourself in your own heart and say, "I forgive you."

It is so painful to put ourselves out of our hearts.

Say "I forgive you" to yourself.

Calling out to yourself in your heart, using your own first name, say "I forgive you" to yourself.

If the mind interposes with hard thoughts, such as that it is self-indulgent to forgive oneself, if it judges, if it touches you with anger and unkindness, just feel that hardness and let it soften at the edge. Let it be touched by forgiveness.

Allow yourself back into your heart. Allow yourself to be forgiven by you.

Let the world back into your heart. Allow yourself to be forgiven.

Let that forgiveness fill your whole body.

Feel the warmth and care that assures your own well-being, seeing yourself as if you were your own child. Let yourself be bathed by this mercy and kindness. Let yourself be loved.

How unkind we are to ourselves. How little mercy. Let it go. Allow yourself to embrace yourself with forgiveness. Know that in this moment you are wholly and completely forgiven. Now it is up to you just to allow it in. See yourself in the infinitely compassionate eyes of the Buddha, in the sacred heart of Jesus, in the warm embrace of God.

Let yourself be loved. Let yourself be love.

And now begin to share this miracle of forgiveness, of mercy and awareness. Let it extend out to all the people around you.

Let all be touched by the power of forgiveness. All those beings who also have known such pain. Who have so often put themselves and others out of their hearts. Who have so often felt so isolated, so lost.

Touch them with your forgiveness, with your mercy and loving kindness, that they too may be healed just as you wish to be.

Feel the heart we all share filled with forgiveness so that we all might be whole.

Let the mercy keep radiating outward until it encompasses the whole planet. The whole planet floating in your heart, in mercy, in loving kindness, in care.

May all sentient beings be freed of their suffering, of their anger, of their confusion, of their fear, of the doubt.

May all beings know the joy of their true nature.

May all beings be free from suffering.

Whole world floating in the heart. All beings freed of their suffering. All beings' hearts open, minds clear. All beings at peace.

May all beings at every level of reality, on every plane of existence, may they all be freed of their suffering. May they all be at peace.

May we heal the world, touching it again and again with forgiveness. May we heal our hearts and the hearts of those we love by merging in forgiveness, by merging in peace.

As a core component of thriving, the intimacy of the father-son connection reveals to us that our intrinsic value as men does not lie merely in achievement, but in the openness of our hearts. We need not be a supreme "doer" to win in this lifetime. I know of no man on his deathbed who bemoaned the fact that he could have worked harder. If there are regrets, they almost always have to do with the absence of close relationships.

Chapter 7

Putting It All Together:
A Program for Thriving

You hit home runs not by chance, but by preparation.

Roger Maris

The dictionary is the only place where success comes before work. Hard work is the price we must all pay for success.

Vince Lombardi

You are really never playing an opponent. You are playing yourself, your own highest standards, and when you reach your limits, that is real joy.

Arthur Ashe

———————————•———————————

Tools for Making Conscious Choices: The Thriving Ladder, List of Program Options, and Timetable

Some scientists will tell you that happiness is predetermined by your genetic makeup and not by the conscious choices that you make in the world around you. They will tell you that a purposeful regimen or action may have a temporary impact for approximately three months, but will disappear entirely by the end of six months when you unconsciously return to your genetic predisposition. Maybe these attitudes depict a cross-section of people who are either unwilling or unaware of how to effect purposeful change in their lives. If this dismal prospect of the tyranny of genetic predisposition were true, you might as well roll over and go back to sleep instead of reading this book. But I don't believe it is true. Nor do my patients, who, by following the program described in this book, have seen a lasting, positive transformation in their lives.

*Thriving results from the **conscious** effort to nurture your body, mind, and spirit.* Implementing a program of thriving requires (1) a consistent effort to change consciously, (2) an openness to working through the fear of this change while becoming more aware of its effects, and (3) the flexibility to adjust or change the program as needed. Structuring a successful program of thriving depends on first knowing what your present state of health is and where you would like it to be.

Thrive Ladder

Condition & Score	Program Options Required for Each Level of Condtion
Thriving 258–288	19 Body 8 Mind 12 Spirit
I Feel Great 228–257	15 Body 7 Mind 10 Spirit
I'm Okay 198–227	13 Body 6 Mind 8 Spirit
I'm Not Sick 168–197	11 Body 5 Mind 6 Spirit
I'm Getting By 138–167	9 Body 4 Mind 4 Spirit
I'm Hangin' In There 108–137	7 Body 3 Mind 2 Spirit
Survival Below 108	5 Body 2 Mind 1 Spirit

You will need to develop a sensitivity to what makes you feel better or worse and consciously choose to practice those options that enhance feelings of well-being.

To get started, let's find out precisely where you are in order to develop a set of practices uniquely suited to you for training to thrive. Take your score from the Thriving Self-Test and locate your current state of health on the Thriving Ladder, at left.

The Thriving Ladder is going to be an important tool because it provides the suggested practices and groupings of options for each level of the training program. As you will see, the program emphasizes building the body first and then the mind and spirit. All practices derive from the three main categories— *body, mind,* and *spirit.* To get an idea of how the program works, let's say your score falls in the Survival category (scoring 108 or below). You would then begin work focusing primarily on ways to strengthen the body. At this level, you have no choices: your practices are all required, consisting of five for the *body,* two for the *mind,* and one for the *spirit.* (These must-do practices are printed in boldface in the lists at left.) For all of the program options, see the lists at left. (To help you schedule these practices into your weekly routine, copy the Weekly Worksheet at the end of the chapter and use it to plan your regimen. Two sample worksheets for Survival and I'm Okay are also provided.)

Training to Thrive Program Options

BODY (Physical and Environmental Health)

BREATHING

1. **Eliminate tobacco smoke,** p. 61
2. **One-Minute Drill, 58**
3. Quiet Five, 59
4. Brain Booster, 59
5. Body Scan, 60
6. Installation of air cleaner or negative-ion generator, 234
7. Installation of good furnace filter and air-duct cleaning, 235
8. Installation of humidifier, 235

DRINKING

9. **Drink $\frac{1}{2}$ oz per pound of body weight of water on days without exercise, $\frac{2}{3}$ oz per pound on days with exercise (160 lbs = ten 8-oz [or thirteen 8-oz with exercise] glasses of water per day), 65**
10. Install a water filter or purchase bottled water, 66
11. Eliminate or reduce alcohol to moderate intake (two beers/day, one glass of wine/day, or one cocktail/day), 75
12. Eliminate or reduce caffeine to moderate intake (two cups of coffee or less/day), 73
13. Eliminate or reduce soda pop to moderate intake (two cans/day), 74

EATING

14. **Conform diet to Thriving Food Pyramid (reduce sugar, fat, red meat; increase fruits and vegetables), 70**
15. Use daily supplements with antioxidants, 82
16. Cook one dinner per week from scratch, 80
17. Take responsibility for food shopping at least twice per month to build dietary awareness, 76

EXERCISING

18. **Schedule at least 15–20 minutes of continuous movement (walking, stationary bike, treadmill, etc.—it needn't be aerobic) five times per week, 84**
19. Regular aerobic exercise 3–5 times per week for 20–30 minutes, 86
20. Regular flexibility-stretching program 3–5 times per week for 20–30 minutes, 91
21. Regular strengthening program 3–5 times per week for 20–30 minutes, 90
22. Engage in a new physical activity or aim for a challenging physical goal in an activity you have already been practicing, 83

SLEEPING & RELAXATION

23. Seven to eight hours of uninterrupted sleep per night, 94
24. Regular naps for 20–30 minutes, 96

25. Engage in some form of sensual or sexual pleasure 2–3 times per week (listening to music, massage, hot tub, steam bath, sauna, or sex), 96, 104, 166

26. Hobbies: 2–3 hours per week, 96

BIOENERGY

27. Regular practice of enhancement of bioenergy 3–5 times per week for 20–30 minutes (being in nature, sun exposure, body work, acupuncture, tai chi, meditation, visualization, etc.), 97, 148

MIND (Mental and Emotional Health)

1. **Develop at least one goal and its corresponding affirmation for every aspect of your health (physical, environmental, mental, emotional, spiritual, and social). Do this monthly, 41**

2. **Write, recite, and/or visualize at least one of these affirmations each day, one for each aspect of your health, 41**

3. Ask yourself at least once daily, "How am I feeling today?" Identify, experience, express, and accept at least two emotions that you have felt that day, 114

4. Identify daily two thought distortions that occurred that same day (115) that affected your actions or feelings

5. Once daily, try to identify and correlate a current physical discomfort with its underlying emotional pain, 117

6. Spend 15–20 minutes 3–5 times per week journaling, 121

7. Spend five minutes daily upon awakening recording your dreams, 122

8. Express your feelings to your spouse or partner daily, 122

9. Engage in weekly sessions of counseling or psychotherapy, 123

10. Self-treat a mood problem using the seven-step program suggested by Dr. Mark Sisti, 124

11. Do at least one anger-release technique daily, 125

12. Choose any form of body work and schedule a session at least every other week, 100

13. Practice the chakra-charging exercise three times per week, 130

14. Identify your two greatest fears or the two areas in which you feel most limited, 114. Create and recite an affirmation that addresses your fear and reduces its limiting effect, 41

15. Effect one change at work that makes your job more enjoyable

16. Work at your income-producing job no more than 50 hours per week, ideally 35–40 hours per week

17. Discover one thing about yourself that you take too seriously and find a way to laugh about it once a day, 127

18. Set one long-term goal for the year in any category—*body, mind,* or *spirit*—and achieve it

SPIRIT (Spiritual and Social Health)

1. **Upon awakening each morning, picture a person, place, or experience (real or imagined) that fills you with exhilaration or happiness just at the thought of it, 145**

2. Engage in regular 10–20 minute meditations at least once a day, 4–7 days per week. Use breathing, chanting, or mantras to structure your meditation, 146

3. Centering exercise to be done three times per week for ten minutes in a quiet place: Assume that your affairs are in order and you have told all of your loved ones good-bye. Now, imagine that you have one hour left to live. With nothing left to be done, allow yourself simply *to be*

4. At least once a week exercise your creativity at work by finding new solutions to old problems, or by giving further expression to a hidden talent

5. Ask yourself once a day: *What have I done today to fulfill my purpose?*

6. Establish a daily practice of prayer or psalms, original or borrowed from conventional liturgy or scripture, 140

7. Daily intuition exercise: Think of an instance in which you had a strong desire that you ultimately manifested as a result of surrendering to it instead of actively pursuing it. Next, think of something that you want badly right now. See yourself enjoying it without worrying about how to achieve it. Let go of the need to know the path of its attainment and listen for your inner voice to tell you how to achieve it, 145

8. Periodically consult a spiritual counselor, depending on your need. A spiritual psychotherapist or clergyman could be seen weekly and a clairvoyant or astrologist annually, 147

9. Spend at least 20–30 minutes daily in nature, 148

10. Visit sacred sites that you consider healing or imbued with higher energy, 149

11. Make a weekly visit to the ocean, a lake, river, hot springs, or soak in a hot tub (more frequently), 149

12. Spend one evening a week by candlelight or in front of a fire, 150

13. Expose yourself to sunlight and/or moonlight for at least 10–20 minutes 3–5 times a week, 99, 150

14. Observe a weekly Sabbath for at least a half-day, indulging yourself and your family in a celebration of life. Abstain from anything even remotely resembling work, 151

15. Engage in a one-day fast once a month, building up to one fast day per week, consisting of liquids only, 151

16. Look at yourself, especially your eyes, in a mirror for five minutes every day, 151

17. Touch or hold a loved one, or pet, 5–10 minutes at least once a day, 151

18. Find some person, action, or experience for which you are grateful every day and give thanks, 154

19. Join a group that meets regularly and supports a vital interest of yours, 159

20. Limit television and computer games to no more than one hour per night, 160

21. Renew an old committed relationship or establish a new one, 161

22. Create a "shared" vision list with your spouse or partner, 163

23. Practice a listening exercise for forty minutes, at least once per week, 163

24. At the beginning of each month, give and receive two requests of your spouse or partner and commit to honoring them, 165

25. Schedule a regular weekly block of time to recreate with your spouse or partner, 165

26. Commit to a program of supersex practices, beginning with a minimum of twenty daily pc contractions, 168

27. Commit to giving each of your children your undivided attention for at least 20–30 minutes each day. If you don't live with your children full-time, spend one day per week with them, 173

28. Take regular steps (at least monthly) to bring yourself and your father closer together, 176

If you scored well enough to qualify for I'm Not Sick (between 168 and 197), the Thriving Ladder calls for at least eleven practices for improving your *body*, five for the *mind*, and six for the *spirit*. Out of these twenty-two practices, eight are the same ones required from the Survival condition. If you are in the Thriving category, you have nineteen *body*, eight *mind*, and twelve *spirit* options. Again, eight of these options consist of the basic Survival requirements.

The Program Options include all the recommendations presented in each of the chapters in Part I. These practices are designed to create a general state of thriving. **However, if you are also treating a chronic disease, consult the appropriate chapter in Part II addressing your specific condition.** Add those recommendations to the number of suggested practices from the Thriving Ladder. Divided into three main areas of concern—*body, mind,* and *spirit*—the program options for each area reflect two aspects of health: **Body** consists of *physical* and *environmental* health. **Mind** includes *mental* and *emotional* health. **Spirit** contains both *spiritual* and *social* health. As an example of how to choose specific program options, let's say your score fell in the Survival category: 107. You smoke a pack of cigarettes a day, you drink the equivalent of a six-pack of beer each evening, you are twenty-five pounds overweight, you don't exercise, and you work in a high-stress job, often as many as sixty hours a week in a "sick" building. Once you have committed to training to thrive, you must start by doing the required five *body* choices from the list and **stick with them for at least three months—ninety days.** (It could take over a month to implement all of the options at your given condition.) As a Survival smoker, you must

- Stop smoking (B-1)
- Perform the One-Minute Drill three times per day (B-2)
- Drink ½ oz per pound of body weight of water (180 lbs = 90 oz or eleven 8-oz glasses of water) (B-9)
- Start conforming to the thriving diet (B-14)
- Schedule fifteen to twenty minutes of continuous body movement (B-18)

With any change you make, the health benefits should soon become apparent. Having quit smoking, you may notice that you have temporarily gained weight. On the other hand, you are probably breathing easier and more efficiently, you have far less mucus and congestion in your nose and lungs, you sleep better, and you have fewer headaches. As you change your diet and continue your moderate program of body movement, within a month you will probably have started to lose your extra weight. You will have gained more energy and you will have experienced a greater sense of optimism. At the Survival level, you also have two required program choices for the *mind* and one for the *spirit*. For the mind, you must develop and write, then recite or visualize daily at least one goal/affirmation for each aspect of health— physical/environmental, mental/emotional, spiritual/social (M-1, M-2). For the spirit, you must visualize or imagine an exhilarating person, place, or experience upon awakening

each day (S-1). As all of these practices become habits over the following months, they will not only feel good, but they will become easier, almost effortless, and you will be ready to add additional practices. Make copies of the weekly Thriving Program Worksheet that appears at the end of this chapter. This will help you schedule your program options and keep you on track. The sample worksheets also should give you some ideas on how to go about organizing your thriving program.

The Thriving Timetable for bringing these options into play is to introduce the recommended and required practices for each level of condition at a rate of two per week, and to sustain them all together for at least three months.

If you are the former smoker scoring 107 (see the Thriving Worksheet for Survival), your eight practices are all required (printed in bold), including stopping smoking. Having chosen two of those requirements the first week, add two more for each following week during the first month. Once you have introduced the required number of practices, you will sustain them for three months. Don't be impatient and try to skip ahead by adding more practices to your list. At the end of your three months of sustained practice, you will take the Self-Test again and evaluate your condition. If your score places you in a higher level, maintain your current list of practices and select additional options to fill out the *body, mind,* and *spirit* requirements for your new level of condition. If you were not nicotine-free until the third week of practice, you would begin counting your three-month consistent practice only from that point.

In addition to the *body* recommendations, it is always helpful to use a *mind* practice such as an affirmation to reinforce your new physical activity or behavior. If you're a former smoker, repeating an affirmation ("I am nicotine-free and feel healthy and more energetic") can enable you to become more consistent in this practice. The *spirit* requirement of visualizing an exhilarating person, place, or experience each morning upon awakening helps to create a more positive outlook, while establishing other sources for the focus and stimulation previously provided by an extended nicotine habit. Having sustained these eight practices together for at least three months, you would retake the Self-Test and, based on your score, could move up to the next rung on the ladder—to I'm Hangin' In There—or perhaps even higher. **Remember: the required practices on each list in bold must be included in every program regardless of your level of condition.**

Training to thrive is a gradual process that you will probably want to continue for the rest of your life. To bring these changes into your daily routine, at a rate that feels right to you, (1) use *the four stages of thriving* as the guiding principles behind each step of this process, and (2) adhere to the **Thriving Timetable.** At each level of health condition, and with every change you make, you will experience *commitment, pain, power,* and *harmony. Commitment* is the necessary first step that provides time, motivation, and consistency of effort. The feedback from this effort is initially transmitted as *pain*—the shock of the new and the accompanying discomfort that occurs with the loss of old habits. *Power* encompasses the heightened vitality and enhanced sense of performance that confers a newfound sense of enjoyment and exhilaration. As this new behavior becomes established as a healthy habit, its effects will resonate *harmoniously* at every level of your being: *body, mind,* and *spirit.* This is true whether the change you are working on is regular aerobic exercise, a new job, or a weekly listening exercise with your wife or partner. In any case, keep your Thriving regimen *manageable* and *fun.*

Conclusion

Depending on your starting condition, it may take several years to reach the "Thriving" level, but don't be in a hurry. Patience is not only a virtue, but a requirement for thriving. This isn't a footrace, and the only object of the game is to learn to enjoy the process. If after sustaining consistent practice of a particular option it still doesn't feel good to you, then discontinue it and choose another one. Each of us is unique and will respond differently to these options. Although we all have a variety of needs and desires, the options in the thriving program were chosen because they have been found to be most effective for the greatest number of people. This book is meant merely to be a guide. I expect that you will supplement my recommendations with your own experience, refinements, and knowledge. Stay committed, and enjoy the trip.

Thriving Program Worksheet

Current Score: 107   *Condition:* Survival   *Body Weight:* 185   *Date:* 10/13/97

Required Program Choices: 5 Body, 2 Mind, 1 Spirit

Body: B-1, B-2, B-9, B-14, B-18   *Mind:* M-1, M-2   *Spirit:* S-1

	Monday	**Tuesday**	**Wednesday**	**Thursday**	**Friday**	**Saturday**	**Sunday**
6–10 A.M.	B-1, B-2, B-9, M-1, M-2, S-1, B-14	B-1, B-2, B-9, M-1, M-2, S-1, B-14	B-1, B-2, B-9, M-1, M-2, S-1, B-14	B-1, B-2, B-9, M-1, M-2, S-1, B-14	B-1, B-2, B-9, M-1, M-2, S-1, B-14	B-1, B-2, B-9, M-1, M-2, S-1, B-14	B-1, B-2, B-9, M-1, M-2, S-1, B-14
10 A.M.–2 P.M.	B-14	B-14	B-14	B-14	B-14	B-14	B-14
2–4 P.M.	B-2	B-2	B-2	B-2	B-2	B-2	B-2
4–8 P.M.	B-18, B-14	B-18, B-14	B-18, B-14	B-18, B-14	B-18, B-14	B-18, B-14	B-18, B-14
8–12 P.M.	B-2	B-2	B-2	B-2	B-2	B-2	B-2

Thriving Program Worksheet

Current Score: 210 Condition: I'm Okay Body Weight: 185 Date: 10/13/97

Required Program Choices: 13 Body, 6 Mind, 8 Spirit

Body: B-1, B-2, B-3, B-6, B-7, B-9, B-11, B-12, B-14, B-15, B-18, B-20, B-23 Mind: M-1, M-2, M-3, M-8, M-11, M-15 Spirit: S-1, S-5, S-8, S-9, S-11, S-13, S-14, S-17

	Monday	Tuesday	Wednesday	Thursday	Friday	Saturday	Sunday
6–8 A.M.	B-1, B-2, B3, B-6, B-7, B-9, B-11, B-12, B-14, B-15, B-18, M-1, M-2, S-1	B-1, B-2, B-3, B-9, B-11, B-12, B-14, B-15, B-18, M-1, M-2, S-1	B-1, B-2, B-3, B-9, B-11, B-12, B-14, B-15, B-20, M-1, M-2, S-1	B-1, B-2, B-3, B-9, B-11, B-12, B-14, B-15, B-18, M-1, M-2, S-1	B-1, B-2, B-3, B-9, B-11, B-12, B-14, B-15, B-20, M-1, M-2, S-1	B-1, B-2, B-3, B-9, B-11, B-12, B-14, B-15, B-18, M-1, M-2, S-1	B-1, B-2, B-3, B-9, B-11, B-12, B-14, B-15, B-18, B-20, M-1, M-2, S-1, S-14
8 A.M.–Noon	M-15	M-15	M-15	M-15	M-15	S-13	S-8, S-11
Noon–5 P.M.	S-9	S-9, S-13	S-9	S-9, S-13	S-9	S-9	S-9, S-13
5–10 P.M.	M-3, M-8, M-11, S-5, S-17	M-3, M-8, M-11, S-5, S-17	M-3, M-8, M-11, S-5, S-17	M-3, M-8, M-11, S-5, S-17	M-3, M-8, M-11, S-5, S-17	M-3, M-8, M-11, S-5, S-17	M-8, S-17
10 P.M.–6 A.M.	B-23	B-23	B-23	B-23	B-23	B-23	B-23

Thriving Program Worksheet

Current Score: Condition: Body Weight: Date:

Required Program Choices:

Body: Mind: Spirit:

	Monday	Tuesday	Wednesday	Thursday	Friday	Saturday	Sunday
6–10 A.M.							
10 A.M.–2 P.M.							
2–4 P.M.							
4–8 P.M.							
8–12 P.M.							

Part Two

The Holistic Medical
Treatment for the Most Common
Chronic Diseases Afflicting Men

Chapter 8

How You Can Practice Holistic Medicine

Holistic medicine is a new medical specialty that addresses the whole person—body, mind, and spirit. Holistic physicians combine conventional and alternative therapies to effectively prevent and treat disease and to create optimal health.

American Holistic Medical Association definition of holistic medicine

The doctor of the future will give no medicines, but will interest his patients in the care of the human frame, in diet, and in the causes of disease.

Thomas Edison

Medicine for the Twenty-First Century

In the latter half of the twentieth century, in the age of modern medicine, physicians have attempted to treat disease through technological and scientific manipulation of the human body. They have operated on the premise that "if it hurts, then eliminate the pain with anal-gesics (pain relievers). If it's infected, inflamed, or allergic, then blast it with powerful antibiotics, corticosteroids, or antihistamines. If it's constricted or obstructed, then open it up with an extensive arsenal of drugs and/or surgical procedures." This approach has been extremely successful at saving lives and in effectively treating acute illness. *But for the most part, modern or conventional medicine as practiced by most M.D.'s* (practitioners of allopathic medicine) *and D.O.'s* (practitioners of osteopathic medicine) *has failed miserably at either healing, curing, or preventing chronic disease.*

Despite the many millions of dollars spent on research, the incidence of cancer continues to increase. In 1996, the World Health Organization predicted that by the year 2020, heart disease and depression would be the world's leading causes of disability, and that tobacco-related disease will become the world's greatest killer. In America today, there are over 100 million people suffering with a chronic illness. In recent years we have developed a number of disorders related to impairment of the immune system. These diseases, which were far less common as recently as twenty years ago, are now turning into epidemics. The Epstein-Barr virus, the cause of mononucleosis, is now in part responsible for chronic fatigue syndrome. The respiratory diseases—sinusitis, allergies, chronic bronchitis, emphysema, and lung cancer—herpes viral infections, prostate cancer, candidiasis, "ecologic illness," multiple sclerosis, lupus, and AIDS are all far more prevalent than just a decade ago. The combination of environmental toxins and emotional stress appears to be most responsible for weakening the human immune system.

According to the 1992 National Health Survey administered by the National Center for Health Statistics, the most common chronic conditions afflicting men are the following (listed in order of frequency):

UNDER 45 YEARS

1. chronic sinusitis
2. allergic rhinitis
3. back pain
4. lower extremity dysfunction (leg, ankle, knee)
5. hearing impairment
6. high blood pressure
7. dermatitis (skin problems)
8. visual impairment
9. arthritis
10. heart disease
11. frequent indigestion
12. hemorrhoids

45–64 YEARS

1. high blood pressure
2. hearing impairment
3. arthritis

4. chronic sinusitis
5. heart disease
6. back pain
7. allergic rhinitis
8. lower extremity dysfunction
9. hemorrhoids
10. tinnitus (ringing in the ear)
11. visual impairment
12. diabetes

65 AND OVER

1. arthritis
2. hearing impairment
3. heart disease
4. high blood pressure
5. chronic sinusitis
6. diabetes
7. visual impairment
8. tinnitus
9. prostate diseases
10. back pain
11. lower extremity dysfunction
12. chronic bronchitis

As effective as medical science is at treating bacterial infections, allergy and asthma attacks, accidents, and life-threatening medical and surgical emergencies, many of these problems represent the *acute* flare-ups of *chronic* conditions. The word *chronic* has become a medical euphemism for *incurable*, while patients suffering with these conditions fill physicians' offices for *symptom* treatment. Americans with a chronic illness spend an estimated $425 billion for treatment and medication. As a result of the prohibitive cost and ineffectiveness of treating these chronic diseases, there is now an unprecedented need for holistic medicine to change our current medical model.

The practice of holistic medicine is primarily focused on the creation of optimal health—the healing of oneself in body, mind, and spirit. Disease is seen as a dis-ease—an imbalance in the whole person that is reflected in the body as physical symptoms. Rather than merely fixing those broken parts, the holistic physician leads patients to the possible causes of their diseases. In this way, he or she facilitates the restoration of balance and harmony to the whole person.

Holistic medicine is predicated on encouraging the miraculous self-healing capacity of the human body. By addressing physical, mental, and spiritual sources of imbalance, it diminishes pain and releases obstructions, allowing the free flow and healing power of life-force energy. Holistic physicians empower their patients to heal themselves. This holistic medical assistance may come in the form of health education, counseling, pharmaceutical drugs, a variety of alternative therapies, surgery, chemotherapy, or a combination of all of these modalities. Sometimes this healing results in a cure of the chronic disease while preventing any further recurrence. At other times it may result in healing the patient's life and enable him to experience peace of mind in spite of still having the physical ailment.

Bernie Siegel, M.D., a clinical professor of surgery at Yale University School of Med-

icine, past president of the American Holistic Medical Association (AHMA), and author of *Love, Medicine, and Miracles,* makes an important distinction between *healing* and *curing.* He says that healing represents "a condition of one's life," and that curing relates to "a physical condition." According to Siegel, "there are *healed* quadriplegics and AIDS patients who, though they may never recover, feel a sense of wholeness in their lives. There are also *cured* cancer patients who are leading fragmented *sick* lives. A healed life may include a physical cure as a by-product." President of the AHMA when I joined the organization in 1988, Siegel first inspired me with the message *"Love heals."* It remains the foundation of the practice of holistic medicine as well as this book.

By reading *Thriving* and following its recommendations, you and I are in a sense practicing holistic medicine together. Think of this book as (1) *a program for self-healing* and (2) *a comprehensive guide to therapeutic options for the treatment of specific chronic diseases.* If you are suffering from a chronic disease or would just like to improve your quality of life, you may want the support of a holistic physician. You can find one in your area by writing to the AHMA, 4101 Lake Boone Trail, Suite 201, Raleigh, NC 27607, or by calling (919) 787-5181 and requesting the *Physician Referral Directory* (the cost is $5). This list includes both active and associate members of the AHMA. To find out more about this new specialty, see the appendix, "The Specialty of Holistic Medicine."

How to Use Part II

Part I of *Thriving* lays the foundation for an effective preventive-medicine program for any of the most common chronic diseases afflicting men. To treat your specific ailment, whether you have been given a diagnosis and are under the care of a physician or not, use Part I as the basis of your holistic medical treatment. With its focus on optimal health, you will be treating and caring for your body, mind, and spirit with an emphasis on your particular disease and its related physical dysfunction. The specific recommendations in Part II will supplement the Part I treatment of your chronic disease. Each disease listed in Part II includes a discussion of the following elements:

- prevalence
- anatomy
- symptoms and diagnosis
- conventional medical treatment
- risk factors and causes
- holistic medical treatment with specific recommendations for body, mind, and spirit:
  - diet
  - vitamin and nutritional supplements
  - herbs
  - specific alternative physical, psychological, and bioenergetic therapies and specific chakra work

Unless you have found a holistic physician, it is advisable to remain under the care of your present doctor and to use Parts I and II as a *complement* to the conventional medical treatment you're already receiving.

For example, if you have a prostate problem, practice the thriving program described in chapters 2 through 7, along with the specific therapies mentioned in chapter 9. A cancerous or chronically inflamed prostate, like any other dis-eased organ, reflects an imbalance in the whole person. To heal it and prevent recurrence, your Part I regimen will teach you to build an awareness of physical, environmental, mental, emotional, spiritual, and social health factors that may have contributed to the cause of the disease. In addition to the recommendations in Part II, building positive attitudes and belief systems in body, mind, and spirit can help reverse the symptoms of disease and create optimal health. *Treatment of all the chronic diseases should include the thriving diet, regular exercise, affirmations, visualization, emotional work, intimate relationships, and prayer.* In the case of prostate cancer, this might also include surgical removal of the prostate and possibly radiation therapy. Conventional treatment should be viewed as part of a larger comprehensive holistic treatment plan.

The best way to cure any disease is to heal your life as well as the physical dysfunction. That's why I strongly suggest you combine Parts I and II with your conventional medical treatment. However, if after careful consideration and consultation with your physician, you believe the liabilities of the conventional treatment (such as toxic side effects) outweigh their potential benefits, commit solely to the holistic approach in Parts I and II. At the very least you will experience significant healing and probably considerable improvement in your physical condition as well. At best, you'll be free of disease and healthier than you've ever been.

One way to monitor the progress of your holistic treatment program is to evaluate your physical symptoms on a weekly basis. You can use a chart similar to the "Symptom Chart" which follows on page 200. This is an example of a "Respiratory Disease" Symptom Chart. It lists the most common symptoms you might experience if you suffered with chronic sinusitis, allergies, or chronic bronchitis. Whatever your particular ailment, list its most frequent symptoms in the left-hand column and rank them from 1 (worst) to 10 (best or no symptom) on a weekly basis. You can also uncover possible emotional factors that contribute to your condition by similarly ranking your emotional stress level as well. You should be able to graphically see a correlation between higher stress and worsening physical symptoms. Also keep track of the medications, herbs, nutritional supplements, etc., that you're taking at the bottom of the chart. The vitamins, herbs, and supplements recommended in Part II are available in most health food stores. The suggested dosages are based upon those I have used extensively in my own practice and upon recommendations from my colleagues contributing to these chapters. These dosages may vary from the "prescriptions" of your own personal holistic physician.

By using the Symptom Chart you can more easily evaluate your progress, what's working and what isn't. As you practice using this chart you'll become quite adept at the early recognition of emotional factors that aggravate your

physical condition, and be able to respond quickly with an effective therapy. This is the basis for the practice of preventive medicine, and as you continue your training you'll develop into a highly skilled self-healer.

Genetic factors play significant roles in the predisposition for almost every chronic disease. For instance, if both your father and grandfather died of heart attacks in their fifties, then your risk of heart disease is significantly higher than that of a man without such a family history. But the hereditary cause is just *one* factor, and it doesn't have to mean that if you've just turned fifty, you need to quit your job, buy a sailboat, and plan to spend your last few years sailing around the world. You can do a great deal to minimize the risk of developing any chronic ailment to which you are genetically predisposed by *training to thrive*. In fact, *I believe strongly that although genetic preconditions are important factors in the formation of disease, the trigger that precipitates every chronic ailment is the repression or denial of painful emotions.*

There are numerous examples of holistic medical treatment used to cure chronic disease, through emphasizing vital emotional-health components. Dean Ornish, M.D., has developed a successful holistic approach for reversing coronary artery (heart) disease. His results are well documented in his book, *Dr. Dean Ornish's Program for Reversing Heart Disease.* Herbert Benson, M.D., has shown how relaxation techniques and prayer can treat high blood pressure, migraine headaches, and many other common and chronic ailments. Bernie Siegel, M.D., has had extra-

Symptom Chart

Began Thriving Program on _____   Rate Symptoms from 1 (worst) to 10 (best = normal)

SYMPTOM	Begin	End week 1	End week 2	End week 3	End week 4	End week 5	End week 6	End week 7	End week 8	End week 9	End week 10	End week 11	End week 12
Head Congestion (fullness)													
Nasal Congestion (stuffy nose)													
Postnasal Drip													
Headache													
Yellow/Green Mucus (from nose)													
Yellow/Green Mucus (back of throat)													
Sneezing													
Itching: Nose, Throat													
Ear Congestion (ears plugged up)													
Sore Throat													
Swollen Glands (in neck)													
Cough—dry													
Cough—wet/mucusy													
Shortness of Breath													
Wheezing													
Fatigue (rate energy level)													
Average # of hours sleep													

EMOTIONAL STRESS

	Begin	End week 1	End week 2	End week 3	End week 4	End week 5	End week 6	End week 7	End week 8	End week 9	End week 10	End week 11	End week 12
Work													
Family													
Other													

MEDICATIONS

	Begin	End week 1	End week 2	End week 3	End week 4	End week 5	End week 6	End week 7	End week 8	End week 9	End week 10	End week 11	End week 12

VITAMINS, HERBS, SUPPLEMENTS

	Begin	End week 1	End week 2	End week 3	End week 4	End week 5	End week 6	End week 7	End week 8	End week 9	End week 10	End week 11	End week 12

ordinary results in treating his cancer patients with holistic medicine. C. Norman Shealy, M.D., a neurosurgeon, founder and first president of the AHMA, and coauthor of *The Creation of Health* with Carolyn Myss, Ph.D. has seen remarkable results for almost twenty years with the holistic treatment of chronic pain. His approach to treating back pain, depression, migraine, and rheumatoid arthritis has also proven highly effective. Longtime AHMA member, and author of the best-seller *Spontaneous Healing*, Andrew Weil, M.D., has effectively treated a variety of chronic diseases holistically. Christiane Northrup, M.D, a gynecologist, past president of the AHMA, and also a best-selling author, documents her holistic approach to treating a number of common chronic women's diseases in *Women's Bodies, Women's Wisdom*. Author of *Conscious Eating* and current member of the board of trustees of the AHMA, Gabriel Cousens, M.D., has been consistently successful in holistically treating arthritis, alcohol and drug addiction, diabetes, and a number of other chronic diseases at his Tree of Life Rejuvenation Center in Patagonia, Arizona. In the ten years that I have been treating chronic sinusitis, allergies, and asthma using the Sinus Survival Program, my patients have experienced consistently good results. Ninety-two percent of those people with chronic sinusitis who have made at least a two-month commitment to this treatment have cured their ailment.

Although they are not physicians, Carolyn Myss, Ph.D., and Louise Hay have contributed a great deal to the holistic treatment of chronic disease. Louise Hay's insight into

the probable emotional causes of disease and her corresponding affirmations have not only helped her to heal her own cancer, but have been an integral part of the treatment program for many of my patients. Her book, *You Can Heal Your Life*, is referenced in many of the following chapters in the "Mental and Emotional Health Recommendations" section.

Carolyn Myss, a gifted medical intuitive, has worked for many years with Drs. Shealy and Northrup, providing diagnostic insight and therapeutic direction. The mental and emotional issues that she believes are associated with each of the seven chakras are discussed thoroughly in her book, *Anatomy of the Spirit*. I've made extensive use of her work with the chakras in treating my patients. She too is frequently referenced in Part II.

The material in Part II was prepared in collaboration with several of my holistic medical colleagues. Each of these healers has contributed significantly to the chapters on the conditions with which they have had consistent success. To my knowledge, most of the information in Part II has never before been synthesized. The contributors, their medical specialty, and their chapters are

- Robert A. Anderson, M.D., family practice, primarily chapters 11, 13, and 14, and secondarily the remaining chapters
- Gabriel Cousens, M.D., psychiatry—chapters 11 and 12
- Mark Hoch, M.D., family practice—chapter 11
- Harriet Ivker, L.C.S.W., psychotherapy—chapter 12

- Edward J. Linkner, M.D., family practice—primarily chapters 9 and 14 and secondarily the remaining chapters
- Joel Miller, M.D., psychiatry—chapter 12
- John Mizenko, D.O., gastroenterology—chapter 15
- Steve Morris, N.D., naturopathic medicine—chapter 9
- Todd Nelson, N.D., naturopathic medicine—chapter 15
- Scott Shannon, M.D., psychiatry—chapter 12

Far more than a collaborator on the chapters that I've just listed for him, Bob Anderson is a coauthor of Part II. He has been practicing holistic family medicine for most of his thirty-five years as a physician and has had many years of experience using holistic treatments for nearly every one of the common chronic diseases in Part II. Much of the information that he's learned is contained in his books, *Wellness Medicine* and *Stress Power!* Bob has been a clinical assistant professor in the Department of Family Medicine at the University of Washington School of Medicine. He is also a cofounder and past president of the AHMA. In my practice and pursuit of holistic medicine, he has been a mentor as well as an inspiration. We hope you find Part II of *Thriving* not only therapeutic, but enlightening and enlivening as well.

G e n i t o u r i n a r y   D i s e a s e

Prostate Cancer
Benign Prostatic Hypertrophy (BPH)
Prostatitis
Impotence
Premature Ejaculation

Prevalence

The most common diseases of the prostate are prostate cancer, benign prostatic hypertrophy (BPH), and prostatitis. The prostate and sexual disorders are probably the greatest health concerns to the majority of men. In 1996, prostate cancer will cause over 40,000 deaths, with about 317,000 newly diagnosed cases. That compares to 244,000 new cases in 1995 and less than 85,000 in 1985. Nearly one of every five American men will develop prostate cancer. After lung cancer, it has become the second most lethal cancer for men. BPH is an enlarged prostate that affects nearly 30 percent of fifty-year-old men, 50 percent of sixty-year-olds, and almost 80 percent of men over seventy. Prostatitis is an inflammation or infection of the prostate usually seen in men between the ages of thirty and seventy.

Impotence and premature ejaculation might well be the most common chronic conditions afflicting men, but we'll probably never know exactly how prevalent they are because most of us aren't discussing these problems—with our physician or, in many cases, with our partner. Of the 20 million American men estimated to be experiencing some form of impotence, only about two hundred thousand per year seek medical attention. It was recently reported in the *Journal of Clinical Practice* that "52 percent of men forty to seventy years old have some degree of erectile inadequacy"; and it is also estimated that 85 percent of men over seventy can't get a firm erection. Impotence is defined as the inability to sustain a satisfactory erection to perform intercourse and ejaculation.

I doubt that many men have never experienced premature ejaculation, which is defined as the inability to exercise voluntary control over one's ejaculation.

Anatomy of the Genitourinary Tract

The male genitourinary tract consists of the penis, testicles, epididymis (a tube along the back side of the testicles where sperm are stored), vas deferens (tube connecting testicle to urethra), prostate, bladder, and urethra.

The prostate gland, about the size and shape of a walnut, lies below the bladder and surrounds the urethra. Its primary function is the secretion of a thin, milky white alkaline fluid during ejaculation that accounts for about 30 percent of the volume of semen. In lubricating the urethra and increasing sperm motility, this fluid enhances delivery and fertility of the sperm, which originate in the testicles. In addition, the prostate also acts as the genitourinary tract's first line of defense against infection and disease.

Prostate Cancer

Symptoms and Diagnosis

The most common cancer in men over fifty is prostate cancer, and, after lung cancer, is the most common malignancy afflicting men. The highest incidence is found in black males, who are 40 percent more likely to be stricken with the disease.

About 20 percent of enlarged prostates are the result of cancer. As long as it's confined to the prostate gland, the cancer is largely curable. About 80 percent of these cancers either do not metastasize (spread beyond the gland to other parts of the body) or are of the slow-growing variety, often causing little or no problem. By one estimate, men with cancers that are in the earliest stages have a 12 percent chance of dying from the malignancy if they leave it untreated for ten years. The highest

estimate of mortality in the medical literature is that about one-fourth of all men who develop prostate cancer will die from it. The lowest estimate is 3 percent (see page 206).

Early detection of cancer of the prostate is difficult, since it is often present without any detectable symptoms. **A rectal exam,** preferably performed by the same physician on an annual basis, is a diagnostic method recommended by urologists (genitourinary-tract physicians). The doctor inserts a gloved finger into the rectum to touch the prostate gland, on which he or she can literally feel cancerous growths, such as bumps or nodules, or an asymmetry from one side of the gland to the other. However, one limitation of the rectal exam is that it's not possible for doctors to feel the tiniest, earliest-stage, most curable tumors. Recent research out of Washington University in St. Louis finds that 60 to 70 percent of cancers detected by rectal exam alone have already spread beyond the prostate.

The Genitourinary Tract

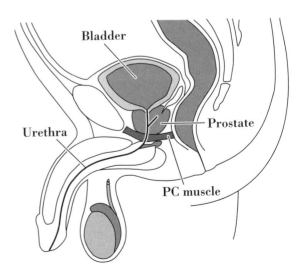

That's the primary reason for the popularity of the prostate specific antigen or **PSA test,** which has been widely used during the past decade and is the biggest factor in the dramatic rise of prostate cancer diagnoses. A PSA test detects cancer much earlier than a rectal exam by measuring the blood level of a protein produced by all prostate cells. In general, PSA readings under 4 indicate that cancer is highly unlikely, while over 22 means highly likely. About 70 percent of cancers detected with the PSA test are still curable—twice as many as those diagnosed with just the rectal exam.

Conventional Medical Treatment

If the PSA is elevated, the next steps may be to take a closer look at the prostate with a transrectal ultrasound probe and then to take needle biopsies from several regions of the gland. If the prostate cancer is diagnosed early and it has not metastasized, men are usually offered two options by conventional medicine—to treat the cancer or pursue a course of "watchful waiting." Treatment usually consists of surgical removal of the entire prostate gland, a procedure called a radical **prostatectomy.** Although this option offers a cure if the cancer has not spread beyond the prostate, it also presents some significant risks. About 1 to 2 percent of prostatectomy patients will have complete lack of urinary control; about 20 to 50 percent will have partial control and stress incontinence—leakage caused by any kind of physical pressure—and more than half will have minimum leakage, only a few occasional

drops. An even greater risk is that of impotence. Until Dr. Patrick Walsh of the Johns Hopkins Hospital in Baltimore developed a new surgical technique, impotence was an inevitable consequence of a radical prostatectomy. Dr. Walsh claims that 90 percent of men under age fifty will regain potency following the surgery. In addition to the huge risk of impotence—estimates still range close to 90 percent in men over fifty—this surgical procedure often requires a weeklong hospital stay, several weeks of depending on an in-dwelling catheter to urinate, and an extended recovery time. A 1994 survey performed by the American Foundation of Urologic Disease found that 16 percent of prostatectomy patients would not choose the treatment again. One distraught patient in San Diego shot his surgeon in the groin after prostate surgery left him impotent.

Another treatment option for prostate cancer is external beam **radiation** (from X rays), requiring a series of exposures over several weeks. But radiation often fails to kill all the cancer cells, and in 75 to 80 percent of these patients, the cancer returns within ten years. That still leaves 20 to 25 percent with a cure.

Cryotherapy (freezing the prostate cells with liquid nitrogen) and hormone therapy are other treatment options with apparent short-term benefits, but with unknown long-range effectiveness. Cryotherapy also leaves 60 percent of patients impotent.

In light of the potential for devastating side effects and the limited evidence that treating prostate cancer actually saves lives, watchful waiting is becoming an increasingly popular option for men diagnosed with this cancer. This option entails frequent blood tests, rectal exams, and an occasional biopsy, but no intervention unless the cancer becomes more aggressive. The answer to the question "Who should be treated for prostate cancer?" is not simple. Experts at the National Cancer Institute in Maryland point out that PSA readings sometimes raise alarms that are misleading, fail to differentiate between fast-growing and less threatening prostate cancer, and can lead to debilitating treatment that may not be necessary. The presence of a few cancer cells may not be a serious problem. Oncologists estimate that by age fifty, as many as four out of ten men have at least some cancerous cells in their prostate, which will cause an elevated PSA reading. But according to Dr. Thomas Stamey of Stanford University, only 8 percent of these men will eventually develop symptoms that affect their quality of life, and only 3 percent will die of the cancer. Most men die *with* prostate cancer, not *of it*.

Some physicians believe that since it usually takes about a decade for prostate cancer to cause symptoms that significantly affect quality of life, any man whose life expectancy is less than ten years (those sixty-five or older) should not be treated.

This controversy about who should be treated will eventually be settled when scientists are able to develop a means of distinguishing (when the cancer is small) between a lethally aggressive and a relatively benign type of prostate cancer. This research is cur-

rently under way, much of it funded by the $25 million pledged by Michael Milken, the infamous junk-bond dealer of the 1980s, who is currently undergoing treatment for prostate cancer.

The American Cancer Society and the American Urological Association both recommend an annual rectal exam and PSA test after age fifty. These should be started at age forty if you are a higher-risk man, such as an African-American or one with a family history of the disease.

Risk Factors and Causes

As with other cancers, the precise cause of prostate cancer is unknown. Genetics and race play a role, as do hormonal factors. Men who enter puberty later than the average male seem to have a higher incidence of prostate cancer. Several studies indicate that men who undergo vasectomies have an increased risk of developing prostate as well as testicular cancer. Environmental toxins from air pollution, chemicals, and especially cadmium (a metallic element used in batteries) have all been implicated as causes of prostate and other cancers as well. One study showed that men with low levels of vitamin A were three times more likely to have prostate cancer than men with the highest levels.

On a *bioenergetic* level, all of the genitourinary conditions are related to the root and lower belly chakras, or first and second chakras. These energy centers are closely connected and I described them briefly in chapter 4. The root chakra is located between the anus and scrotum. It is associated with feelings of security, survival, and vitality. Root chakra energy connects us to the earth and to our "tribe," which might consist of our family, other men, our country of origin, ethnic background, and/or religion. Most American men have become so urbanized and competitive that to a great extent we've lost our close connection to the earth and to our fellow male tribesmen.

Sexual energy is also a component of the root chakra and can overlap with the lower belly chakra. The second, lower belly or sex, chakra is located four finger widths below the navel. As the body's natural center of balance and movement, the second chakra provides a focus of concentration and energy for martial artists, dancers, and athletes. It is the center of creative energy and of feelings of pleasure. According to Carolyn Myss, in her book *Anatomy of the Spirit*, the mental/emotional issues related to these chakras include family and group physical safety and security, ability to provide for life's necessities, ability to stand up for oneself, feeling at home, and social and familial law and order.

Holistic Medical Treatment and Prevention

Physical Health Recommendations

The holistic treatment and prevention program for genitourinary disease is directed at loving, nurturing, and restoring balance to the prostate gland and the entire pelvic area. This program is composed primarily of the comprehensive approach for optimal physical fitness described in chapter 3. Those recommendations such as diet, water, vitamins, minerals, and exercise can be applied to all of the conditions of prostatic dysfunction, impotence, and premature ejaculation. In addition, I would include some of the following therapeutic measures:

Diet. Several studies have found that decreasing the consumption of sugar leads to lower levels of prostate cancer. It has also been shown that cultures that consume higher amounts of red meat have a higher incidence of cancer of the prostate. In China and Japan, where low-fat diets of vegetables and fish are the norm, the incidence of prostate cancer is extremely low. However, prostate cancer rates for first- and second-generation Japanese-Americans are considerably higher than in Japan.

Vitamins, minerals, and nutritional supplements. The following regimen, although designed primarily for BPH and prostatitis, can only improve the health of the prostate and is therefore beneficial for prostate cancer as well.

In addition to the daily regimen of antioxidant vitamins and minerals in the dosages listed in chapter 3, **essential fatty acids (EFAs)** and **zinc** are particularly helpful in reducing the size of an enlarged prostate. EFAs are found in large amounts in sunflower oil, safflower oil, flaxseed oil, and in lesser quantities in soybean and other oils. Either take one to two tablespoons per day of any of these oils, or the equivalent amount in capsules (six 1000-mg capsules of flax oil is equal to one tablespoon). I take one tablespoon per day of flaxseed oil preventively. Zinc should be taken in the form of zinc picolinate, 15 to 30 mg three times a day. If you take this high an amount (90 mg) of zinc, then blood electrolyte levels should be checked every three to six months. I take 30 mg daily as preventive medicine. If you are taking these increased amounts of EFAs and zinc, it will also increase the body's need for vitamin E and copper. Therefore in addition to the daily regimen of vitamins and minerals in the dosages listed in chapter 3, take at least

- Vitamin C, 2,000 mg 3x/day
- Vitamin E, 400 IU 2x/day
- Vitamin B_6, 100 mg 2x/day (both B_6 and vitamin E can reduce prolactin levels; prolactin increases testosterone uptake by the prostate); B_6 should be taken in the form of pyridoxine hydrochloride (100 mg 2x/day) or pyridoxine 5-phosphate (15 mg 2x/day)
- A daily multivitamin high in B vitamins and magnesium
- Copper sebacate, 4 mg 2x/day for both BPH and prostatitis

High doses of intravenous vitamin C, B complex, and zinc have been used with some success in the treatment of prostate cancer.

Herbs. **Saw palmetto, *Pygeum africanus***
(see BPH herbs for a detailed description of these two herbs), *Conium maculatum, Berberis aquifoliam, Echinacea angustifolia, Arctium lappa, Hydrastis canadensis* (goldenseal), and *Arctostaphylos uvaursi,* can all be used as part of a complementary program to help treat cancer of the prostate. The first two can decrease swelling and increase blood flow to the prostate, while the rest of the herbs stimulate the immune system in a variety of ways.

Homeopathy, Chinese medicine, and Ayurvedic medicines.
Homeopathic remedies, Chinese herbs and acupuncture, and Ayurvedic herbs have been used successfully in treating each of the prostatic disorders and impotence. But they should be administered by a trained practitioner of these healing arts.

Empty the prostate.
Every organ in the body works more efficiently and is healthier when it is being used regularly and when fluids are able to flow through it without obstruction. From this physiologic common-sense perspective comes the recommendation of ejaculation about three times per week for both prevention and treatment of BPH. A recent study in England reported that men who ejaculated five times a week had a significantly lower incidence of prostate cancer. Even with prostatitis, once the painful symptoms have decreased, ejaculation or sex using a condom may help the infection leave the body more efficiently.

Mental and Emotional Health Recommendations

Together with the medical (urologic) community, most men share the beliefs that

- An enlarged prostate with its concomitant symptoms is an inevitable consequence of aging.
- Our ability to maintain strong erections and engage in enjoyable sexual intercourse diminishes greatly as we get older, until eventually we are unable to function sexually at all.
- There is a growing threat of prostate cancer and that if we live long enough, we will get it.

Statistically, it is true that 80 percent of men over the age of seventy will develop BPH, that one out of five men will contract prostate cancer, and that most of us will eventually experience some degree of impotence. To thrive, however, it is essential that we change our limiting beliefs and attitudes. To be holistically healthy and prevent these conditions that most men will develop, or to treat them if you are already afflicted, it is essential that you believe it's possible to be free of these disorders. After all, 20 percent of us will not develop enlarged prostates; four out of five will never have cancer of the prostate; and millions of us are not and will not ever be impotent. To me, these are comforting thoughts, and I fully expect to be among the fortunate "few." Do you? That doesn't mean that merely having this expectation is sufficient to make it a done deal. Optimism is a key ingredient of holistic health, but I plan to continue practicing the preventive medicine that I describe in this chapter and in the remainder of Part II.

If you already suffer from prostate cancer or from one of the other common male conditions, then I would first determine what your goals are for treatment. Do you want to cure it, learn to live with it, or prevent it from getting any worse? When your goals have been established, write them down, then reword them into the form of **affirmations.** (Refer to chapter 2 for a "refresher course" on the use of affirmations.) "My prostate is strong and healthy" is a good basic affirmation. You can be creative with these and think about them in visual terms.

Bioenergy. Parts of the body or organs that are malfunctioning are related to a weakness in the chakra closest to that damaged organ. The male genitourinary tract corresponds to the first two chakras—**the root and sex chakras.** Any therapeutic measure that helps to strengthen the energy of these chakras will benefit any of the five conditions discussed in this chapter. These energy centers have to do with sexuality, our connection to the Earth, and our tribal connections. Some methods of strengthening these chakras might include

- visualizations that send light and energy into these chakras (you might see it originating deep in the earth, coming up through your legs, and filling your pelvis)
- spending more time in nature or in contact with the earth
- feeling more connected to other men

- counseling to emotionally heal family wounds

Working at this root level of dis-ease can empower men and ultimately create a sense of security, pleasure, and potency far greater than any other therapeutic measure.

In treating prostate cancer, I recommend that the holistic approach be used as a complement to the conventional treatment. Over the age of fifty, periodic PSA tests and rectal exams by a family physician or urologist are still considered good preventive medicine for cancer of the prostate.

Benign Prostatic Hypertrophy (BPH)

Symptoms and Diagnosis

By the age of fifty, about 30 percent of all men will experience some difficulty with urination related to enlargement of the prostate—BPH. The most common *symptoms* of prostatic hypertrophy are

- increased frequency (especially at night), urgency, and hesitancy with urination
- a reduction in the force and caliber of the urine stream.

This enlargement, caused by an abnormal overgrowth and/or swelling of the tissue of the prostate, creates a blockage of the bladder outlet (urethra). If left untreated, this could cause complete obstruction of urine. The following Prostate Enlargement Test was developed by the American Urological Association to help men determine if they are candidates for treatment of prostate enlargement. A **digital rectal**

exam performed by a physician, along with suggestive symptoms, is still considered a reliable method for *diagnosing* BPH.

Conventional Medical Treatment

Depending upon how much trouble the symptoms are causing, urologists are *treating* men with BPH with pharmaceutical drugs, surgery, or just **watchful waiting.** In one recent study of six hundred men with BPH who were treated with the latter approach, only 10 percent requested medical treatment at study's end. It was learned that men could control many of their symptoms simply by limiting fluids before bedtime, especially anything that irritates the prostate, such as caffeine and alcohol. **Regular ejaculations** (three times a week) also helped some men find symptom relief. Currently the most popular drug being used to treat BPH is **Proscar.** It works by preventing the buildup of dihydrotestosterone, a testosterone-like compound that appears to promote the development of BPH. However, recent clinical studies have shown it to be only marginally effective. Proscar also causes impotence in about 4 percent of men who take it and decreases libido in 7 percent. Other commonly used drugs are Hytrin, Minipress, and Cardura. They work by relaxing small muscles in the prostate and are also used to treat high blood pressure. They only relieve symptoms, but do not slow the progress of the condition. They may also produce side effects such as dizziness and fatigue, and in unusual cases, impotence. If a man's symptoms don't respond

Prostate Enlargement Test

If you think you might have an enlarged prostate, then take the following test developed by the American Urological Association. It will give you and your doctor an approximate idea of how troublesome the symptoms of prostate enlargement have become.

With a score of 0 to 7, symptoms are considered **mild** and usually no conventional treatment is indicated, just watchful waiting. However, this would be a good time to begin the holistic treatment plan (see page 212) preventively. A score of 8 to 35 would reflect **moderate** to **severe** symptoms which might indicate a need for medication, or surgery, in addition to the holistic regimen. This test is just one element of the diagnostic evaluation of the prostate.

Circle one number for each of the following questions. Add up the seven numbers to get your AUA symptom score _____ 0–7 = mild 8–19 = moderate 20–35 = severe	Not at all	Less than 1 time in 5	Less than half the time	About half the time	More than half the time	Almost always
1. Over the past month, how often have you had a senstation of not emptying your bladder completely after you finished urinating?	0	1	2	3	4	5
2. Over the past month, how often have you had to urinate again less than 2 hours after you finished urinating?	0	1	2	3	4	5
3. Over the past month, how often have you found you stopped and started again several times when you urinated?	0	1	2	3	4	5
4. Over the past month, how often have you found it difficult to postpone urination?	0	1	2	3	4	5
5. Over the past month, how often have you had a weak urinary stream?	0	1	2	3	4	5
6. Over the past month, how often have you had to push or strain to begin urination?	0	1	2	3	4	5
7. Over the past month, how many times did you most typically get up to urinate from the time you went to bed at night until the time you got up in the morning?	0 (none)	1 (1 time)	2 (2 times)	3 (3 times)	4 (4 times)	5 (5 + times)

to drug treatment, transurethral resection (TUR) of the prostate—removal of a portion of the prostate gland—is the option offered by most urologists. Although the risk of incontinence (loss of urinary control) is greater than with drugs, the relief from symptoms is also more significant. Unfortunately this surgical procedure is the choice most readily offered by urologists, who, as surgeons, clearly have a bias. Of the 350,000 prostate operations performed each year, many could be avoided if physicians offered the simple and safe natural remedies described in the "Holistic Medical Treatment and Prevention" section.

Risk Factors and Causes

As men age, their hormone levels change. After the age of fifty, free testosterone levels in the blood begin to decrease, while at the same time testosterone levels are increasing in the prostate gland. Within the prostate, testosterone is converted to an even more potent compound called **dihydrotestosterone.** This hormone causes cells to multiply excessively, eventually leading to prostate enlargement.

The increased uptake of testosterone by the prostate appears to be the result of another hormone, prolactin, secreted by the pituitary gland in the brain. Prolactin also increases the activity of the enzyme that converts testosterone to dihydrotestosterone. Since alcohol in excess and emotional stress increase prolactin levels, both may be significant contributors to causing BPH.

Holistic Medical Treatment and Prevention

Diet. For treating BPH, prostatitis, and impotence, and preventing prostate cancer, especially avoid foods that are high in fat and refined carbohydrates, as well as caffeine, alcohol, and tobacco. Each of them can negate the beneficial effects of vitamins C and E, and zinc, which are all essential components of prostatic tissues and are necessary for the formation of seminal fluid. One handful per day of nonrancid raw pumpkin seeds is also helpful in treating BPH.

Vitamins, minerals, and nutritional supplements. See recommendations for prostate cancer.

Herbs. Perhaps the most exciting addition to the treatment of BPH has been the extract of **saw palmetto berries** (*Serenoa repens*). Multiple studies have shown that the fat-soluble (liposterolic) extract of these berries prevents the conversion of testosterone to dihydrotestosterone, thus preventing prostate enlargement. This mechanism is similar to the way in which Proscar works, but clinical studies suggest that saw palmetto berries are more effective. In one controlled study, as many as 89 percent of men taking saw palmetto berries improved after one month of treatment. Unlike Proscar, saw palmetto berries do not cause impotence. In fact, it has a reputation for being an aphrodisiac (although I have to admit, I haven't noticed that effect). It is much less expensive than

Proscar and has been used safely for many decades with no significant side effects reported. The clinical results have been impressive in improving the symptoms of frequency of nighttime urination and urine flow rates for hundreds of men with BPH. These results were obtained after usually two to three months. For the treatment of BPH, the recommended dosage for a liposterolic extract of saw palmetto berries containing 85–95 percent fatty acids and sterols is 320 mg per day (either 160 mg 2x/day or 80 mg 4x/day). One-half of that dosage (160 mg/day) can also be effective as a maintenance dose for treating or for preventing BPH.

The powdered bark of the tree **Pygeum africanus** has been shown to promote the regression of symptoms associated with BPH, with no toxic side effects. Many health food stores currently have products that combine saw palmetto and *Pygeum africanus*—a great daily dose of preventive medicine. A saw palmetto berry a day might keep the surgeon away. The herb *Aletrius farinosa* is also beneficial.

Empty the prostate. As in the treatment of prostate cancer, it may be even more important to empty the prostate through frequent ejaculation for both prevention and treatment of BPH. See "Empty the prostate" in prostate cancer.

Prostatic massage and the PC muscle. Regular prostatic massage has been shown to be an effective therapy for relieving pressure and discomfort due to BPH. It is usually ad-

ministered by a physician, who inserts a gloved finger into the rectum to massage the prostate directly. I'd like to suggest a much simpler method for achieving a similar result. In addition to emptying the prostate, which also relieves pressure, you can massage your own prostate by regularly **contracting or tightening your PC muscle,** which I described in chapter 6. When you squeeze this muscle, it pushes against, or "massages," the prostate.

Mental and emotional health recommendations. See the prostate cancer section.

Bioenergy. See the prostate cancer section.

Prostatitis

Symptoms and Diagnosis

Prostatitis is usually seen in younger men than BPH and falls into three categories:

1. bacterial prostatitis—an infection of the gland that causes swelling
2. nonbacterial prostatitis—swelling of the prostate without an infection
3. prostadynia—a general irritation of the prostate without infection or swelling

Symptoms of prostatitis might include
- difficulty, frequency, and urgency of urination
- burning sensation or pain during urination

- a discharge from the penis after bowel movements
- postejaculatory pain

These symptoms can be intermittent and range from mild to severe, with the prostate gland being susceptible to both acute and chronic infection or inflammation. An acute infection is noted by severe pain and tenderness in the area of the prostate, at times extending into the genitals, pelvis, and back. Fever, chills, and extreme fatigue might also be present with acute prostatitis. Chronic prostatitis has similar symptoms, but more mild. If this condition goes untreated, which it often does, there is an increased risk of transmitting the infection to a sexual partner, as well as more severe complications such as kidney infection, epididymitis (inflammation of the epididymis), and orchitis (a painful swelling of the testicles). Other possible consequences of untreated chronic prostatitis are bladder obstruction and prostate stones.

Conventional Medical Treatment

Medical *treatment* for both acute and chronic prostatitis consists almost exclusively of **antibiotics.**

Risk Factors and Causes

Prostatitis may result from
- a weakened immune system
- depletion of prostatic glandular elements such as zinc, ascorbic acid (vitamin C), and proteolytic enzymes

- increased amounts of sexual activity, particularly with multiple partners, which depletes the prostate of zinc and enzymes

Both zinc and proteolytic enzymes sterilize the urethra and protect the gland from infection. Excesses of caffeine and alcohol also contribute to a lack of glandular nutrition, which ultimately adds to depletion of the prostate and lowered immune function.

Bacteria in the urine, as it passes through the urethra, can settle in the prostate. Chlamydia, an intracellular parasite transmitted through sexual contact, is also believed to be a common cause of prostatitis. The noninfective or inflammatory causes of prostatitis may be associated with autoimmune disorders, resulting from a depleted glandular environment.

Holistic Medical Treatment and Prevention

Herbs. The evergreen plant **Chimaphila umbellata,** or **pipsissewa,** is especially effective for chronic prostatitis. It helps provide the prostate and urinary tract with increased blood flow and nutrition. Horsetail is an herbal medicine used to treat acute prostate infection. The herbs, *Delphinium staphysagria, Thuja occidentalis*, and *Anemone pusatilla* are also used for inflammation of the prostate gland. They act to decrease pain, vesicle irritation, swelling of the prostate, and impotence associated with prostatitis. **Echinacea angustifolium,** an effective herb for treating any infection, can be a valuable part of the treatment program for both acute and chronic prostatitis.

Medications. I will usually prescribe an antibiotic as part of the holistic medical treatment of acute and chronic prostatitis.

Exercise. Follow the suggestions for regular aerobic exercise in chapter 3. Avoid long bike rides with a full bladder and jarring exercise such as jogging or rope jumping. Special bicycle seat covers made of sorbathane gel, which diminish prostate impact, are available. Swimming is probably the most gentle and effective means of exercising your entire body.

For the remainder of the holistic medical treatment and prevention, see BPH and prostate cancer sections.

Impotence

Symptoms and Diagnosis

Impotence is defined as the inability to sustain a satisfactory erection to perform intercourse and ejaculation.

Conventional Medical Treatment

Impotence may be the health problem that is most disturbing to men and for this reason might possibly be one of the most well-researched problems in medical science. Conventional medicine, along with its two primary therapeutic weapons of drugs and surgery, has added a third—mechanical devices—for the treatment of impotence. Vacuum erection devices, available from most urologists for about $400, are used to assist a man who's having trouble initiating or sustaining his erections. Vacuum pumps are basically clear cylinders that you put over your penis and pump until a vacuum is created, then you wait three or four minutes until you develop an erection. The vacuum causes the blood that creates an erection to rush into the penis. Once the penis is erect, you fasten an occlusion band around the base of the penis to maintain the erection for as long as half an hour. Penile prosthetic devices, silicone implants, and an inflatable hydraulic model are also being used for impotence.

The most successful drug treatments are papaverine, phentolamine, or prostaglandin E-1 administered through self-injections into the penis. Regular use of injections can improve your capacity for natural erections not only because they can improve the efficiency of penile blood flow, but probably more so because of the mental boost resulting from knowing you are capable of having erections. The most successful oral medication is called Erex and works about 30 percent of the time for psychogenic (emotionally caused) impotence.

The surgical procedure most often performed for treating impotence is penile revascularization. In this procedure, blood from abdominal arteries is directed into the penis, bypassing the damaged or dysfunctional arteries that contribute to impotence. It might be more appropriate to call it "penile bypass" surgery. Unfortunately, it's not nearly as successful as the far more common heart bypass surgery. In one recent study, only 38 percent of those men who had had the surgery were able to have spontaneous erections six months later.

Risk Factors and Causes

Although impotence has long been associated with aging, it is not an inevitable consequence of growing old. The adage "If you don't use it, you lose it" is also applicable to our sexual capability. As I mentioned in chapter 6, Masters and Johnson, authors of *Human Sexual Response,* found couples in their eighties who were still enjoying regular sexual intercourse. However, older men who had not been sexually active for a number of years, often due to the death of a spouse, were frequently impotent if they entered into a new relationship. As men age, the amount and force of ejaculation decreases, and the recovery time between ejaculations becomes longer, but our physiologic ability to have erections is still present. (Thank you, God!) We simply have to continue to exercise that capability while adding some of the holistic recommendations in the following section.

Although the vast majority of physicians believe that impotence is usually **psychologically induced,** a growing number of physical factors have also been identified.

Medications, especially those used to treat high blood pressure and depression, are most commonly associated with impotence. Some endocrine disorders, such as hypothyroidism and hypopituitary function, and vascular disease, including diabetes, may diminish blood flow to the penis. Some neurologic conditions, such as Parkinson's disease and multiple sclerosis, might also affect a man's ability to have an erection.

Other physical causes of impotence or erectile inadequacy include low testosterone levels, high cholesterol (for every ten points above normal cholesterol levels, there is a 32 percent increase in the risk of impotence), low zinc intake (zinc indirectly stimulates testosterone production), and the activation of specific nerves in the brain. When these neuroreceptors in the brain are activated, they can prevent blood from flowing into the penis.

Impotence, however, most often results from a multitude of emotional causes; this is called psychogenic impotence. Depression, performance anxiety, and boredom are probably the feelings most men are aware of, at least to a minimal extent. But shame, guilt, fear of intimacy, and low self-esteem are usually the unconscious emotional factors underlying impotence. Many men with alcohol and drug addictions can be sexually active when they're under the influence of the drug, but when sober they become impotent. For these men, shame is almost always the feeling connected with sexuality. As infants, the majority of us were traumatized through circumcision. The emotional wound inflicted by that routine surgical procedure is often much deeper than most men realize. From the time we were young boys, most of us were aware that our penis was the body part most associated with shame and with the greatest fear of exposure. Yet for men this hidden appendage and its functional status have come to symbolize our masculinity and our power, because without the ability to have an erection, we are "impotent"—without power or strength. The usual reaction to any instance of "erectile dysfunction" is so devastating that it creates intense pressure and worry during subsequent sexual encounters. This can easily lead to mounting performance anxiety and greatly worsen the condition.

In addition to impotence, **shame** can be a frequent but usually unconscious contributor to any of the prostate problems. Of these other conditions, I'm most familiar with shame as an emotional cause of prostatitis. Louise Hay, in *You Can Heal Your Life*, describes the probable emotional causes of impotence as "sexual pressure, tension, guilt; social beliefs; spite against a previous mate; fear of mother." For prostate problems: "mental fears weaken the masculinity; giving up; sexual pressure and guilt; belief in aging." In this age of feminism and male-bashing, the emerging independence and power of women has left millions of men feeling emasculated, guilty, and impotent. In an attempt to behave "appropriately," many of us have learned to keep our sexuality so well hidden that we've lost much of it. We've learned to contain our sexual energy so tightly that we've squeezed the passion and vitality right out of it.

Holistic Medical Treatment and Prevention

Physical Health Recommendations

Vitamins, minerals, and nutritional supplements. For impotence, **zinc** may be the most valuable nutritional supplement. According to clinical studies conducted at the University of Rochester School of Medicine, the testosterone levels of men given zinc supplements rose dramatically. At the University of Virginia Medical School it was discovered that zinc can also diminish the pituitary gland's production of prolactin—a hormone that stops testosterone production. You can also take *beta-carotene*, 25,000 IU twice a day, *magnesium*, 500 mg per day, and *essential fatty acids* (EFAs) for treating impotence.

The hormone DHEA has been successfully used in treating impotence. Although it is available in some health food stores, it is recommended that this treatment be administered by a physician, after obtaining blood levels of DHEA.

Herbs. Perhaps the most powerful sexual stimulant ever discovered comes from a tree in Cameroon, Africa, called ***Pausinstalia yohimbine.*** A study conducted by Dr. Robert Margolis, published in the journal *Current Therapeutic Research*, found that in ten thousand impotent patients taking yohimbine, 80 percent of them reported good to excellent results. Almost 55 percent of the patients were from fifty-five to eighty years of age. A. J. Riley, M.D., a specialist in sexual medicine, has concluded from the extensive testing of yohimbine that "it is now possible to restore usable erections for up to 95 percent of men with erectile inadequacy." Most patients using yohimbine reported that overall sexual pleasure increased with more intensive orgasms. It also decreases the latency period between ejaculations and can stimulate blood flow to the penis, just as **Gingko biloba** is capable of doing. Scientists believe that the most profound therapeutic effects from yohimbine are a result of its blocking the activation of the nerves in the brain (alpha-2-adrenergic receptors) that interfere with erection. *Siberian ginseng* or *Pax ginseng* is believed to be an aphrodisiac and has been effective in treating impotence. *American ginseng, Eleuthrococcus senticosus,* although not quite as beneficial, is safer to use on a long-term basis. *Aletris farinosa,* or true unicorn root, is another effective herbal medicine for impotence, as is *Turnera aphrodisiaca,* or *Damiana.*

Mental and emotional health recommendations. Use **affirmations** for treating impotence. Be creative and use vivid imagery for the greatest effect. For example: "My magic mushroom is full and erect" or "There is an infinite supply of energy filling my wand of light." Mental imagery or **visualization** in conjunction with reciting and/or writing these affirmations is extremely helpful. To shrink an enlarged prostate, you might picture a ball or balloon being slowly deflated. In treating impotence, it helps to imagine some type of

fluid (representing blood) filling an empty space (limp penis). Or you might imagine an attractive woman who happens to be a master in the art of the blow job, gently, slowly, and lovingly stimulating the largest erection you've ever had.

After all of the possible physical causes for impotence have been ruled out, you might consider seeing a psychotherapist, or possibly a sex therapist, as part of the holistic treatment program. You could also begin the regular practice of journaling, which I described in chapter 4. The longer the problem persists, the more difficult it can be to treat on your own.

Social health recommendations. It is particularly helpful to **discuss your feelings** about your impotence with your spouse or sexual partner. If she's agreeable, try being physically intimate while knowing beforehand that you will not attempt to have intercourse. This relieves a lot of psychological pressure to perform and can eventually help to restore normal function. I have already mentioned the value of openly discussing the problem of premature ejaculation with your spouse or partner. Men are usually reluctant to acknowledge either of these sexual problems to their significant other. But their fears are almost always exaggerated, and once you "break the ice," the outcome is usually beneficial.

Bonding with other men in meaningful ways is important for first chakra health. Being able to share feelings and spending enjoyable "play" time with your son, another young boy, your father, a close male friend, or relative, or joining a men's group, might allow you to more closely connect and bond with other men or feel your maleness more deeply.

Bioenergy. See the bioenergy section in prostate cancer.

Premature Ejaculation

Symptoms and Diagnosis

A man with good ejaculatory control can usually decide approximately when he will ejaculate. A lack of this degree of control, premature ejaculation, doesn't necessarily cause a problem. If a man and his partner are content, there is no reason for change. I found it interesting to note that the first major study of human sexuality, called the *Kinsey Report,* performed in the late forties, reported that 75 percent of the men interviewed ejaculated within two minutes of beginning intercourse. According to Barry McCarthy, author of *Male Sexual Awareness,* one out of three men today is an involuntary ejaculator, and the average length of intercourse is two to four minutes.

Conventional Medical Treatment

To my knowledge, conventional medicine has no prescribed treatment for premature ejaculation. It is another of the many chronic conditions that we are told we'll have to learn to live with.

Risk Factors and Causes

Neil Rosenthal, M.A., a marriage and family therapist in Denver, believes the reasons that men experience rapid, early, or premature ejaculation include the following:

- He may be bored, repelled, or otherwise turned off by his partner. If he doesn't want to be there, for whatever reason, he may be giving his body the message "Get out of there in a hurry."
- The woman may have resentments or fears about him or about sex. If so, knowingly or not, he may be trying to be responsive to her by finishing quickly.
- He may fear intimacy and closeness.
- He may be physically, mentally, or emotionally tense.
- He may be trying to build his pleasure too quickly. He may need to slow the process down.
- He may be angry at his lover. Anger kills desire and performance.
- Unresolved conflicts may cause him mixed feelings about his lover.
- He may be afraid his partner will criticize or judge him. Fear inhibits sexual desire.
- He may be withholding his emotions from his partner. If so, he will tend to ejaculate more quickly.
- He may be feeling guilty about something, which will lower his libido and may make him want to finish quickly.

- Thinking kills desire. Thoughts such as "Tomorrow I've got to . . . ," "Earlier today I should have . . . ," "I wonder if she still finds me attractive?" will quash desire. If he is thinking too much, he is unlikely to be fully present during lovemaking. He needs to relax mentally.

- Worrying about his ejaculatory control may lead to his not having good control.

- His religious training or upbringing may lead him to believe that he is doing something wrong.

- He might be trying to tell his partner he is upset or dissatisfied.

- He may have low pleasure tolerance. Some people simply cannot tolerate much pleasure.

- Past experience with premature ejaculation may make him tense and anxious during lovemaking, thereby causing him to lose control more rapidly in the present.

Holistic Medical Treatment and Prevention

PC contractions. If you tighten and relax the muscle quickly, as you would during orgasms, it can allow you to maintain stronger erections and to have better control over your ejaculations. The regular practice of PC contractions is, in fact, an effective component in the treatment for premature ejaculations. Begin with fifteen to twenty contractions per day and you can gradually work up to fifty to a hundred contractions. (Or try doing ten contractions at a time, six times a day.) After

practicing this exercise for a few months, your PC muscle will be strong enough to prevent ejaculation if you contract it tightly just before the urge to come reaches the "point of no return." This exercise is great preventive medicine for a healthier prostate, it increases blood flow to the penis, which is good for preventing impotence, and it will add an exciting new dimension to your sex life. Other options for treating premature ejaculations might include

- frequent sexual encounters, such as once or twice a day, which will help you gain more voluntary control over ejaculations, but also requires a willing partner

- breathing abdominally to help you relax if you're tense while making love

- masturbation on the same day as anticipated intercourse

- pinching or squeezing the head of the penis at the junction of the glans and the shaft when you're close to ejaculation

- the "stop-start" technique—before ejaculation becomes inevitable, stop thrusting or slow down for a short time, then begin again

- become more aware of the sensations just before the point of ejaculatory inevitability, while you still have voluntary control of ejaculation; this occurs about one to three seconds before ejaculation

- identifying and discussing with your partner any persistent emotional issues affecting your relationship

- counseling if the problem stems from a fear of intimacy

Summary of Holistic Medical Treatment of Genitourinary Disease

Prostate Cancer

- low-fat diet
- antioxidants: vitamins C and E, zinc picolinate
- essential fatty acids (EFAs)
- high doses of intravenous vitamin C, B complex, and zinc
- saw palmetto berries and *Pygeum africanus*
- regular aerobic exercise
- pc contractions
- affirmations and visualization
- bioenergy: strengthen root chakra with connections with nature and other men
- homeopathy and Chinese medicine

BPH

- diet low in fat, refined carbohydrates, caffeine, alcohol, and tobacco; add raw pumpkin seeds
- EFAs: flaxseed, sunflower, or safflower oil
- zinc picolinate, magnesium, copper
- antioxidants: vitamins C and E, B_6, B complex, beta-carotene
- Saw palmetto berries and *Pygeum africanus*
- regular aerobic exercise
- ejaculate 3x/week
- pc muscle contractions
- affirmations and visualization
- bioenergy: root chakra strengthening

Prostatitis

Same as BPH except:
- herbs: pipsissewa and echinacea
- exercise: avoid jogging or other jarring exercise
- avoid ejaculation with acute prostatitis
- antibiotics

Impotence

- zinc picolinate
- beta-carotene, magnesium, and EFAs
- yohimbine, *gingko biloba*, Siberian ginseng, *Damiana (Turnera aphrodisiaca*
- regular aerobic exercise
- pc contractions
- affirmations and visualization
- communication with wife or sexual partner; intimacy without intercourse
- bioenergy: connect with other men and nature

Premature Ejaculation

- consistent PC contractions
- frequent intercourse
- masturbation prior to intercourse
- squeeze technique
- stop-start technique

The holistic physicians contributing most to this chapter are Edward J. Linkner, M.D., a family physician in Ann Arbor, Michigan, and Steve Morris, N.D., a naturopathic family physician practicing in Mukilteo, Washington.

R e s p i r a t o r y   D i s e a s e

Chronic Sinusitis
Allergic Rhinitis (Hay Fever)
Chronic Bronchitis

Prevalence

The most common group of diseases afflicting men, and women too, are those of the respiratory tract. As a result of the environmental plague of air pollution, most urban dwellers are breathing unhealthy air. The nose and sinuses are under a relentless assault from a barrage of pollutants. The EPA says that 60 percent of Americans live in areas where breathing is a risk to one's health. A 1993 study performed by the EPA and the Harvard School of Public Health reported that fifty thousand to sixty thousand deaths a year are caused by particulate air pollution. A subsequent study in 1995 bolstered the earlier findings while concluding that people who live in highly polluted cities die earlier (15 percent or about ten years sooner) than they would have had they been breathing healthier air.

Air pollution has become such a significant health hazard that four of America's most common chronic diseases are now respiratory ailments: chronic sinusitis (#1), allergies (#5), chronic bronchitis (#8), and asthma (#9). Ninety-two million of us, or one out of every three people, suffers from at least one of these respiratory diseases. Although men are not especially prone to asthma, they suffer heavily from the other three conditions. For men under forty-five years of age, among their most common chronic conditions, sinusitis and allergies rank first and second; forty-fix to sixty-four they are fourth and seventh; and over sixty-five, sinusitis is fifth and bronchitis twelfth. Acute sinusitis (sinus infection) may have already replaced the common cold (the most common respiratory-tract infection) as our nation's most prevalent acute illness. In a study performed at the University of Virginia in 1993, students who thought they had a *cold* were evaluated with CT scans—the most accurate diagnostic test for sinusitis. The scans revealed that 87 percent did not have a simple cold, but in fact had a *sinus infection*. The mounting scientific evidence documenting the health risks of breathing polluted air is presented in my book *Sinus Survival: The Holistic Medical Treatment for Allergies, Asthma, Bronchitis, Colds, and Sinusitis.* Most of the information in this chapter comes from that book.

Anatomy

The respiratory tract, whose chief function is breathing, consists of the nose, sinuses, and lungs. The nose and sinuses serve as the body's primary air filter and protector of the lungs. The respiratory tract works ceaselessly to provide every cell in the body with an adequate supply of oxygen and to expel carbon dioxide. Nothing is more important to optimal physical well-being than the quality of our air and our ability to breathe it. During the past twenty years, both of these critical aspects of health have drastically diminished.

Chronic Sinusitis

Symptoms and Diagnosis

Acute sinusitis is an infection of one or more of the sinus cavities. It often begins as a cold and is usually accompanied by most or all of the four primary symptoms of head congestion, headache or facial pain, green/yellow mucus, and fatigue. (Since **acute sinusitis** is so often confused with a cold or allergies, please refer to the table on page 225 to differentiate between them.) If this problem recurs three or more times within six months or never goes away completely, then it is called **chronic sinusitis.**

The Respiratory Tract

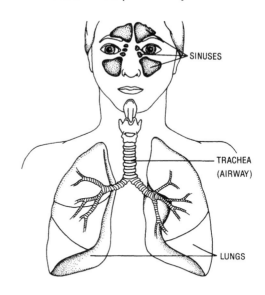

SINUSES

TRACHEA (AIRWAY)

LUNGS

Conventional Medical Treatment

Most people with sinus infections first visit their primary care physician—family doctor or internist—for treatment. In almost every instance that consists of a prescription for a **broad-spectrum antibiotic.** Amoxicillin is most often the first choice. If after ten days to two weeks the infection has not cleared, then a more powerful drug is prescribed:

Second-Step Antibiotics for Sinus Infections—After Amoxicillin

Best drugs for killing both *Streptococcus pneumoniae* and *Hemophilus influenza* (most common bacteria causing sinusitis); drugs are listed in order of efficacy; those on the same line are roughly equivalent:

Augmentin
Ceclor, Ceftin, Lorabid
Biaxin
Bactrim, Septra, Cotrim
Vibramycin, Vibra-Tabs

Best for killing staphylococci:

Augmentin
Ceclor, Ceftin, Lorabid
Duricef, Ultracef, Keflex, Cefanex,
     Anspor, Velosef
Bactrim, Septra

In addition to antibiotics, doctors often prescribe a **decongestant** or recommend an over-the counter (OTC) alternative. The most common ingredients in both choices are pseudoephedrine, phenylpropanolamine, and phenylephrine. Each works in much the same way to shrink swollen mucous membranes and reduce nasal and sinus congestion. These should be avoided if you have high blood pressure. They can also cause insomnia.

If the head and nasal congestion is severe, a **nasal decongestant** spray might be recommended. The OTC sprays include Afrin, Dristan, Sinex, Neo-sinephrine, and Vicks. These should be used with great caution and only for three days at most. They can easily become addictive! They produce what is called a rebound effect, which means that as their decongestant effect wears off and the head and nasal congestion return, the feeling of stuffiness is worse than it was before using the spray. This elicits a strong desire to spray

again, and a vicious cycle begins. Be careful with these sprays.

Depending upon the symptoms accompanying the sinus infection, such as headache, cough, or sore throat, other OTC-drug recommendations might include analgesics (pain relievers), antitussives (cough suppressants), or combinations of these two with decongestants.

If repeated courses of antibiotic are not successful in treating the sinus infection (an increasingly common occurrence), then **surgery** is often recommended. Through the use of the endoscope (a tiny telescope inserted into the nasal cavity), sinus surgery has improved dramatically over the past decade. **Endoscopic surgery** usually involves enlarging the ostia, the sinus drainage ducts, so the sinuses will be able to drain more effectively. Sinus surgery has quickly risen to almost half a million procedures per year, costing anywhere from $3,000 to $10,000. Unfortunately it is still a long way from a guaranteed cure for chronic sinusitis. Many people experience short-term improvement, six months to one year, then begin the cycle of sinus infections and antibiotics all over again. The surgery is most successful when it eliminates one or more of the obstructive causes of sinusitis, such as polyps, cysts, an enlarged or distorted nasal turbinate (turbinate hypertrophy), or a deviated septum. But even in these cases, the surgery is still treating the symptom, not the cause. What is responsible for stimulating the growth of the polyps, cysts, or swollen turbinates in nasal mucous membranes to such an extent that a congenitally deviated

Diagnosing and Recognizing the Symptoms of Colds, Sinusitis, and Allergies

Primary symptoms—almost always present Secondary symptoms—frequent but less often present

The Common Cold

Primary

- preceded by high stress; too much going on at once
- preceded by a sore throat
- nasal congestion
- runny nose
- thin, clear/white nasal mucus
- fatigue
- mild muscle aching
- lasts for four to seven days

Secondary

- headache
- sore throat
- cough
- low-grade fever

Sinus Infection (Acute Sinusitis)

Primary

- preceded by the common cold
- preceded by unexpressed anger
- head congestion (facial or head fullness)
- head or facial pain (headache, cheek, tooth, or eye pain)
- thick green/yellow nasal or especially postnasal mucus drainage (down back of throat)
- extreme fatigue
- lasts for two or more weeks

Secondary

- preceded by allergies or by prolonged exposure to air pollution, smoke, or toxic fumes
- fever
- sore throat
- cough
- hoarseness
- nasal congestion
- lasts for several months

Allergies, Hay Fever, or Allergic Rhinitis

Primary

- preceded by personal or family history of allergies, eczema, or asthma
- intermittent symptoms: either seasonal (pollen), food-related, environmentally or emotionally triggered
- positive allergy skin tests
- thin, clear/white nasal mucus
- nasal congestion
- sneezing
- itching of nose, eyes, or throat
- symptoms relieved with antihistamines, food elimination, environmental clearing, or stress reduction

Secondary

- persistent or perennial symptoms
- postnasal drip with intermittent sore throat, cough, or hoarseness
- wheezing, difficulty breathing
- skin rash
- allergic "shiners" (dark circles under eyes)

septum is now all of a sudden obstructing the sinus from draining? Most ENT surgeons claim that there is no known cause for these phenomena. They just happen. Until conventional medicine addresses the multiple causes of chronic sinusitis, this symptom-focused treatment means the ailment will remain largely incurable with the prognosis "You're going to have to learn to live with it."

Risk Factors and Causes of Respiratory Disease

The outermost lining of the entire respiratory tract is one continuous **mucous membrane.** Like an extension of the skin covering the external surface of your entire body, this membrane is a connected porous protective shield for the air portal of your body. It serves as your first line of defense against bacteria, viruses, pollen, animal dander, cigarette smoke, dust, chemicals, automobile exhaust, and any other potentially harmful air pollutants. Far beyond the protective capability and breathability of Gore-Tex or any similar high-tech material, this membrane also has the job of humidifying dry air and warming cold or cooling hot air. The bulk of the job of filtering, humidifying, and temperature-regulating occurs in the nose and sinuses—the entrance and vestibule of the respiratory tract. If the membrane breaks down, the immediate consequence might be a cold or sinus infection. Since the lungs are the site of oxygen/carbon dioxide exchange, they need the protection provided by the nose and sinuses to do their best in carrying out this vital life-giving function. Unfortunately, the front-line nose/sinus defense is giving way to a massive assault by a barrage of air pollutants.

Air pollution appears to be the leading cause of America's first environmental epidemic. Every respiratory disease is impacted by air quality, and as I pointed out in chapter 3, the condition of our air—both indoor (see the table on page 63 in chapter 3) and outdoor—is deteriorating. **Particulates** have been identified as the most unhealthy outdoor pollutant. They are tiny particles of dust, sand, cinders, soot, smoke, and liquid droplets found in the atmosphere. They come from a variety of sources, including roads, farm fields, construction sites, factories, power plants, fireplaces, wood-burning stoves, wind-blown dust, and diesel and car exhaust. While our mucous membranes are overloaded with too much to filter, they are also being injured, irritated, and abraded by the pollutants themselves. Imagine rubbing a piece of fine sandpaper across the back of your hand twenty-three thousand times per day! Can you picture the condition of your skin and how difficult it would be for that skin surface to ever heal? That is comparable to the assault your mucous membranes are subjected to daily from merely breathing. The longer this insidious barrage of pollution persists, the greater the irritation of the membranes, and the higher the risk of subsequent inflammation and swelling. With persistent swelling of the membranes, usually resulting from colds and/or allergies, the openings of the sinus ducts that drain into the nose can easily become blocked. This can leave a pool of stagnant mucus in a sinus that might look like an oasis to invading bacteria. People suffering from allergies and/or chronic sinusitis have diminished protection of the lungs and increased vulnerability of its mucous membrane to cigarette smoke and any other air pollutant. The inflammation and swelling that might ensue in the lungs can then cause narrowing of the airways and excessive mucus, which can in turn create a greater susceptibility to the lung diseases asthma and bronchitis. The EPA has concluded that air pollution is the primary cause for the nearly 50 percent increase over the past decade in the incidence of asthma, chronic bronchitis, and emphysema.

The leading causes of **chronic sinusitis** are

- *air pollution*—indoor and outdoor
- *overuse of antibiotics*—causing antibiotic-resistant bacteria and yeast (candida) overgrowth
- emotional stress—especially *repressed anger and sadness* ("unshed tears")
- dry air
- cold air
- allergies—pollen, animal dander, mold, and food (wheat and dairy products are most common)
- occupational hazards—for auto mechanics, construction workers, airport and airline personnel
- dental problems—especially with upper teeth

The first three risk factors on this list are the most significant. Although antibiotics are the mainstay of conventional medical treatment for sinusitis, they are not absolutely necessary to successfully treat sinus infections. Unfortunately they have been prescribed so indiscriminately that we are now seeing a growing number of **antibiotic-resistant bacteria,** called supergerms. Besides the prescriptions, our diets are filled with antibiotic-laden meat and dairy products. Many people suffering from chronic sinusitis are still sick because their sinuses are infected with antibiotic-resistant bacteria.

Another problem resulting from antibiotics is that they can destroy the friendly bacteria in our digestive tract, which allows for the **overgrowth of yeast** or **candida** organisms. The subsequent infection of the sinuses by candida may be creating another epidemic. Although it's more common in women, over the past ten years the male patients I've treated with the most severe cases of chronic sinusitis have almost all been suffering with candidiasis. Not only can this problem weaken the immune system, but it can also cause a multitude of food and mold allergies that further aggravate the sinusitis.

As with every chronic disease, **repressed emotions** contribute to weakening the immune system. Many of my patients with chronic sinusitis are high achievers and perfectionists. They often have a strong need for control. Anger often results from their perception of mistakes made by themselves or others, or from a perceived loss of control. I also now believe that a deep sadness exists in most of these patients. The many tears that have not been shed can result in congestion of the tear glands, which surround the eyes and are in close proximity to the sinuses as well. Perhaps this swelling and congestion is also a contributor to congested sinuses.

Allergic Rhinitis (Hay Fever)

Symptoms and Diagnosis

See the table on page 225 for a complete list of symptoms.

Conventional Medical Treatment

The conventional medical treatment for **allergic rhinitis, allergies,** or **hay fever,** besides removing the offending allergen, consists of **medication** and **allergy desensitization injections.** Eliminating the allergen is usually a bit of a challenge. Avoiding allergenic foods can be relatively simple, but getting rid of the family pet if you're allergic to cats or escaping from pollen is much more difficult.

You can minimize pollen exposure by taking refuge in sealed, air-conditioned office buildings and houses, where filters cleanse most of the offending pollen from incoming air. For those allergy sufferers unconcerned with domestic decor, the NIH recommends the following: Remove carpeting, upholstered furniture, heavy curtains, venetian blinds, fuzzy wool blankets, and comforters stuffed with wool or feathers. Empty the room, scrub it and everything that is to be returned to it, and thereafter thoroughly clean the room every week. If replacing curtains, hang some that are lightweight and can be laundered

weekly. Replace the comfortable chairs with wooden or metal ones that can be scrubbed, keep clothing in plastic zippered bags, and shoes in closed boxes off the floor.

For temporary relief of mild allergies, doctors usually prescribe **antihistamines.** For years these drugs almost always caused drowsiness, but now a few do not have this inconvenient side effect. Seldane, Hismanal, and Claritin are all nonsedating prescription options. There are a number of OTC antihistamines (most will cause some drowsiness), either alone or in combination with decongestants.

Many allergy sufferers also derive significant benefit from the antiallergic and anti-inflammatory effects of the **prescription corticosteroid nasal sprays** such as Beconase, Vancenase, Nasalide, and Nasacort. Cromolyn sodium has a similar action and is available as a nasal spray (Nasalcrom) and as an eyedrop (Opticrom). A seasonal pollen allergy sufferer, especially one who is also prone to sinus infections, should use the spray on a maintenance schedule throughout most of the allergy season, about one to two months. Long-term use of these cortisone sprays, beyond three months, can cause chronic irritation, inflammation, and increased mucus secretion.

If you are not satisfied with the symptomatic relief you have received from antihistamines and steroid nasal sprays, your next step will often be a visit to an allergist. Depending upon the results of a battery of **allergy skin tests,** you might then be considered a candidate for allergy **desensitization injections.** These shots, containing small amounts of the offending allergen(s), will often be given a few days apart early on and progress to monthly injections that could last for several years. People with severe pollen allergy seem to benefit most from this treatment, while those with mold, dust-mite, and animal-dander allergies do not fare as well. Why the shots do and sometimes don't work remains a mystery. Whether or not they do, however, they are consistently an expensive treatment option.

Conventional medicine continues to develop better diagnostic tools and more effective medications to both identify the allergen and nullify its effects. But a guaranteed or permanent cure for the sneezing and stuffy and drippy nose of allergic rhinitis is still a long way off.

Risk Factors and Causes

Possibly even more than chronic sinusitis, allergic rhinitis has a strong genetic component. Often at least one parent or a sibling has had a history of allergies or hay fever, eczema, or asthma. However, I believe that both air pollution and emotional factors are the primary *triggers* for precipitating the allergy symptoms. Polluted, dry, and cold air can act as an irritant that over the years can cause the nasal mucous membrane to become extremely sensitive and potentially react to pollen, mold, dander, dust, smoke, etc. The foods that most commonly cause allergies are cow's milk and all dairy products, wheat or any grain, chocolate, corn, white sugar, soy, yeast (brewer's and baker's), oranges, toma-toes, bell peppers, white potatoes, eggs, fish, shellfish, cocoa, onions, nuts, garlic, peanuts, black pepper, red meat, aspirin, artificial food coloring, coffee, black tea, beer, wine, and champagne.

The emotion I've identified most often in my allergic patients is fear. It is probably more important to determine who or what circumstance in your life you are "allergic" to (are afraid of or feeling insecure about) than what food or airborne allergen is causing your symptoms. The next time you have a sneezing spell, pay attention to your thoughts, images, and feelings that immediately preceded the onset of the symptoms. Your sneezing, itching, and congestion can become an emotional barometer that helps you to identify the deeper and hidden causes of allergic rhinitis.

Chronic Bronchitis

Symptoms and Diagnosis

Bronchitis can be either an infection (acute bronchitis) or an inflammation (chronic bronchitis) of the bronchi, the two large tubes that branch off into the lungs from the windpipe or trachea. The typical person suffering from chronic bronchitis is a smoker over the age of forty-five. Acute bronchitis often occurs in conjunction with acute sinusitis, an infection called sinobronchitis. This results from the postnasal drainage of infected mucus from the sinuses into the lungs. The primary symptom of acute bronchitis is a persistent (day and night), deep, wet, and green/yellow mucousy cough. In chronic bronchitis, excessive mucus is secreted from the inflamed respiratory mucosa lining the bronchi. To qualify as chronic bronchitis, there must be a cough that produces thick white or gray mucus for at least three months, and the cough must recur for at least two consecutive years (according to the American Lung Association). In addition, there may be shortness of breath and wheezing, similar to the breathing problems experienced by people with asthma. Other frequent *symptoms* of chronic bronchitis include:

- difficulty breathing
- frequent episodes of acute bronchitis
- weakness
- weight loss

Conventional Medical Treatment

Just as with acute sinusitis, the treatment of acute bronchitis is an antibiotic. However, the first choice may be erythromycin, or its newer and stronger derivatives, Zithromax and Biaxin. The basic conventional medical treatment for chronic bronchitis begins with stopping smoking, otherwise there can be no effective treatment.

The primary objective is to open and drain the bronchi of its thick and/or infected mucus. Steam can be helpful. Steaming in the shower, steam room, or with a device called a Steam Inhaler® (available in many pharmacies) is recommended at least once a day. This should be followed by postural drainage to loosen and remove the trapped mucus

blocking the airways (see diagrams on following pages). Drinking plenty of water daily; avoiding the use of cough suppressants; regular use of a humidifier that puts out warm moisture; and avoiding highly polluted, cold, or dry air will also help to thin and loosen the mucus. If you must be in an area with highly polluted air or strong fumes, wear a special protective mask over your nose and mouth. Some pharmacies and bike shops sell them. There is also a mask called the Brinks chemical respirator, which is effective in filtering fumes and other indoor pollutants. Try to stay away from anything that you know can cause an allergic reaction.

The conventional medical approach for treating chronic bronchitis can mitigate the symptoms to the extent that you adhere to the program. It is a chronic disease and requires daily persistent treatment. If this is not strictly maintained, as is often the case, the bronchitis slowly progresses. The bronchial walls eventually thicken, and the number of mucous glands increases. The bronchitis sufferer becomes increasingly susceptible to lung infections—acute bronchitis and pneumonia—and the bronchial mucosa becomes more inflamed and secretes a higher volume of thicker mucus. Chronic bronchitis can be incapacitating, often leading to emphysema and eventually death. Chronic lung disease, consisting primarily of bronchitis, emphysema, and asthma, is currently the fourth leading cause of death in the United States. Each year it is relentlessly gaining ground on the conditions that hold the top three positions: heart disease, cancer, and stroke.

Postural Drainage

Each of the positions shown in the following diagram, either sitting or lying, is designed to allow gravity to assist in draining the mucus from each part of the lungs. Each lung has three parts: an upper, middle, and lower lobe. In each position an arrow indicates where an assistant would tap or cup the chest to help jar the mucus loose. This procedure involves cupping the hands as if you were about to clap, then lightly to moderately striking the chest wall, while alternating hands. The rate at which you tap the chest is similar to an average clapping speed. If you are unsure about how to perform this procedure, consult with a respiratory therapist.

UPPER LOBES—A TO F

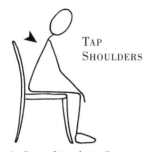
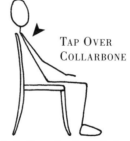

TAP
SHOULDERS

TAP OVER
COLLARBONE

A. Seated in chair. Lean forward about 20°.

B. Seated in chair. Lean backward about 20°. You can support lower back with a pillow.

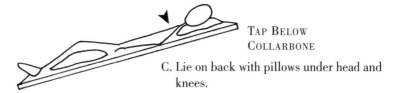

TAP BELOW
COLLARBONE

C. Lie on back with pillows under head and knees.

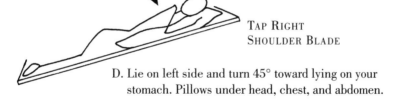

TAP RIGHT
SHOULDER BLADE

D. Lie on left side and turn 45° toward lying on your stomach. Pillows under head, chest, and abdomen.

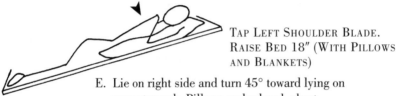

TAP LEFT SHOULDER BLADE. RAISE BED 18″ (WITH PILLOWS AND BLANKETS)

E. Lie on right side and turn 45° toward lying on your stomach. Pillows under head, chest, and abdomen.

TAP JUST IN FRONT OF LEFT ARMPIT, SLIGHTLY HIGHER ON WOMEN (NOT DIRECTLY OVER BREAST). RAISE BED 12″

F. Lie on right side and turn 45° toward lying on your back. Pillows under head and back.

MIDDLE LOBE—G

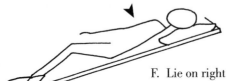

TAP JUST IN FRONT OF RIGHT ARMPIT, SLIGHTLY HIGHER IN WOMEN. RAISE BED 12″

G. Lie on left side and turn 45° toward lying on your back. Pillows under head and back.

LOWER LOBES—H TO L

TAP LOWER RIBS. RAISE BED 18″

H. Lie on your back. Pillows under head and knees.

TAP LOWER LEFT RIBS. RAISE BED 18″

I. Lie on your right side. Pillows under head and waist.

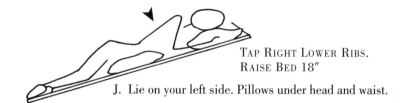

TAP RIGHT LOWER RIBS.
RAISE BED 18″

J. Lie on your left side. Pillows under head and waist.

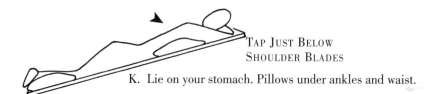

TAP JUST BELOW
SHOULDER BLADES

K. Lie on your stomach. Pillows under ankles and waist.

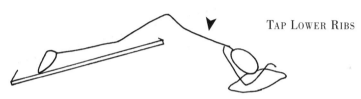

TAP LOWER RIBS

L. Hang over edge of bed with hips bending 60°.

Risk Factors and Causes

The most important risk factor for causing chronic bronchitis is cigarette smoking. All of the physical and emotional causes for chronic sinusitis, especially air pollution, can also contribute to this condition.

In her book *You Can Heal Your Life,* Louise Hay suggests other probable emotional causes of respiratory diseases such as:

- Sinus problems: Irritation with one person, someone close.
- Allergies: Whom are you allergic to? Denying your own power.
- Bronchitis: Inflamed family environment. Arguments and yelling. Sometimes silent.

- Candidiasis: Feeling very scattered. Lots of frustration and anger. Demanding and untrusting in relationships. Great takers.

These may or may not fit for you, but give them some thought before deciding that they don't apply.

The Holistic Medical Treatment and Prevention for Respiratory Disease

Because the holistic medical treatments for each of the chronic respiratory diseases are so similar, they are grouped together in this section. In recognizing how the nose, sinuses, and lungs are connected by one continuous mucous membrane, you can not only appreci-ate their intimate relationship, but also under-stand how one affects another; why certain factors, especially colds, cigarette smoke, and air pollution can adversely affect all three parts simultaneously; and how an effective treatment program directed at one condition can benefit your entire respiratory tract. The primary goals of the holistic treatment for res-piratory disease are (1) to heal the mucous membrane lining your nose, sinuses, and lungs; and (2) to strengthen your immune sys-tem. If you suspect candida is involved with your condition, then its elimination will re-quire a major commitment and will become your third goal. I have devoted an entire chap-ter to that subject in the current (third) edition of *Sinus Survival*. The holistic treatment pro-gram is directed at loving and nurturing your body, particularly the respiratory tract, and specifically the injured, inflamed, and irri-tated mucous membrane. I call it the Sinus Survival Program.

Physical and Environmental Health Recommendations

Air. The simplest and most effective way to heal the damaged mucous membrane is to stop breathing unhealthy air. (For most urban Americans that would mean to stop breath-ing.) If you haven't already done so, the first step is stop smoking, followed by the prohibi-tion of cigarette smoking in your home and workplace. Although it will be many years before we're able to see a substantial change in our outdoor air, technology has now made it possible for us to breathe optimal *indoor* air. Healthy air is clean (can't see or smell it), moist (40 to 60 percent relative humidity), warm (between sixty-five and eighty-five de-grees), negative-ion and oxygen rich (100 percent saturation). Negative air ions can create a profound difference in indoor air quality. Optimum levels for good health are between 3,000 and 6,000 ions/cu cm, and the EPA reports that the average indoor environ-ment in the United States contains only 200 ions/cu cm.

Negative-ion generators are potentially the most efficient air-cleaners—they attract dust, pollen, mold, animal dander, and even bacteria, then precipitate these particles out of the air. They have also been shown to help re-store the damaged mucous membrane by stim-ulating the cilia (microscopic hairs that act as a filter) that line its surface. Negative-ion gener-ators, for use as room air-cleaners, are becom-ing much easier to find. Look for one that puts out a minimum of one trillion ions/second.

If you're unable to locate one of these, or if you've found a weaker model, the next best thing to use is an air-cleaner with a **HEPA filter,** along with the lower-strength ion gen-erator, or an air-cleaner that combines both. Place the ion generator or air-cleaner in your bedroom and, if you spend a great deal of time there, in your office as well. There will soon be efficient air-cleaners for your car too. I describe the ion generator that I use and recommend to my patients in *Sinus Survival.* I list it along with all of the other products in the Sinus Survival Program and where they can be obtained in the product index at the end of that book. Since it is not yet available in stores, it may be obtained through the manufacturer at (303) 530-3934. It is called the Sinus Survival Air Vitalizer.

A **good furnace filter** on a forced-air heating and air-conditioning system is also important. Look for a pleated filter in the $15 to $25 range—3M makes a good one. Remember too that while air-conditioning cools and dries the air, it also depletes it of negative ions.

Humidifiers are essential, even in humid climates. During the winter months, while the windows are closed and the heat is on, it's usually extremely dry. A warm-mist room humidifier is best. Central humidifiers attached to the furnace can also be helpful. Be sure to install a flow-through type, one without a tray of standing water.

Plants can also add moisture to your home, as well as oxygen. Spider plants, aloe vera, philodendron, and chrysanthemums all function as effective air filters.

Don't forget the value of **good ventilation** as your primary source of more oxygen and fresh air. Adequate ventilation also helps to reduce indoor air pollution. Air-duct cleaning and carpet cleaning (without using toxic chemicals) are both valuable steps in creating healthy indoor air. Following all these steps can lead to indoor air that I describe as Hawaii-like! This is air that not only does no harm, but can actually help your mucous membranes heal.

Water. In chapter 3, I discussed the value of **drinking good-quality water** for optimal physical fitness. The mucous membrane of the respiratory tract also benefits from drinking an adequate amount of water. The wetter the membrane the thinner the mucus, and the easier it can flow and drain. When mucus dries, it tends to get thicker and plug things up, such as a nose, sinus, or lung. Other than herbal tea, water is our only healthy beverage. Besides drinking it, you can also bathe your mucous membranes in water. One of the best ways I know of to nurture your entire respiratory tract is to breathe steam. I recommend a device called a Steam Inhaler® to all of my patients. It's not as hot and is more direct than holding your head over a pot of boiling water, and it is also more efficient than a steam room. Available in some pharmacies, it can also be purchased by calling 1-800-544-6425. If you really want to treat your mucous membranes well, then add a couple of drops of eucalyptus oil to the hot water.

Nasal irrigation with salt water—using a rubber ear syringe, a Neti pot, or a Grossan nasal attachment to a Water Pik—is extremely helpful for flushing infected sinuses or for cleansing the membranes of the nose and sinuses. For people with chronic sinusitis, I recommend this procedure at least once daily, preferably in the evening. It's even more effective if you use the Steam Inhaler® just before irrigating. To make your irrigating solution, mix one third teaspoon of noniodized salt into an eight-ounce glass of nonchlorinated water and add a pinch of baking soda. This same saltwater mixture can also be added to a nasal spray bottle to be used frequently throughout the day, especially when the air is dirty and/or dry. A **saline nasal spray** acts as an irrigant, washing out the tiny particles of pollution, and as a humidifier, keeping the membranes moist. Be sure that the spray comes out of the bottle as a mist, not a stream. I've recently formulated my own saline spray that also contains several medicinal herbs. Called the Sinus Survival Spray, it is available in many health food stores or by calling 1-800-933-9440.

Diet. The recommended **diet** for treating and preventing respiratory disease is essentially the same healthy diet that was described in chapter 3. The foods to avoid if you have a respiratory condition are milk and dairy products, sugar, caffeine, and alcohol. Milk and dairy can increase and thicken mucus and may cause food allergy; sugar can weaken immunity and is a primary fuel for candida, as is alcohol; while caffeine has a multitude of potentially harmful side effects (see table on page 73). If you suspect you have candidiasis, then I recommend that you read the chapter entitled "Candida" in *Sinus Survival* and adhere to the candida-control diet.

A **food allergy** may be one of the primary causes of your nasal allergies or chronic sinusitis (most often milk and wheat). The best way to confirm this diagnosis is to eliminate from your diet for at least three weeks all of the foods that are most often responsible for food allergies (listed on page 229). Then begin to reintroduce each of these foods into your diet at the rate of one every three days. Pay attention to your body and note any new symptoms such as headache, nasal congestion and itching, increased mucus secretion, nausea, diarrhea, gas, or mental fog. It should be obvious to you which food, if any, causes your body to react.

Vitamins, minerals, herbs, and nutritional supplements. Most of the vitamins and minerals that I recommend for sinusitis, allergies, and bronchitis were discussed in chapter 3. They consist primarily of the **antioxidants**—vitamin C, E, beta-carotene, grape seed extract, zinc, and selenium. All of them are listed with their dosages for both treatment and prevention in the table on pages 238–39.

There are also **herbs** that can strengthen the immune system and act as a natural antibiotic. I usually recommend them only for treating the acute respiratory conditions and for whenever you feel as if you might be getting sick. Both acute sinusitis and acute bronchitis usually begin with a cold. Therefore, if you can prevent the cold, you can often prevent the sinus and/or lung infection. The following herbs and supplements are best taken right at the beginning of your symptoms (most colds begin with a sore throat) and throughout the illness (if you can't totally prevent it, you'll at least be able to minimize the symptoms):

- *Yin chiao:* used only for colds, this is a Chinese herb to be taken along with the rest of this entire cold regimen; it's great for knocking out a cold before it ever gets bad. Take 5 tablets 4 or 5x/day for 2 or 3 days.
- Garlic: a nonodorous variety in a liquid or capsule; take 3 capsules 3x/day. It can be effective as an antibacterial (sinusitis,

bronchitis), antiviral (colds), and antifungal (candida) agent.

- Echinacea: liquid is best (or capsule); 1 dropperful 3x/day. A true natural antibiotic, antibacterial, and antiviral, it is also an anti-inflamatory. Take it regularly throughout an infection.
- Goldenseal: liquid is best; 1 dropperful 3x/day. It enhances the function of the mucous membranes. Avoid with pregnancy or with ragweed allergy.
- Bee propolis: in liquid or capsules; 500 mg 3x/day. Not an herb, but also appears to strengthen immune function.

In addition to this regimen for preventing and treating colds, I would

- get more rest and sleep
- gargle with salt water, use saline spray and Sucrets or throat lozenges
- drink lots of warm or hot liquids
- take a hot bath and get steam exposure
- diet: eliminate dairy products and eat lighter foods with less protein

Beyond what I've just listed, more vitamins, herbs, and supplements for **allergies** are listed on the table on pages 240–41.

NATURAL QUICK-FIX SYMPTOM TREATMENT

Cough

gargle, then drink lemon juice:honey (1:1) with a tablespoon of vodka
licorice-based tea
ginger tea

wild cherry bark syrup
Bronchial drops (a homeopathic)

Fatigue

ginseng
antioxidants, especially vitamin C
folic acid
vitamin B-12 500mcg 2x/day
vitamin B-6 75 to 100mg/day
pantothenic acid 500mg 1 or 2x/day
meditation
exercise
sleep
pace yourself between activity and rest
rule out anemia

Headache

adequate water intake
negative-ions
steam
eucalyptus oil
acupressure/reflexology points
hydrotherapy—alternate hot and cold shower
garlic or horseradish (chew it)
calcium/magnesium
quercetin 2 caps 3x/day
Fenu/Thyme (Nature's Way) 2 caps 3x/day
Gingko biloba 40mg 3x\day
Feverfew avena 20 drops 3x/day

Runny Nose

adequate water intake
saline spray
ephedra (not with high blood pressure)
nettles 1 cap 3x/day
quercetin 2 tabs 3x/day
vitamin C 6,000 to 10,000mg/day

The Physical and Environmental Health Components of the Sinus Survival Program for Treating and Preventing *Sinusitis*, *Bronchitis*, and *Colds*

COMPONENT	PREVENTIVE MAINTENANCE	TREATING AN INFECTION
Sleep	7–9 hrs/day; no alarm clock	8–10+ hrs/day
Negative ions or air-cleaner	Continuous operation; use ions especially with air-conditioning	Continuous operation
Humidifier, warm mist	Use during dry conditions, especially in winter if heat is on and in summer if air-conditioning is on	Continuous operation
Saline nasal spray (SS spray)	Use daily, especially with dirty and/or dry air	Use daily, every 2–3 hours
Steam	Use as needed with dirty and/or dry air	Use daily, 2–4x/d
Nasal irrigation	Use as needed with dirty and/or dry air	Use daily, 2–4x/d after steam
Water, bottled or filtered	Drink $\frac{1}{2}$ oz/lb body weight; with exercise, drink $\frac{2}{3}$ oz/lb	$\frac{1}{2}$–$\frac{2}{3}$ oz/lb body weight
Diet	Increase fresh fruit, vegetables, whole grains, fiber Decrease sugar, dairy, caffeine, alcohol	No sugar, dairy
Exercise, preferably aerobic	Minimum 20–30 mins, 3–5x/week; avoid outdoors if high pollution	No aerobic; moderate walking only
Postural drainage[1]	—	—

This chart was created in 1995 by Robert Ivker, D.O., Steve Morris, N.D., and Todd Nelson, N.D.

[1] Postural drainage for chronic bronchitis only
[2] Use the higher dosages on days of higher stress, less sleep, and increased air pollution
[3] Use this dosage for maximum of one month
[4] Dosage depends on brand
[5] Use with caution if you have ragweed allergy
[6] Use only for preventing and treating chronic bronchitis
[7] Use only at *onset* of a cold and influenza
[8] Use only if candidiasis is suspected
[9] Take this preventive acidophilus for only two weeks, 3x/year
[10] Antibiotics—an option for sinusitis and bronchitis if taken infrequently, i.e., 1 or 2x/year

Component	Adults	
	Preventive Maintenance[2]	For Sinusitis, Bronchitis, or a Cold
Vitamin C (polyascorbate or ester C)	1,000–2,000 mg 3x/d	4,000–6,000 mg 3x/d
Beta-carotene	25,000 IU 1 or 2x/d	50,000 IU 2x/d[3]
Vitamin E	400 IU 1 or 2x/d	400 IU 2x/d
Proanthocyanidin (grape seed extract or pycnogenol)	100 mg 1 or 2x/d	100 mg 3x/d
Multivitamin[4]	1–3x/d	1–3x/d
Selenium	100–200 mcg/d	200 mcg/d
Zinc picolinate	20–40 mg/d	40–60 mg/d
Magnesium citrate or aspartate	500 mg/d	500 mg/d
Calcium	1,000 mg/d	1,000 mg/d
Chromium picolinate	200 mcg/d	200 mcg/d
Garlic	—	1,200–2,000 mg 3x/d
Echinacea	—	200 mg 3x/d or 25 drops 4–5x/d
Goldenseal[5]	—	200 mg 3x/d or 20 drops 4–5x/d
Bee propolis	—	500 mg 3x/d
Grapefruit seed extract	—	100 mg 3x/d or 10 drops in water 3x/d
Flaxseed oil (or omega-3 fatty acids in fish oil)	2 tbsp/d	2 tbsp/d
N-acetylcysteine[6] (NAC)	500 mg 3x/d	500 mg 3x/d
Yin chiao (1 bottle = 8 tablets)[7]	—	5 tablets—4/5xd for 2 days
Acidophilus (*Lactobacillus acidophilus* and *bifidus*)[8]	½ tsp in ½ cup water 2x/d (A.M. + P.M.)[9]	½ tsp 3x/d or 2 caps 3x/d
Antibiotics[10]		

The Physical and Environmental Health Components of the Sinus Survival Program for Treating and Preventing *Allergies*

COMPONENT	PREVENTIVE MAINTENANCE	TREATING ALLERGIES
Sleep	7–9 hrs/day; no alarm clock	8–10+ hrs/d
Negative ions or air-cleaner	Continuous operation (neg. ions, esp. if air-conditioner is in use)	Continuous operation (esp. during allergy season)
Humidifier, warm mist	Use during dry conditions — in winter if heat is on, in summer if air-conditioning is on	
Saline nasal spray (ss spray)	Use daily, several times/day, especially with dirty and/or dry air	—
Steam	Use as needed with dirty and/or dry air	Use daily, 2–4x/day
Nasal irrigation (allergies only)	Use as needed with dirty and/or dry air	Use daily, 2–4x/day after steam
Water, bottled or filtered	Drink ½ oz/lb of body weight,	—
Diet	Increase fresh fruit, vegetables, whole grains, fiber Decrease sugar, dairy, wheat, and alcohol; do food elimination diet to determine any food allergy	
Exercise, preferably aerobic	Minimum 20–30 min, 3–5x/week; avoid outdoors if high pollution and/or pollen	No aerobic; moderate walking OK. Avoid outdoors if high pollution and/or pollen

Component	Adults	
	Preventive Maintenance[1]	Treating Allergies
Vitamin C (ester C)	1,000–2,000 mg 3x/d	3,000–5,000 mg 3x/d
Beta-carotene	25,000 IU 1 or 2x/d	25,000 IU 3x/d
Vitamin E	400 IU 1 or 2x/d	400 IU 2x/d
Proanthocyanidin (grape seed extract or pycnogenol)	100 mg 1 or 2x/d	100 mg 3x/d
Multivitamin	1–3x/d	1–3x/d
Selenium	100–200 mcg/d	200 mcg/d
Zinc picolinate	20–40 mg/d	40–60 mg/d
Magnesium citrate or aspartate	500 mg/d	500 mg 2 or 3x/d
Calcium	1,000 mg/d	1,000 mg/d
Chromium picolinate	200 mcg/d	200 mcg/d
Vitamin B_6	50 mg 2x/d	200 mg 2x/d
Garlic	—	1,200–2,000 mg 3x/d
Ephedra or ma huang[2]	—	12.5–25 mg 2 or 3x/d
ALLERGY SEASON[4] — Licorice (*Glycyrrhiza glabra*)[3]	—	10–20 drops 3x/d
Nettles, freeze-dried	—	300 mg 1–3x/d
Quercetin + bromelain	—	1,000–2,000 mg/d (into 3–6 doses/d)
Pantothenic acid	—	500 mg 3x/d (after meals)
Hydrochloric acid	—	1 or 2 after protein-based meals
Antihistamines	—	OTC or Rx
Corticosteroid nasal spray	—	Rx
Allergy desensitization injections	Physician supervised	
Flaxseed oil (or omega-3 fatty acids)	2 tbsp/d	3 tbsp/d

This chart was created in 1995 by Robert Ivker, D.O., Steve Morris, N.D., and Todd Nelson, N.D.

[1] Use the higher dosages on days of higher stress, less sleep, more pollen, and increased air pollution
[2] Do not use with high blood pressure
[3] Do not use with high blood pressure or an enlarged prostate
[4] Allergy season only—take these only during your allergy *season;* natural products may be taken with or without Rx's

Sneezing

adequate water intake

acupressure/reflexology points

nettles 2 caps 2 to 3x/day

quercetin + bromelain 2 caps 2 to 3x/day
   before meals

Sore Throat

gargle with lemon juice:honey (1:1)

gargle with pinch of cayenne + 1 tsp. salt in
   8 oz water

licorice-based tea (Long Life, Traditional
   Medicinals, or Throat Coat)

lozenges (Zand Eucalyptus, Holistic brand
   Propolis)

zinc picolinate 30mg 3x/day

zinc lozenges, 20–25 mg, 3–4 x/day

garlic 2 caps 3x/day

Zand Throat Spray

Stuffy Nose

adequate water intake

hot tea with lemon

steam

hydrotherapy (hot water from shower)

eucalyptus oil

horseradish

acupressure/reflexology points

massage

orgasm

exercise

garlic

onions

cayenne pepper

Breathe™ Right—External Nasal Dilator

no ice-cold drinks

no dairy

no gluten: wheat, rye, oats, barley

ephedra 20 to 30 drops 4x/day for 2 to 3
days (max.)

rule out allergies

For **chronic bronchitis** the amino acid N-acetylcysteine (NAC) has been useful in reducing mucus viscosity. The dosage is one 500-mg capsule three times per day. This is included on the table on pages 238–39 and should be taken along with everything else in this table. The herbal bronchodilator ephedra can be used if wheezing accompanies the bronchitis. Otherwise this condition can be treated in much the same way as chronic sinusitis.

Homeopathic drugs and nasal sprays, and Chinese herbs and acupuncture, can also be helpful for treating all three of the respiratory diseases. It is preferable to be evaluated by a homeopathic physician or a licensed practitioner of Chinese medicine (O.M.D.) rather than to self-administer any of the above. Acupressure and reflexology points (refer to the figures opposite) can be another valuable addition to a holistic medical treatment plan. Apply direct pressure to these points for twenty to thirty seconds, two or three times a day.

Exercise. In treating respiratory diseases, exercise presents a unique challenge. In people with these conditions, the mucous membrane is often the weakest part of their body, and they may also have diminished lung function. Exercise can potentially harm both even more. Strenuous running or bike riding in polluted air can easily precipitate a sinus

Finger Acupressure

Reflex Points

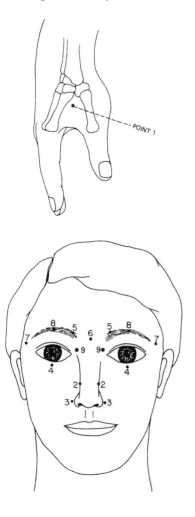

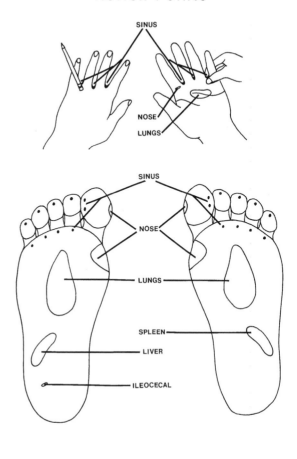

infection or allergy attack, or the flare-up of a bronchitic cough. Therefore, with respiratory conditions, there is an especially fine line between strengthening and further damaging the respiratory tract and immune system with aerobic exercise. When the proper precautions are taken, it can be the most beneficial of all forms of exercise. That's why I continue to recommend that my respiratory patients gradually walk that fine line by beginning an aerobic

exercise program with brisk walking. Even for those who are already used to more demanding forms of exercise, I ask them to pull back in order to heal the mucous membrane and strengthen the immune system.

For **aerobic exercise** guidelines, see chapter 3, page 86.

After starting your exercise program with brisk walking, you can vary it with hiking, jogging, swimming, and cycling. Treadmill, rowing, stair-climb, and cross-country-ski machines are excellent indoor alternatives. Having an **indoor option** for aerobic exercise is especially important for respiratory disease sufferers. Given the highly polluted air of most cities, there might be days when you would be doing yourself (and your mucous membranes) more harm than good by exercising outdoors. Since the 1970s, Boulder, Colorado, has been a training center for many world-class runners and cyclists. During the past several years, however, Boulder has seen an exodus of many of these athletes due to their growing number of asthma, bronchitis, and sinus problems resulting from air pollution. Extremely dry and/or cold air are the other air-quality factors to consider before exercising outdoors. Also try to avoid main roads when you plan your walking, biking, or jogging route.

It is best to schedule exercise around the rise and fall of pollution levels. In the winter, cold night air can trap a layer of particulates, carbon monoxide, nitrogen dioxide, and sulfur dioxide that lingers into the early morning. In the summer, ozone builds up during the morning, reaches its maximum late in the afternoon, and then ebbs in the evening. A good general practice is to restrict outdoor exercise to evenings during the winter and mornings during the summer.

Ultimately you must learn to listen to your body to determine whether you're doing too much or the air quality is hurting you. If you experience a wheeze, cough, tightness in your chest, or sinus pain during your workout, then it might be time to head indoors for aerobic exercise. Ozone levels in most homes, gyms, and pools are about half that of the outdoors— even less with a good air-conditioning system.

If you have a chronic respiratory condition and you exercise regularly, then try the following. After your heart rate has dropped to its pre-exercise level, get five to ten minutes of exposure to wet steam. This can be done either in a steam room at a health club, in the bathroom of your home, or with the Steam Inhaler that I mentioned earlier. Breathe in slowly and deeply through your nose and exhale through your mouth. Do this as often as you can following exercise, whether it's indoor or outdoor.

Mental and Emotional Health Recommendations

Whether they suffer from bad sinuses, allergies, or bronchitis, most people with chronic respiratory disease have consistently heard the message "You're going to have to live with it," either from their physician or from themselves. This belief will often add to already existing feelings of anger, sadness, fear, and possibly hopelessness. Louise Hay recommends specific **affirmations** for a variety of ailments. I've used many of them in my practice, with excellent results. They are the following:

Allergies: *The world is safe and friendly. I am safe. I am at peace with life.* Bronchitis and sinusitis (the same for both): *I declare peace and harmony are within me and surround me at all times. All is well.*

Candidiasis: *I give myself permission to be all that I can be, and I deserve the very best in life. I love and appreciate myself and others.*

There are many other affirmations that you can create on your own. For example:

I am breathing freely and easily.

The air that I breathe is strengthening and nurturing me.

My mucous membranes are healing with every breath I take.

My sinuses (lungs or allergies) are getting better every day.

My sinuses are now completely healed.

Remember to be as specific as possible with the affirmations and try to visualize what you want. In picturing healthy mucous membranes, it may help to look in the mirror and pull your lower lip down. The glistening pink tissue lining the inside of your lip resembles a healthy mucous membrane. This image will help in healing your nose, sinuses, or lungs.

Imagery can also be helpful in reducing allergic responses to sensitizing substances. The following is an "allergy walk" taught by Jack Schwartz, an Oregon naturopathic physician.

Begin by placing yourself in a state of relaxation using abdominal breathing. Once relaxed, imagine yourself traveling to seven allergy-producing sites.

1. An animal farm with a large variety of domesticated and wild animals and fearlessly petting and talking with them all;
2. A family farm in springtime with everything covered with deep layers of tree, flower, and grass pollen;
3. An old abandoned Victorian house in which you descend to the basement filled with dust, cobwebs, and mildew;
4. An industrial park replete with strong odors of chemical solvents, polluted air, and heavy smog;
5. A department store, walking up and down aisles filled with cologne and perfume, Naugahyde, new rugs, and potent detergents;
6. A banquet hall with a large smorgasbord of a large variety of foods, sampling each;
7. A large well-appointed room in which you find every person you have ever disliked, greeting each briefly, wishing them well and moving to the next.

In each of these scenes, imagine that you are breathing fully and deeply through your nose and bronchial passages without restriction, feeling energetic and confidant.

Suppressed anger, fear, and sadness seem to be a common theme causing respiratory diseases. Safely **releasing anger** on a regular basis has done more for many of my sinus patients than years of antibiotics or multiple sinus surgeries. Punching, stamping, screaming, or any combination of sound (exhaling) plus body movement for even a minute or two a day would be sufficient. Giving yourself permission to cry allows the tears to flow while also helping your sinuses to drain. Any of the recommendations for emotional fitness in chapter 4 are helpful in treating and preventing sinusitis, allergies, or bronchitis.

Bioenergy. Physical problems with the nose and sinuses are related to the **sixth chakra.** According to *The Anatomy of the Spirit* by Carolyn Myss, the mental and emotional issues associated with this chakra are self-evaluation, truth, intellectual abilities, feelings of adequacy, openness to the ideas of others, ability to learn from experience, and emotional intelligence (the ability to identify experience and express feelings). Lungs are related to the fourth chakra, and the concomitant issues of the "heart chakra" are love and hatred, resentment and bitterness, grief and anger, self-centeredness, loneliness and commitment, forgiveness and compassion, hope and trust.

Any **energy medicine modality,** such as therapeutic or healing touch, *reiki, qi gong,* or the chakra-charging visualization described in chapter 4, can be beneficial in treating and preventing the respiratory diseases. These therapies can be directed at the specific chakra associated with your condition. It is also helpful to work on the specific mental and emotional issues related to that chakra that you feel apply to you. For instance, the perfectionism and strong need for control present in many people with chronic sinusitis would apply to the issues of self-evaluation, feelings of adequacy, openness to the ideas of others, and the ability to learn from experience. Just in becoming more aware of these possible factors that might be contributing to your dis-ease, you can begin the process of healing.

All of the information in this chapter came from my book *Sinus Survival: The Holistic Medical Treatment for Allergies, Asthma, Bronchitis, Colds, and Sinusitis* (Tarcher/Putman, 1995).

M u s c u l o s k e l e t a l   D i s e a s e

---■---

Osteoarthritis (Arthritis)
Back Pain
Knee Pain

---■---

Prevalence

The musculoskeletal diseases are ailments affecting the bones, joints, muscles, and connective tissue. The National Center for Health Statistics uses the category "lower extremity dysfunction" to include knee, leg, and ankle problems, but the majority of these involve the knee. Therefore in this chapter I will focus on knee pain, along with back pain and arthritis. These conditions are among our most common health problems. For men under forty-five, back pain is the third most common chronic ailment, lower extremity dysfunction is fourth, and arthritis, ninth. For men forty-five to sixty-four years of age, arthritis isthird, back pain sixth, and lower extremity/knee is eighth. And for men over sixty-five, arthritis is first, while back and knee pain drop to tenth and eleventh. Up to 40 percent of everyone over the age of sixty-five is estimated to have some degree of arthritis.

Osteoarthritis

Symptoms and Diagnosis

Osteoarthritis, or arthritis, is an inflammatory joint disease that causes a breakdown in the cartilage covering the bone inside the joint. Cartilage is a softer (than bone), cushionlike material that acts as a shock absorber and prevents the bones from rubbing against one another. A clear, thick liquid in each joint lubricates the cartilaginous surfaces and allows for smooth motion. Although diagnosis can be made from an examination, an X ray, fluid withdrawn from a joint, and especially from the medical history, there are no definitive laboratory diagnostic tests for arthritis. The primary *symptoms* of arthritis are

• pain
• stiffness
• swelling of the joint

Although arthritis can occur in any joint in the body, the most common sites are the fingers—particularly the last two joints—the knees, and the hips. The degenerative changes of osteoarthritis can often be seen in the spine on X rays, but the majority of people with these changes do not have back pain.

The two major forms of arthritis are osteoarthritis and rheumatoid arthritis. (Whenever the word *arthritis* is used in this chapter it refers to osteoarthritis.) Rheumatoid arthritis is an autoimmune disease ("allergic to oneself") and is seen most commonly in women. The joints most often affected are the knuckles closest to the hand.

Conventional Medical Treatment

- *Reduction of stresses* on joints is usually advised. Physical therapy is often recommended, including exercises, hot and cold packs, diathermy, and paraffin baths.
- *Drugs.* Treatment usually includes nonsteroidal anti-inflammatory drugs (NSAIDs), which may either be prescription or over-the-counter. The OTC NSAIDs currently available are ibuprofen (Advil, Nuprin), Naprosyn, Tolectin, Indocin, and Feldene. Tylenol is often the first drug of choice. The NSAIDs do not stop joint deterioration, and long-term use can lead to a significant incidence of kidney and liver damage. They can also be a major cause of stomach and small-bowel irritation.
- *Surgery,* which may be used as a late-stage intervention, might include reconstruction or replacement of knees, hips, knuckles, and other joints.

Risk Factors and Causes

- Heredity—there is often a genetic predisposition to develop arthritis.
- Severe or recurrent joint injury, skeletal postural defects, and congenital joint instability can predispose one to the development of arthritic changes in the affected joints.
- Overweight—total body weight and body mass index are significant predictors of osteoarthritis of the knee. The risk for arthritis of the knee in men is 50 to 350 percent *greater* in men who are the heaviest compared to those of normal weight. This principle probably relates to other joints as well.
- Exercise—there is some evidence that only the most violent joint-pounding activities (long-distance running, basketball, etc.) performed over many years will predispose to the development of arthritis.

Holistic Treatment and Prevention

Like any other chronic condition, arthritis is a systemic (whole body) disease. It is not usually just a local disease of a particular joint. If there is no major joint degeneration, it can be cured using a holistic approach.

Physical Health Recommendations

The first step in the deterioration of the arthritic joint is inflammation and subsequent swelling. This may be a result of an excess of acid in the body, which can cause excessive amounts of calcium, minerals, and acid toxins to be deposited in the joint. This causes inflammation and pain.

Many other systemic disorders are often associated with the pathophysiological changes of arthritis, including digestive disorders, constipation, fatigue, emotional stress, nutritional deficiencies, endocrine disorders, and low-grade infections. A successful treatment program for arthritis will also address these other problems as well.

Diet. The first step in treating arthritis is to remove all inflammatory causes. Many people with arthritis have food allergies that cause joint inflammation. Dairy products, wheat, and nightshade plants such as potatoes, tomatoes, eggplant, bell and jalapeno peppers, are most often responsible for these food allergies. Eliminating all of them from your diet for at least one month and then gradually reintroducing them (one new food every three to four days) will help to determine if a food allergy, and which specific food, is contributing to your arthritis.

The next step is to remove the excess calcium, mineral deposits, and acid out of the joints. A raw food vegetarian diet and fasting is highly successful. This is not a new idea. For more than fifty years, fasting clinics throughout Europe have had outstanding results with juice fasting. Gabriel Cousens, M.D., at his Tree of Life Rejuvenation Center in Patagonia, Arizona, has administered a juice fasting program followed by a vegetarian diet for treating arthritis, and has been consistently successful. Fasting enhances the eliminative and cleansing capacity of the lungs, skin, liver, and kidneys. It also rests and restores the digestive system and helps to relax the nervous system and mind. If you're considering fasting as a therapeutic option, it is best to do it under the supervision of a well-trained physician.

Weight reduction, through diet and exercise, can relieve the stress on affected joints and is also recommended in treating arthritis.

Vitamins, minerals, and nutritional supplements. The antioxidants—vitamin C, 1,000–6,000 mg/day; vitamin A, 10,000–25,000 IU/day; and vitamin E, 400–1,200 IU/day—have all demonstrated benefits in treating arthritis. Proanthocyanidin (grape seed extract or Pycnogenol), in a dosage of 100–300 mg/day, can act as a strong anti-inflammatory. The minerals zinc picolinate, 30–50 mg/day; selenium, 200 mcg/day; copper aspirinate, 2 mg/day; magnesium, 400–800 mg/day; and manganese, 10–20 mg/day should also be taken.

Glucosamine sulfate is a building block of cartilage and can be used to repair damaged cartilage or to grow new cartilage. It usually takes four to eight weeks to get significant benefit from this supplement. Glucosamine sulfate is available in most health food stores and the recommended dosage is 500 3x/day or 750 mg 2x/day.

Niacinamide is a type of B vitamin, similar to niacin, that has been beneficial in treating arthritis. The dosage for most men should be 500 mg 4x/day, but some will have benefit with 250 mg 3x/day. The only possible harmful side effect is that on rare occasions it can be harmful to the liver. A periodic liver profile (blood test) through your doctor's office can monitor your liver function.

Essential fatty acids in the form of evening primrose oil, black currant seed oil, borage oil, and omega-3 oils from fish and flaxseed oil have been effective in treating arthritis. Flaxseed oil should be taken in a dosage of 2 tbs/day.

Bovine cartilage and supplements containing condroitin sulfate may also be helpful, and could be used in conjunction with glucosamine sulfate.

Herbs. Ginger (0.5–1.0 grams of powdered ginger), feverfew *(Tenacetum parthenium),* thunder vine, and licorice root *(Glycyrrhiza glabra)* have all shown significant anti-inflammatory effects in treating arthritis. Licorice used long term can elevate blood pressure. Reasonable doses of licorice are $\frac{1}{8}$ to $\frac{1}{4}$ of a tsp of a 5:1 solid extract up to 3x/day.

Acupuncture. Traditional Chinese medicine, using acupuncture and Chinese herbs and administered by a highly skilled practitioner, can be quite effective in treating arthritis by relieving inflammation and increasing circulation through arthritic joints.

Osteopathy. An osteopathic physician who is highly skilled in osteopathic manipulative therapy, can insure that skeletal alignment is optimal. This reduces strain on the joints.

Mental and Emotional Health Recommendations

In her book *You Can Heal Your Life,* Louise Hay relates the probable emotional cause of arthritis to feeling unloved, criticized, or resented. She recommends the affirmation "I am loved. I now choose to love and approve of myself. I see others with love."

Arthritis is associated with low energy in the **third** or **solar plexus chakra.** The mental/emotional issues related to this chakra, according to Carolyn Myss in *Anatomy of the Spirit* are

- trust
- fear and intimidation
- self-esteem, self-confidence, and self-respect
- care of oneself and others
- responsibility for making decisions
- sensitivity to criticism
- personal honor

You could create a number of **affirmations** focused on the joints affected by arthritis or to the activity the arthritis prevents you from doing. For example: "My fingers move freely and easily." "My hands are filled with energy and vitality as I _____ (write, type, work at my computer, paint, sculpt, play the piano)." Remember that you cannot use negative words. So don't say, "I am _____ (writing, painting, etc.) *without* pain. You could say, "My hands are free of pain," but that still focuses your attention to some extent on the *pain.* Try to make the affirmations as *positive* as possible.

In addition to writing and reciting the affirmations, don't forget to visualize them. In addition to seeing your own affirmations, another effective **visualization** for arthritis is to picture the surface of your arthritic joint as if it were healed. The cartilage covering a joint resembles the smooth, grayish-white, glistening cartilaginous tissue that you have seen in the joint of a chicken or turkey drumstick. Using this image, take a few minutes each day to picture an irregular, inflamed, discolored cartilaginous surface being transformed into this perfectly healthy joint surface.

Bioenegy recommendations. Since arthritis is associated with a weak *third or solar plexus chakra,* any of the **energy medicine therapies—chakra-charging visualization, healing touch,** *reiki*—could be directed specifically at this chakra, as well as on the affected joints.

Back Pain

Back pain describes a variety of conditions. Most instances of back pain occur in the lower back. The most common types of chronic **low-back pain** are associated with **muscle strain, sciatica,** and other causes. Although we often think of the back as a single entity, it is actually a complex connection of many parts:

- *Bones,* including the vertebrae at each level of the spine; the sacrum or last five bones of the spine before the tailbone, which sit between the bones of the pelvis and the back; and the pelvic bones themselves.
- *Nerves* of the low back, which includes a pair of nerves that leave the spinal cord at each level, one on each side below each vertebra. These later join together to form the nerves of the low back, the pelvis, and

the legs. Several nerves come together in the buttocks and run down the back of the leg as the sciatic nerve. This nerve later divides and innervates the entire leg all the way down to the tips of the toes.
- *Muscles,* which connect the spine and pelvis to the lower back, upper back, ribs, hips, legs, and abdomen, and muscles that connect the pelvis to the low back.

The *functions* of these different structures are as follows:
- *Bones* provide support and form for the body and protect the internal organs.
- *Nerves* carry signals from the brain and spinal cord to the muscles to allow for movement, sensations of pain, pleasure, heat, cold, pressure, and sharpness, and also to send information back to the nervous system as to the position of the body, how far it is bent, how fast it is moving, and where it is in space.
- *Muscles* allow for the various movements, including bending, squatting, rotating, walking, standing, sitting, and rising up.

Together, all of these parts of the back allow us to do a variety of activities, to comfortably remain in one position, or to balance ourselves and perform complex movements.

The following section describes two of the most *common chronic back problems,* their symptoms, diagnosis, causes, and conventional and holistic medical treatment.

Muscle Strain

Muscle strain or **torn muscle or tendon** often results from lifting something too heavy or moving too quickly or awkwardly. It can cause both acute and chronic back pain. Symptoms may include a sharp, burning pain at the time of the injury that later becomes worse. Muscle strains may also lead to muscle spasms. Other symptoms can manifest as changes in posture and limited mobility and activity. Normal healing takes about three to four weeks, and pain usually starts to decrease after a few days or a week.

Conventional Medical Treatment of Back Pain Caused by Muscle Strain

- *Bedrest,* usually for no more than two days, and/or limited activity.
- *Ice* to the affected area for the first two days. It can be applied hourly for twenty minutes at a time to help decrease swelling and pain.
- *Sleeping on the back* with a big pillow under the knees or on the side with a big pillow between the knees.
- After two days, change to *moist heat* to help loosen the muscles and decrease spasm. Begin gentle stretching to the point of tolerance (no pain). It is very important to listen to your body and not overstretch it. The intensity of the stretches may be increased daily, gradually until a return to full motion (or even better motion than originally) is attained. If you're not patient with this healing, you may reinjure the muscle and have to start over. An excellent guide for stretching is a book entitled *Stretching* by Bob Anderson.
- *Pain medications* might include Tylenol,

one or two extra-strength, 500-mg tablets, four times a day (maximum eight per day); aspirin, one to two tablets every four hours; ibuprofen, 200-mg tablets, two tablets, three or four times a day; or naproxen sodium, 220 mg, one tablet, two or three times a day. The Tylenol has fewer potential side effects than the other medications but may not provide as much pain relief. For short periods of time, all of these medications are relatively safe. The exceptions are for persons with stomach ulcers or kidney and liver problems. None of them should be taken with alcohol, including the Tylenol. These medications can be purchased over the counter, or similar stronger versions can be prescribed by a physician.
- *Muscle relaxants* may be prescribed if muscle spasm is a significant component of the back pain. These medications are often effective, but are not meant for long-term use. Most of them can cause drowsiness.
- Other conventional treatments include taking time off from work and learning proper lifting and carrying techniques. Please see the section on chronic back pain on page 254.

Risk Factors and Causes of Back Pain Caused by Muscle Strain

Physical

- Poorly conditioned muscles due to lack of exercise, flexibility, and coordination, and high-risk activities, such as lifting heavy objects, especially with a twisting motion.

• Rushing through one's activities and trying to do too many things at one time.

• Poor nutrition, especially low protein intake and inadequate magnesium, can lead to poor health of muscles.

Mental and Emotional

• Emotional stress and lack of sleep, leading to increased tension and decreased blood flow to the muscles.

• According to Louise Hay, the mental and emotional causes of back pain are:
  • lower back: fear of money; lack of financial support
  • middle back: guilt; stuck in all that "stuff" back there; get off my back
  • upper back: lack of emotional support; feeling unloved; holding back love

Chronic *low-back pain* is associated with low energy in both the root and sex chakras. The mental/emotional issues related to these chakras are:

Root Chakra

• physical family and group safety and security
• ability to provide for life's necessities
• ability to stand up for self
• feeling at home
• social and familial law and order

Sex Chakra

• blame and guilt
• money and sex
• power and control

• creativity
• ethics and honor in relationships

Middle-back pain is associated with the third or solar plexus chakra. This was described in the holistic treatment for arthritis.

Upper-back pain is associated with low energy in the fourth or heart chakra. Its mental/emotional issues are love and hatred; resentment and bitterness; grief and anger; self-centeredness; loneliness and commitment; forgiveness and compassion; hope and trust.

Holistic Treatment for Chronic Back Pain Caused by Muscle Strain

Physical health recommendations. Consider a brief course of **structural treatments,** such as osteopathic or chiropractic manipulation, which can speed healing and decrease pain. **Acupuncture** can decrease pain, spasm, and swelling and speed healing. Some **herbs** may be helpful with pain. These include **bromelain,** which is an extract from pineapple, 500 units, three times a day. **Ginger,** 100 mg, two times a day, may also be helpful. The advantage of the herbs is that they are safe to take even if one has ulcers or has an allergy to the standard medications. A possible disadvantage is that they may not be as effective in relieving this type of pain.

Mental/emotional health and bioenergy recommendations. These will be discussed in the holistic treatment section for chronic low-back pain (page 256), which is essentially the same as for muscle strain.

Sciatica and Chronic Low-Back Pain

Sciatica refers to the irritation of the sciatic nerve, causing pain or tingling in the lower back, lower buttocks, or back of the leg, which may radiate down to the foot. **Symptoms** of chronic **low-back pain with sciatica** can be either mild and intermittent or severe and persistent. As a result of the chronic pain, other symptoms might include severe fatigue, inability to sleep, irritability and increased anger, and loss of ability to perform typical activities of daily living. Sometimes, severe depression can also be present, including feelings of extreme sadness and hopelessness, crying spells, sleep problems, and loss of appetite. These symptoms can occur even without a prior history of depression and should be treated by a physician.

With symptoms of chronic low-back pain and sciatica, it is important to be examined and diagnosed by a well-trained physician. A thorough history will include a careful accounting of all of your symptoms: the type of pain and its location, body positions that relieve or aggravate the pain, activities you were engaged in just before the onset of the pain, and the current stressors affecting your life. This evaluation, coupled with a careful, well-focused physical examination, is often all that's necessary to make a **diagnosis.** Many primary care physicians are capable of evaluating back pain, especially more recently trained family physicians or an osteopathic physician (D.O.) who has maintained his or her skills in osteopathic manipulation.

If a severe nerve injury is suspected following the physical exam (symptoms may include the loss of reflexes and true muscle weakness), then tests, such as an MRI or CAT scan, may be warranted. Otherwise, these tests often reveal many "incidental" or common minor abnormalities that are not significant and are probably not related to the pain. These findings may create unnecessary anxiety for the patient and could lead to further testing and procedures, including surgery. Bulging intervertebral disks, minor "degenerative joint changes," and flattened, narrowed disks, especially at the L5-S1 level, are all common on MRI scans, especially in older people. These changes are also frequently seen in people with *no* back pain.

Conventional Medical Treatment of Chronic Low Back Pain and Sciatica

- Use of *pain medications,* including Tylenol, ibuprofen, naproxen sodium, and other similar products in over-the-counter or prescription strength.
- *Narcotic medications,* such as codeine, hydrocodone, or oxycodone.
- *Physical therapy* and home exercise programs.
- Addressing *posture,* the *ergonomics* of the workstation, and proper instruction in *lifting* and carrying. Lifting should be done by bending the hips and knees, while keeping the back straight and the spine

and shoulders over the hips. It is best to grab the object, pull it as close to your body as possible, then stand up by straightening the knees and hips while keeping the spine straight. Follow this same procedure when putting a heavy object down—all the bending should be done with the hips and knees and not with the back. It is also important when moving heavy objects to turn the entire body by turning the feet and legs, to avoid twisting the back. If the back is twisted while lifting, it is much more prone to injury.

- *Injections* into muscle trigger points. This procedure often gives temporary and sometimes long-lasting relief.

- *Nerve blocks*—injections into the joints of the spine or near the spinal cord—can sometimes offer dramatic relief. However, it is a high-risk procedure because the injections are given in close proximity to the spinal cord and other vital structures. Therefore it must be performed by a trained physician skilled in this procedure.

- *Surgery* on the spine or disks between the bones of the spine, called laminectomies and discectomies, in some instances can be helpful and afford immediate relief from pain. Surgery should only be done if the abnormalities seen on tests and scans correspond well to the exact location of the symptoms. For some back problems arthroscopic surgery can be performed through a small instrument inserted into the back by either an orthopedic or neurosurgeon. Some of the potential problems with surgery include a long

recovery period even if the surgery is successful, scarring near the spinal cord, and rarely, infections of the spine. It is essential to consider the potential benefits before choosing surgery, since many procedures are performed with no resulting pain relief. When performed in the right circumstances, surgery can work quite well.

- *Pain clinics* may do further testing and are often helpful in combining a program of physical therapy and learning to cope with the psychological effects of chronic pain.

- A *support group* can be helpful but only if it is based on a positive attitude and works to improve the situation. If the support group becomes a complaining session, then it could be detrimental.

Risk Factors and Causes of Chronic Low-Back Pain and Sciatica

Physical

- Accumulation of injuries that have not completely healed, chronic muscle tension from poor posture or stress, loss of motion at the joints of the lower spine, particularly the sacroiliac joint or the spine joints of the pelvis, and tight muscles in the hip area such as the piriformis muscle, that can press on the sciatic nerve.

- Ruptured disks in the low back that can push against nerves.

- Severe degenerative osteoarthritis of the spine (mild and even moderate degrees of osteoarthritis usually do not cause pain).

- Inflammatory types of arthritis, such as spondylitis and rheumatoid arthritis.
- Other types of bone disease, including cancer of the bone or cancer that has spread to the bone.
- Poor nutrition, including inadequate intake of certain minerals, such as magnesium, and other nutrients, such as protein. A magnesium deficiency may be accompanied by chronic muscle pain or cramps. Diuretics, often used to treat high blood pressure, heart medications, diabetes, and high alcohol intake can cause a loss of magnesium.
- Inadequate activity leading to poor posture and poorly conditioned muscles, and a decrease in normal coordination and balance.
- Inadequate sleep.
- Uncomfortable bed, especially a mattress that is too soft.
- Uncomfortable workstations, such as chairs with improper support or having to sit or be in contorted positions, such as turning to a telephone or computer, or working under an automobile or with heavy equipment.

The following types of back pain need the *urgent attention of a skilled physician.* If you have any of these symptoms, have them evaluated immediately.

- Sudden severe back pain associated with pain in the abdominal area and shortness of breath, especially when there is no injury. This could be an aneurysm in the aorta (large blood vessel in the back).
- Weakness or inability to move your leg or

legs, with or without back pain, could be a stroke or a severe ruptured disk.
- Persistent back pain in one place could be a sign of bone disease or cancer. X rays or other tests may be helpful in making the diagnosis.

Mental and Emotional

For sciatica, Louise Hay believes the probable emotional cause to be "fear of money and of the future. Being hypocritical." All of the mental/emotional issues associated with the root and sex chakras listed above under the causes of back pain from muscle strain would apply to sciatica and any other cause of chronic low-back pain.

Holistic Treatment of Chronic Low-Back Pain and Sciatica

Physical health recommendations. Holistic treatment includes a comprehensive medical history of the mental, emotional, and social status of the patient. It would also include the same thorough physical examination and diagnostic tests that would be performed conventionally. Less testing might be done if the practitioner is more comfortable with a structural examination.

Maintaining the **structural alignment** of the muscles, tendons, joints, bones, and fascia (the lining of muscles) is an essential component of the holistic treatment for back pain. Several treatments may be needed. Lasting benefit is most likely with the more indirect types of treatments, such as **myofascial release, craniosacral osteopathy,** muscle energy, and strain/counterstrain techniques. The more direct or high-velocity thrusting techniques, which force areas that are out of alignment back into alignment, are usually more helpful with acute injuries than they are with chronic back pain. However, other forms of **osteopathic** or **chiropractic** treatments, which usually consist of high-velocity techniques, can be helpful in some cases of chronic pain. But if these modalities or any other form of therapy do not offer noticeable improvement after three to six treatments, it is important to evaluate whether to continue.

Physical therapy performed by a highly skilled therapist using a variety of modalities, such as heat, ice, ultrasound, and electrical stimulation, is often helpful. However, these are adjunct therapies and are not substitutes for structural treatment. When used alone, they are unlikely to provide lasting relief with chronic pain. Standard physical therapy often utilizes strengthening exercises to overcome areas of weakness or malalignment. A holistic treatment program is designed to help the body realign itself, thus healing the weakness and directly treating the cause of the problem.

Two highly effective injectable treatments include:

1. Soft tissue injections of sarapin, a derivative of *Sawacenia purpurea* (North American pitcher plant), by a holistic physician, offers long-lasting relief of pain of neuromuscular or neurogenic origin. Injections offer pain relief for up to three weeks with no reports of undesirable side effects.

2. A series of intravenous injections of colchicine (a drug used in treatment of gout) has been used successfully in chronic low-back pain due to a ruptured disk. The injections must be carefully given. Pioneered by a Nevada complementary physician Michael Rusk, colchicine was reported in 6,000 cases to give 85 % good to excellent results.

Several other **body-based therapies,** also called **body work,** may be helpful in treating chronic back pain. These therapies utilize methods to retrain the nervous system to improve posture, alignment, balance, coordination, and self-awareness. In addition to helping you to move more efficiently, they build awareness of your body and how it works. Some of the more common body-based therapies include **Trager® psychological integration, Feldenkrais® awareness through movement, the Alexander® technique,** and **Rolfing® structural integration.** For several years I have been working with a practitioner who uses the **Loren Berry® method** of body work. His results with my patients suffering chronic back pain have been outstanding. These approaches often involve both hands-on treatments and instruction from the practitioner for exercises to be done by the patient at home. These exercises can directly address the cause of the back pain by helping the body to integrate its functions and resolve areas of dysfunction. These practitioners are becoming much easier to find. You can either evaluate them on your own (see chapter 3, page 101) or you can obtain a referral from a holistic physician.

Yoga has demonstrated remarkable success in treating chronic low-back pain. Find a teacher, a class, or a videotape and start out *very* gradually. Remember—*don't push yourself*. If you keep it slow and steady, practicing every day, you might well end up with a healthier back than you had prior to the onset of your back pain. *Tai chi* can also be helpful.

Acupuncture may be helpful both for acute injuries and chronic back pain. It can offer substantial and long-lasting relief and often works well in combination with structural approaches. The sooner the problem is addressed with acupuncture, the better the chance that it will work.

With any of these therapies for treating chronic back pain, you need to continually evaluate their benefit. If you are receiving the same treatment repeatedly without lasting results, the therapy is probably not addressing the underlying cause. Not only can continuing this course of treatment become expensive, but it can also create a dependence upon the practitioner. Remember, holistic medicine addresses causes while empowering you to learn to heal yourself.

Mental and emotional health recommendations. Affirmations can provide powerful messages to the subconscious to help relax constricted muscles, improve posture, and enhance spinal alignment. Louise Hay recommends the following affirmations for back problems:

Low back: *I trust the process of life. All I need is always taken care of. I am safe.*

Middle back: *I release the past. I am free to move forward with love in my heart.*

Upper back: *I love and approve of myself. Life supports and loves me.*

Sciatica: *I move into my greater good. My good is everywhere, and I am secure and safe.*

According to Hay, the back represents the support of life. As a preventive measure, she suggests the affirmation "I know that life always supports me." As with any other malfunctioning part of the body, you can create your own affirmations that picture a healthy, fully functioning back. Remember to be as vivid as possible. Here are a few more examples: "My back is strong and flexible." "I am sitting, standing, bending, and lifting easily with full range of movement." "My back is now completely healed." "I am stretching every day and my back continues to heal."

Visualizations that represent healing are powerful. Regardless of your knowledge of the physiological cause of your back pain, visualizations create positive imagery that program the body for healing. For irritation of your sciatic nerve, picture red, inflamed tissue surrounding the ganglia of the sciatic nerve as it emerges from the spinal cord into the hip. Gradually visualize that tissue turning pink as it shrinks down to normal size. If the precise cause of your back pain is unknown, then allow a healing image to come to you and use it every day while doing Quiet Five (page 59). As each breath fills your abdomen, imagine its energy radiating to your low back with light and energy. Perhaps you can picture a concentrated beam of light zeroing in on your aggravated tissue or painfully contracted muscle. Sense the light's gentle warmth as it heals the tissue or relaxes the muscles and allows the spine to realign itself. Be consistent, be vivid, engage as many of the senses as possible, and most important—be committed. If the regular practice of visualization has been shown to successfully dissolve cancerous tumors, it can certainly help to relax tight muscles and move bones and vertebrae.

Counseling or any of the other emotional health recommendations in chapter 4 are helpful in treating chronic low-back pain. The focus of your emotional work will be on one or more of the emotional issues associated with the first (root) and second (sex) chakras that were listed under risk factors and causes of back pain caused by muscle strain. A useful book for treating back pain is *Healing Back Pain* by John Sarno, M.D.

Bioenergy recommendations. **Energy medicine,** using healing or therapeutic touch, *reiki,* or more advanced techniques can also be helpful in treating chronic low-back pain. They work similarly to acupuncture, but instead of the specific meridians used by acupuncturists, these modalities should be directed toward the root and sex chakras. Practicing your visualizations while being treated by a practitioner of energy medicine can further enhance the healing potential of the therapy.

Knee Pain

Although this chapter will focus on chronic knee pain, it's worth briefly mentioning **acute** or **sudden onset** knee pain, which usually results from an injury. The most common knee injuries are

- sprain—a torn ligament, a structure that connects bone to bone and helps stabilize a joint; the pain usually begins at the time of the injury.
- strain—an injury to a muscle or tendon, which connects the muscle to the bone; causes a sudden burning pain at the time of the injury.
- tendinitis—is swelling and inflammation of a tendon, usually resulting from overuse of the knee.
- torn cartilage (meniscus)—the menisci are disks that sit between the two bones (femur and tibia) in the knee. Pain is usually gradual in onset and may be accompanied by swelling and/or locking of the knee.

Pain may be both acute and chronic. Acute knee pain that is not related to an injury, with swelling, severe pain, or fever, requires an immediate medical consultation—it may be an infection.

The most common cause of chronic knee pain is **osteoarthritis,** the central focus for this chapter. Other causes of chronic knee pain include rheumatoid arthritis, gout, pseudogout, and infection.

The most common **symptoms** of arthritis of the knee include

- pain that is worse after activity and at the end of the day

- possible swelling or creaking (a noise with movement) of the knee
- stiffness of the knee after rest, but this should not last more than thirty minutes
- usually occurs after age fifty
- gradual onset, becoming progressively worse over weeks, months, and years. If knee pain begins suddenly and severely, it is probably not due to arthritis.

Conventional Medical Treatment for Arthritis of the Knee

- **Exercises** designed to strengthen the muscles around the joint, such as swimming, bicycling at seventy to ninety cycles per minute at a relatively low resistance, or leg-extension exercises. It may take two months before a major benefit is seen from the strengthening exercises. If pain lasts for more than two hours after an exercise, that exercise should be avoided or shortened in the future. **Support** around the knee, such as an elastic or neoprene-type sleeve, may be helpful. In severe cases, the use of a cane in the hand of the opposite side of the pain may also be helpful.
- Climbing stairs, bending, and kneeling are best avoided.
- A good **cushioned insole** or insert into the shoe can act as a shock absorber when walking. This can protect the knee.
- **Weight loss,** including decreasing fat and calories in the diet.

- **Ice** applied for twenty minutes after exercise.
- **Medications,** such as capsicum cream applied three times a day for several days, may be helpful. Side effects include a burning sensation in the skin after each application, which may last for a few days. You also need to wash your hands carefully to avoid getting the ointment into your eye or on other sensitive places on the body.
- Medicines by mouth. One or two extra-strength **Tylenol** up to four times a day is a good first choice. Advantages of Tylenol are that it is safe for persons with ulcers and that generic brands are rather inexpensive. Surprisingly, Tylenol is often as effective as the anti-inflammatories. If Tylenol is not helpful, you might consider ibuprofen, 200 mg, one to two tablets, 3x/day, or naproxen sodium, 220 mg, one tablet, 2x/day. If these offer some relief, but not lasting benefit, you may consider obtaining a prescription from your physician.
- Injections of **cortisone** into the joint up to four times a year is an accepted conventional treatment. Benefits include relatively long-lasting relief of the pain, especially with flare-ups. The side effects can include a multitude of problems as cortisone can affect many different parts of the body after repeated injections.
- Another technique that rheumatologists and orthopedic surgeons might use includes **flushing the knee joint** with

large amounts of fluids. This can sometimes be helpful.

- Finally, as a last resort for older men with severe debilitating arthritis of the knee, **surgery** can replace the entire joint. Advantages include long-lasting benefits; disadvantages include a major operation with several months before full recovery, potential problems with the prosthesis, and some limitation in function after surgery, although this is usually minimal compared to the problems before surgery. This procedure is not recommended for younger men who have had traumatic injuries or for those grossly overweight. Physically active younger men often have chronic pain and swelling after a knee replacement. Joint replacements are not permanent and may need redoing after several years.

Risk Factors and Causes of Arthritis of the Knee

The risk factors and causes are the same as those mentioned earlier in this chapter for osteoarthritis. However, since the knee is the largest weight-bearing joint in the body, being **overweight** is a significant risk factor. Louise Hay believes that the knee represents "pride and ego," and that knee pain reflects "stubborn pride and ego, inability to bend, fear, inflexibility, won't give in." Emotional issues related to either the first (root) or third

(solar plexus) chakras can be associated with arthritis of the knee. These emotions have all been listed earlier in this chapter.

Holistic Medical Treatment of Arthritis of the Knee

This treatment program includes all of the therapies described for the holistic treatment for osteoarthritis. There is a particular emphasis on weight loss if you are overweight. Louise Hay's affirmation for knee pain is "I bend and flow with ease, and all is well. Forgiveness. Understanding. Compassion." She also suggests "I am flexible and flowing." Other affirmations with visualizations that represent a healthy knee to you can be extremely helpful. In addition to Ms. Hay's affirmations, one that I've used with my patients is "My knee is completely healed," while picturing themselves running, jumping, skiing, or any other favorite physical activity that they are presently unable to do as a result of their knee pain.

The energy medicine techniques should be applied directly to the knee and to the **root and solar plexus chakras.**

The holistic physicians contributing to this chapter are Robert Anderson, M.D., Gabriel Cousens, M.D., and especially Mark Hoch, M.D., a family physician practicing in Phoenix, Arizona.

P s y c h o l o g i c a l   D i s e a s e

●

Depression
Anxiety
Addictions

●

Prevalence

Depression, in its various forms, currently afflicts an estimated 11 million people in the United States each year. This disorder does not distinguish between social classes or occupations—it is pervasive in all echelons of society. Only half as many men are treated for depression as women, but it is not known whether this is because women are more likely to be depressed or whether men tend to deny their depression. The estimated cost to the country from depression is $43 billion per year (1990 statistics). According to the World Health Organization (WHO), depression is currently the fourth leading cause of disability in the world. By the year 2020, WHO estimates that depression will be second only to heart disease as the world's leading chronic disease.

Anxiety is defined as excessive fear or worrying and often accompanies depression. According to Alan Caruba, executive director of the National Anxiety Center, Americans live in the "age of anxiety," with the level of fear in our country rapidly rising. Mood disorders are a significant health problem and need to be addressed with an open mind.

D e p r e s s i o n

Symptoms and Diagnosis

Depression is an all-inclusive term covering many types, from painful "blues" to a disabling "major depression." Before the diagnosis of depression is made, a complete physical examination by a primary care physician is recommended. It should include thyroid and adrenal function tests, a complete blood count (CBC), and a stool analysis for parasites and candida (a rapidly increasing cause of depression). In general, the **diagnosis** of depression is made when a negative change occurs in one's thoughts, mood, behavior, and physical responses, as indicated below.

According to *DSM-4*, the handbook of the American Psychiatric Association, one needs to display five of the following nine symptoms for at least two weeks to be diagnosed with depression:

- depressed mood for most of the day
- markedly diminished interest in usual activities
- insomnia or excessive sleep nearly every day
- significant loss of weight or appetite
- agitated or markedly slowed movements
- loss of energy or fatigue nearly every day
- feelings of worthlessness or inappropriate guilt
- diminished ability to think or concentrate
- recurrent suicidal thoughts or plans

Typically, if you're depressed, you will experience severe sleep disturbance, with difficulty falling asleep, early-morning awakening, or both. Other typical symptoms include significant fatigue, crying spells, self-loathing, extreme pessimism, and a sense of futility. There is a general tendency to withdraw, pull down the shades, and vegetate. In that condition, it is often difficult to get out of bed and get oneself dressed. There is often either an increase or decrease in both appetite and weight. Other features of depression include excessive irritability and a short-fused temper. This often causes erratic behavior. In time, irritability and anger often turn into generalized apathy, with a lack of interest in sex, hobbies, and people.

The milder and more "normal" forms of depression can be considered the blues or blahs. When the symptoms increase in frequency, intensity, and duration, they become more disabling to the individual. Their relationships, work, and general functioning be-

come more impaired. At that point, when one's symptoms and functioning are clearly perceived as distressing, one has a major depression and treatment is required. However, it is usually more effective if therapy is begun before reaching the crisis stage. The spectrum of depression from the blues to a major depression is broad, with many names and categories.

Conventional Medical Treatment

The most common treatment modalities for depression are **medication** and **psychotherapy.**

Medications. For treating depression, two commonly used groups of antidepressant medications are **tricyclics** and **SSRIs.** Of the tricyclics, the most common medications are nortriptyline (Pamelor), desipramine, imipramine (Tofranil), and amitriptyline (Elavil). Although tricyclics encourage sleep, improve depressive symptoms, create a mild antianxiety effect, and improve general functioning, they can cause dryness of the mouth, constipation, and drowsiness. They can also take up to four weeks to become effective and possibly cause problems with heart rhythm.

SSRIs (selective serotonin reuptake inhibitors) are a "new generation" of antidepressants that includes Prozac, Zoloft, Paxil, and Effexor. This second group of antidepressant medications has fewer side effects than the tricyclics and takes only two to four weeks to be effective. The disadvantages of

SSRIs can include frequent sexual dysfunction, insomnia, indigestion, headache, and increased anxiety.

One of the new antidepressants, Wellbutrin, is in a class by itself. It has fewer sexual side effects, but seems to have a greater incidence of headache and insomnia.

None of the antidepressant medications are addicting, but they can become psychologically habituating. They generally have few withdrawal effects; however, they can become a psychological crutch. In my own practice, I have found that the combination of medication and conventional psychotherapy alone, without treatment of the body and spirit, is usually *not sufficient* to effectively treat moderate to severe depression.

Psychotherapy. The term *psychotherapy* literally means "healing of the mind" and includes all forms of psychological therapy. **Conventional psychotherapy** is generally limited to *talking* forms of treatment. In the current era of managed care, these talking therapies have become more focused and goal-directed, as therapists strive for **symptom relief** in the most expedient manner possible. Deeply rooted issues often require more time. The conventional therapist frequently uses a psychodynamic model, which emphasizes the primary importance of early childhood programming on all subsequent adult issues and behavior. Chapter 4, page 123 discusses the more common types of psychotherapy.

Psychotherapy has changed dramatically during the past few decades. Only a few years ago, the most effective form of psychotherapy was considered to be **psychoanalysis.** This form of therapy required that the patient spend four or five days per week with the analyst, free-associating to allow patterns of psychic behavior to emerge. A typical course of psychoanalysis could last for five years or longer. Today's *conventional* psychotherapist usually asks three essential questions: (1) What are the problems of this client? (2) How did these problems start? (3) How should I treat the problems? Many conventional psychiatrists usually answer this third question with drug therapy alone and little effective counseling.

Risk Factors and Causes

The most significant factors which can contribute to depression are classified in the following categories to identify their specific impact on the body, mind, and spirit:

Body: Physical (Medical) and Environmental

- heredity
- candidiasis (yeast overgrowth)
- hypothyroidism
- hypoadrenalism
- obesity
- metabolic deficiency/poor diet
- drugs and medications: Tagamet, Inderal, benzodiazepines (see anxiety section), prednisone, alcohol, marijuana
- lack of exercise

- biochemical—low levels of the neurotransmitters serotonin and norepinephrine
- air pollution—decreased negative ions, increased positive ions
- decreased sunlight (seasonal depression)
- overcrowding
- lack of grounding in the earth
- nutritional deficiencies
- inhalant and food sensitivity reactions

Mind: Mental and Emotional

- distorted thinking (See list of thought distortions in chapter 4, page 115)
- grief—feelings of disconnection or loss
- feelings of failure
- lack of stimulation
- addiction to work
- low root chakra energy—sense of helplessness
- low throat chakra energy—lack of self-expression
- low solar plexus chakra energy—sense of powerlessness
- emotional traumas as a child: history of abuse or violence

Spirit: Spiritual and Social (Bioenergy)

- lack of purpose or meaning in life
- low heart chakra energy—feelings of isolation; lack of compassion or a committed loving relationship
- low crown chakra energy—disconnection from God

- spiritual issues are more prominent with severe or chronic depression

Holistic Medical Treatment and Prevention

Physical and Environmental Health Recommendations

Clean air and *exposure to nature* can benefit both depression and anxiety. In addition to **clean air, negative-ion-filled air** at levels above 3,000 ions/cu 1cm has been shown in various studies to enhance mood. **Sunlight** and **beautiful natural settings** can provide both a sense of grounding and relaxation.

Diet. There is a dynamic interaction between the foods that we eat and our mood. Although the brain is only 2 to 3 percent of our total body weight, it consumes more than 20 percent of our total energy supply! The brain has a voracious and continual appetite for a multitude of nutrients—vitamins, minerals, amino acids, carbohydrates, essential fatty acids, and accessory factors. It is often heard that "we *are* what we eat." We certainly *feel* what we eat.

The basic dietary recommendation for treating depression is a diet high in **protein** and **low in fat.** The frequent use of the spices **red pepper, garlic,** and **ginger** may also be helpful. It should also include one or two servings of **cold-water fish,** such as salmon or herring, per week, as they contain high amounts of essential fatty acids—see below. Caffeine, alcohol, and sugar should be eliminated.

Vitamins, minerals, and nutritional supplements. In many cases, natural products can have an effect upon mood that is greater than or equal to antidepressants. Although you should start out slowly and carefully consider your unique "biochemical individuality," the following amino acids, vitamins, minerals, and essential fatty acids are usually effective in treating depression.

L-phenylalanine (LPA) is an amino acid considered a most important and effective nutrient for treating depression. It is a precursor (directly on the formative pathway) to norepinephrine, one of the main neurotransmitters that govern mood. Many pharmaceutical antidepressants, such as desipramine and Wellbutrin, also work by raising the level of norepinephrine in the brain. In addition, LPA strengthens the entire metabolic pathway that produces the norepinephrine neurotransmitter, and it also enhances dopamine release at the pleasure centers in the brain. Unlike medications, it replenishes this pathway naturally. *Recommended dosage:* One should begin with 500 mg (one capsule), 2x/day, *on an empty stomach with juice.* This can gradually be increased by 500 mg per day, to two or three capsules, 3x/day. For maximum effect, it is best to take 50 mg of vitamin B_6 at the same time as well as niacin 500 mg per day and 1 gram of vitamin C. Vitamin B_6 is particularly important in regulating the absorption, metabolism, and utilization of amino acids.

L-tyrosine is an amino acid formed from phenylalanine and is one step closer than LPA to norepinephrine, the "excitatory" neurotransmitter that is so important in mood disorders. L-tyrosine is also quite effective in strengthening this entire metabolic pathway, as well as releasing dopamine at the pleasure centers in the brain. It is also important in the production of epinephrine, the "stress" neurotransmitter. *Recommended dosage:* As with LPA, it is recommended that one start with 500 mg (one capsule) of L-tyrosine, 2x/day, *on an empty stomach with juice.* This can also be increased by increments of 500 mg per day, up to two or three capsules (1,500 mg), 3x/day. It is also recommended that this be taken with 50 mg of vitamin B_6 to facilitate its absorption and 1 gram of vitamin C. **Note:** Some nutritional companies formulate both L-tyrosine and glutamine together. Glutamine is another excitatory amino acid that seems to combine quite well with L-tyrosine to improve its effectiveness. This combination capsule contains the correct ratio of both and may be taken up to six capsules per day in divided doses, on an empty stomach.

With both LPA and L-tyrosine, one needs to be watchful for increased blood pressure, headaches, or insomnia. These side effects are indications that an excessive stimulation of the nervous system has occurred. **DO NOT take these amino acids if you are currently taking standard antidepressant medications, especially MAO inhibitors. Also, avoid with the following conditions: phenylketonuria (PKU), hepatic cirrhosis, or melanoma.**

Like other essential amino acids, **tryptophan** cannot be manufactured by the body. Tryptophan must come directly from food or supplements. It is the building block for *serotonin,* the same neurotransmitter that Prozac influences in depression. When properly taken, tryptophan is extremely useful as a natural antidepressant as well as a sleep aid. Recently, the FDA lifted its ban on tryptophan, although it must be prescribed. Decades of previous use have already proven this amino acid's broad therapeutic effectiveness. *Recommended dosage:* For depressive symptoms, take 2 grams (2,000 mg) of tryptophan 2 or 3x/day. It should be taken between meals, with fruit or juice (simple sugars) to improve its utilization. It should not be taken with a protein meal, because tryptophan competes poorly with other amino acids for absorption. To convert tryptophan to serotonin the body must have adequate levels of folic acid, vitamin B_6, magnesium, niacin, and glutamine.

The amino acids LPA, L-tyrosine, and tryptophan should be tried one at a time. If after six weeks at a high dosage there is no improvement, then you should take a different amino acid.

The **B-complex vitamins,** along with **vitamin C** and **folic acid,** are critical cofactors in the production of neurotransmitters. Folic acid deficiency is a frequent cause of depression. With mood disorders in general, the addition of folate to one's diet often provides dramatic results. Vitamin C is also quite essential in the production of neurotransmitters, as well as for numerous other functions. *Recommended dosage:* In the case of a depressive

or anxiety disorder, it is suggested that one take 50 mg, twice per day, of **B-complex** (containing all of the B vitamins). Additionally, one needs to take more vitamin B_6 (150 mg per day) and vitamin B_{12} (1,000 mcg per day). **One should never take B_6 at doses higher than 100 mg per day for longer than two months (possibility of nerve damage). Folic acid** may be taken up to 5 mg (5,000 mcg) per day for one month, then 800 mcg per day. It is suggested that one take 1,000 mg of **vitamin C,** 3x/day. For an even greater effect on depression, one could take up to 500 mg per day of **niacinamide** (vitamin B_3). This is highly recommended by "orthomolecular" physicians. (This field of medicine uses high doses of natural nutrients to treat disease.)

Minerals are crucial micronutrients that can often be the source of a mood disorder. Of particular note is **magnesium,** which is necessary for the production of neurotransmitters and is frequently deficient in the American diet. **Zinc, calcium,** and **selenium** are additional micronutrients that are required in the metabolic pathways for mood regulation. These minerals are also quite important for one's immune and antioxidant systems. *Recommended dosage:* **Magnesium** and **calcium** should be taken in a one-to-one ratio—1,000 mg of each per day. The dosage of **zinc** for a mood disorder is 30–40 mg per day, and selenium 200 mcg per day.

Although still somewhat controversial, certain **essential fatty acids (EFAs)** have been shown to balance prostaglandin production and thereby improve depression. These fatty acids are necessary for healthy metabolism and cannot be synthesized by the body. Excellent sources of these precursor EFAs are evening primrose oil (omega-6) and flaxseed oil (omega-3). For men, EFAs are quite essential for sound prostate health, as well. *Recommended dosage:* Flaxseed oil can be taken in liquid form (one tablespoon per day) or capsule form (two capsules, 3x/day with meals). The dose of evening primrose oil should be two capsules (500 mg each), 3x/day, with meals.

Herbs. **St.-John's-wort (*Hypericum perforatum*)** is a natural herb and one of the most widely prescribed antidepressant medications in Europe. Various clinical studies have shown it to be as effective as standard antidepressants (amitriptyline and imipramine). The herb also has far fewer side effects. It is postulated that St.-John's-wort acts like a monoamine oxidase inhibitor, thereby increasing the amount of norepinephrine in the brain. This herbal remedy has been of interest to healers since early Greek times. *Recommended dosage:* The active ingredient in St.-John's-wort is hypericin. The dosage to be taken is 300 mg, 3x/day. (The extract should have a hypericin content that is standardized to 0.3 percent.) When using an herb, one should always note its potency, because it varies a great deal with each brand. A trial period of one month is adequate to determine its potential benefits.

Ginkgo biloba is one of the most well-researched herbs in the world and has been used for over five thousand years by healers in China and other countries. Widely pre-scribed by physicians in Europe, ginkgo improves cerebral circulation, improving memory and often benefiting depression, although this varies with each individual. Generally, ginkgo is not as effective as St.-John's-wort for depression, but it can be taken along with other herbs and nutrients to bolster one's overall mood. Ginkgo has also been found to enhance the effectiveness of pharmaceutical antidepressants when taken in combination with them. *Recommended dosage:* As with all herbs, the potency should be carefully noted. *Ginkgo biloba* should be in an extract that is standardized to contain 24 percent ginkgo flavoglycosides. The usual dose is 40 to 80 mg, 3x/day. Benefits with herbs and other nutrients often require more time than standard drugs. An advantage, however, is the safety in long-term use and absence of reported side effects.

Yohimbine is an herb that comes from the bark of trees found in West Africa. Used for decades in treating male impotence or diminished sexual interest, recent research indicates that yohimbine can also improve the overall effectiveness of standard antidepressant medications. It activates the central nervous system in ways that are not fully understood. In some cases, yohimbine can be used by itself to both stimulate sexual functioning in men and relieve mild depression. *Recommended dosage:* For mild depression and enhanced sexual functioning, take 5.4 mg of standardized yohimbine extract, 3x/day. Unfortunately, most of the commercially available products of yohimbine do not specify the actual content of the active yohimbine alkaloids. Prescribed yohimbine is easier to monitor. A suggested trial period for this yohimbine regimen would be two to three weeks. Yohimbine can then be taken periodically, as needed. **Note: For some individuals, yohimbine can cause increased anxiety or uncomfortable cardiac stimulation. It should be taken under the supervision of a health professional.**

Exercise. The beneficial effects of regular aerobic exercise in the treatment of depression are well documented. (See chapter 3 for more details.) Some psychotherapists believe **aerobic exercise,** through its powerful release of **endorphins,** may be the most effective as well as the most readily available antidepressant. It's especially important for depressed men to engage in some form of exercise that feels like fun! Studies have shown that 35 to 50 percent of depressed patients need no other treatment than aerobic exercise.

Traditional Chinese medicine—acupuncture and Chinese herbs—and homeopathic medicine. With a highly skilled practitioner, both of these therapies can be helpful in treating depression.

Mental and Emotional Health Recommendations

Psychotherapy. In addition to helping the patient see into his psychological problems, the **holistic psychotherapist** tries to raise the patient's awareness of life-force energy or spirit. The holistic psychotherapist will typically help the patient to discover his purpose and unique talents, interests, dreams, and desires in life. This orientation can also be described as **spiritual psychotherapy.** Providing the encouragement and motivation to change are the hallmarks of a skilled therapist. This can only be done by bringing out the assets and gifts in each person, as well as focusing on their current problems. Psychotherapy is most successful when the client establishes a comfortable therapeutic rapport with the therapist. Although this connection and trust is more important than the treatment model itself, several other psychotherapeutic options can be helpful in treating depression:

- cognitive/behavioral therapy—multiple studies have demonstrated its effectiveness in treating depression (discussed in chapter 4). Affirmations and visualization are an integral part of this form of therapy.
- psychosynthesis—a type of spiritual psychotherapy
- Hakomi therapy—a body-centered form of psychotherapy
- solution-focused/brief therapy—a goal-oriented form of psychotherapy
- spiritual psychotherapy—described above

Stress-reduction techniques. Each of the following can be helpful in treating both depression and anxiety.

Meditation is a sitting technique for calming the mind. A sound or mantra can be used as an "object of meditation." Transcendental meditation (TM) uses a repetitive phrase to focus one's attention. Another method is to focus attention on the breath or other body sensations, a technique used in Vipassana or Zen meditation. Whatever the specific method, the goal is to empty the mind of thoughts and to transcend feelings. Thus, the feedback loop—consisting of depressive thinking→anxiety→hopeless feelings→more depressive thinking—is diminished. This method of attaining inner peace and clarity has become increasingly popular in the West. It is discussed in greater detail in chapter 5.

Relaxation training teaches you to relax the body by progressively tensing and then relaxing various muscle groups. Variations include tensing the fists while rolling the eyes upward and holding your breath. You then sequentially relax the eyes, exhale, and release the tension in your fists. This produces a "letting go" effect that can then be enhanced by focusing on counting down from five to one, picturing each number in a different color. Unlike meditation, this method emphasizes physical relaxation. Since you can't think depressing thoughts while relaxing, this method is effective for relaxing the mind as well.

Breath techniques include various breathing methods derived from yoga and various forms of meditation. More recently, these practices have been used with good effect by patients of psychotherapy to calm the mind and body. Sometimes called **breath therapy,** these breath techniques include quickly paced, connected (no pause between inhalation and exhalation) mouth breathing (to evoke emotions). Breath therapy allows repressed emotions to surface and release. Alternating mouth-nose breathing is useful for centering, and alternating-nostril breathing enhances creativity (see Brain Booster in chapter 3, page 59). Some of these breathing techniques can be enhanced with imagery and music. All breathing methods have their own intention and rationale and can be quite helpful in treating depression and anxiety. To get started, work with a qualified breath therapist. These methods are quite easy to learn and highly effective.

Biofeedback training teaches you to control your physiology through the use of various visual or sensory cues. By allowing you to refocus energy in a more self-empowering way, it gives you a greater feeling of control over physiological response. With the help of a biofeedback technician, you are hooked up to an apparatus that measures physiological responses (heart rate, muscle tension, brain waves) while you focus on a sensory cue to help you relax. If you need technical confirmation that something is happening, this technique is for you. A variety of sounds, dials, and numbers document your deepening state of relaxation. Once you are familiar with your body's responses, you can effect those changes on your own without equipment.

Discussed in chapter 4, **journaling** is a technique for recording your emotions and understanding patterns of action based on your feelings. To begin to focus on positive happenings, try keeping a **gratitude journal.** This consists of writing each day about something for which you can be grateful. By making a daily gratitude entry each evening before bed, you neutralize the mind-set that focuses on what's wrong in your life—the depression cycle—and you begin to appreciate what's right.

Bioenergy. Depression (and anxiety) can commonly be associated with low energy in nearly every one of the **chakras** (see above "Risk Factors and Causes" for depression). Refer to the chakra diagram in chapter 4 (page 131) and try to determine which of the mental and emotional issues associated with each chakra apply to you. Therapeutic touch, healing touch, and *reiki* are **energy medicine therapies** that apply hands-on techniques to strengthen the most depleted chakras. The essence of this healing energy is love.

Qi gong is another effective way of treating both depression and anxiety. It is a moving meditation that strengthens the energy of each of the chakras. I don't know what the incidence of depression and anxiety is in China, but over 300 million Chinese practice *qi gong*.

Regular exposure to **sunlight** or **full-spectrum lights** that simulate sunshine can help treat depression, especially with people suffering from seasonal affective disorder (SAD). This condition is most prevalent during the winter months in places with little sunshine during this time of the year.

Hypnosis (hypnotherapy). This form of treatment can be quite effective with milder types of depression and anxiety. Hypnosis is an **altered state of consciousness** (ASC) in which certain senses are heightened and oth-

ers seem to fade into the background. It is *not* a state of sleep. While in a hypnotic trance, you become more aware of words and suggested images, and they grow more intense. Bodily sensations and time are often distorted. One does not require a deep trance for benefit to occur. A light trance is often adequate. Images of calm, relaxing scenes are often suggested for clients with anxiety. Although visual imagery is quite effective, much hypnotic benefit for anxiety is obtained by the simple act of learning to relax. It is often a revelation to learn that one *can* relax.

Progressive muscle relaxation is another form of hypnotherapy that is effective for anxiety. The client is instructed to start by tensing, then relaxing the muscles of the feet, then repeating this process up through the body, with each muscle group, all the way to the face and forehead (similar to relaxation training, described above).

Depression is often a pattern of seeing yourself and your life with a bleak sense of entrapment. Hypnotherapy can be used to imagine, while in a heighened state of suggestibility, more hopeful options and better methods of dealing with painful issues. While in a hypnotic state, one can visually rehearse newer ways to perceive oneself.

Self-hypnosis, which can easily be learned from a skilled therapist (and even from books), provides simple and effective methods for training yourself to enter hypnotic states. Audiotapes are also an excellent source of training in self-hypnosis and learning strategies to relax and reprogram habits of mind.

NLP (neurolinguistic programming) has proven extremely successful with intractable phobias and certain forms of anxiety. It utilizes transformational imagery to modify behavior and help reshape emotional patterns.

Body-work therapies. A multitude of hands-on techniques can help to release deeply held or repressed emotions. Some of these methods are described as **body-centered psychotherapy** and often combine deep-tissue body work, such as **Rolfing,** with types of **body movement,** such as **yoga** or **Feldenkrais.** Some of these therapies are described in chapter 4. Depression and anxiety are frequently more amenable to physical touch than verbal therapies. These therapies are particularly important for men with a history of physical abuse, somatic complaints, or poor body image.

Spiritual and Social Health Recommendations

Any of the recommendations made in chapters 5 and 6 are helpful in treating depression. However, of the spiritual practices, meditation, prayer, and altruism (volunteering) are possibly the most beneficial.

Joining or maintaining your connection to a **men's group,** or sustaining **individual friendships** with other men, is especially helpful for depressed men in strengthening their social health. Working on your committed relationship with a spouse or partner can often mitigate depression.

Anxiety

Symptoms and Diagnosis

Often called generalized anxiety disorder, anxiety is characterized by excessive worry (over work, finances, relationships, or health) that occurs chronically for at least six months. Men with this disorder find it difficult to control their worry, and their anxiety, with its physical symptoms, can cause significant distress or impairment in social, occupational, or other important areas of functioning. Typically anxiety is associated with three (or more) of the following six symptoms:

- restlessness or feeling keyed up or on edge
- being easily fatigued
- difficulty concentrating or mind going blank
- irritability
- muscle tension
- sleep disturbance (difficulty falling or staying asleep, or restless, unsatisfying sleep)

Conventional Medical Treatment

Conventional medical treatment for anxiety consists of **medication** and **psychotherapy.**

The medications for anxiety that are most often prescribed belong to the class of drugs called **benzodiazepines.** These include Xanax (alprozalam), Klonopin (clonazepam), Ativan (lorazepam), and Valium (diazepam). Although these medications act rapidly and effectively, relieve panic attacks and general anxiety, they can be addictive, impair memory, and increase tiredness. When carefully used, however, these medications can be quite helpful for a short time. Increasingly, psychiatrists are using SSRIs to treat anxiety, since anxiety and depression are so closely related.

Psychotherapy for anxiety includes those treatments described in the above section on psychotherapy for depression.

Risk Factors and Causes

The causes of *anxiety* include

- fearful relationships and situations that contribute to insecurity
- excess caffeine
- excess sugar, chocolate, NutraSweet
- stimulants—decongestants, No Doz, tobacco, asthma medications
- hyperthyroidism
- hyperadrenalism
- hypoglycemia
- nutritional deficiencies of B vitamins and magnesium
- history of trauma: physical or sexual abuse

Holistic Medical Treatment and Prevention

Physical and Environmental Health Recommendations

Air. Same as for depression.

Diet. The recommended diet for treating anxiety is high in **complex carbohydrates** (grains, pasta, vegetables), high in foods containing **L-tryptophan** (sunflower seeds, bananas, milk), and low in protein, fat (30 percent of calories), and spices. Avoid caffeine and alcohol.

Vitamins, minerals, and nutritional supplements. **Gamma amino butyric acid (GABA):** Most tranquilizers (Xanax, Ativan, Valium, etc.) work by stimulating the natural GABA receptors in the brain. This creates a calming effect. Occasionally, one does not have enough of this nonessential amino acid and requires GABA supplements. This "natural tranquilizer" has also been found to be quite useful for sleep. *Recommended dosage:* For daytime relaxation, take 750 mg of GABA, 3x/day. For sleep, take 1,500 mg before bed.

As with depression, **tryptophan** is often quite effective in dealing with anxiety. This amino acid is readily converted into **serotonin,** which is a calming neurotransmitter, as well as an antidepressant. It requires a carbohydrate such as fruit juice to facilitate its absorption and conversion, as well as vitamins B_3, B_6, and C. *Recommended dosage:* For anxiety, a 500-mg capsule of tryptophan, twice a day between meals, is often sufficient. As a sleep aid, tryptophan is also excellent. One can take 2 or 3 grams before bedtime, with a carbohydrate.

Vitamin C, at least 1,000 mg, 3x/day; **vitamin B complex** 50 mg, 2x/day; and **vitamin E,** 1,200 mg/day, can all contribute toward easing anxiety.

Magnesium, calcium, and **essential fatty acids** (EFAs) are all helpful in treating anxiety. Their daily requirements are the same as for depression.

Inositol is a unique B vitamin that has been found through research to reduce anxiety when taken in high doses. Its exact mode of action is unknown. Inositol may be an important nutrient, along with **choline,** for healthy brain-cell metabolism. *Recommended dosage:* To reduce anxiety or promote a more calm state of sleep, take inositol at doses of 4–6 grams. The dose can be adjusted upward until relief is obtained. There is no known toxicity to inositol, even at doses as high as 50 grams.

Herbs. **Kava kava** *(Piper methysticum)* is a botanical herb that has been successfully used by herbalists since the discovery of its use in Polynesia by Capt. James Cook. It is used for treating anxiety and promoting sleep. Kava kava is one of the new herbal "stars" that are becoming much more widely known and utilized as health practitioners discover their effectiveness. *Recommended dosage:* Kava kava is available in both liquid and capsule form. The standardized extract of its active ingredient, kavalactone, should be 30 percent or 15 mg per capsule. For daytime relief of anxiety, take 250 mg (one capsule or one-half dropperful), 3x/day with meals. One can take four to six capsules for sleep (up to 1,500 mg). As with all other medications and nutrients, each individual has his own biochemical individuality and needs to take responsibility for finding his own unique level. Kava kava should not be taken continuously for a prolonged period (over four months).

For over two hundred years the plant extract **valerian** has been the treatment of choice throughout the world for anxiety and insomnia. Although it is quite safe to take for short periods, its long-term effects are not known. *Recommended dosage:* For daytime anxiety, take 150 mg (standardized extract of 0.8 percent valeric acid), 3x/day. For difficulty with sleep, start with 150 mg, forty-five minutes before bed. If that dose is insufficient, gradually increase valerian to 600 mg.

Other herbs that can be used for treating anxiety **include passionflower, lemon balm,** and **skullcap.** The latter two are best for acute anxiety.

Exercise. Longer, low-intensity aerobic exercise requiring greater endurance, such as jogging, swimming, and hiking, is best for relieving anxiety.

Traditional Chinese medicine and homeopathy. As with depression, the treatment needs to be individualized and administered by a skilled therapist.

Mental and Emotional Health Recommendations

Almost every mental and emotional health technique recommended for depression is also effective for anxiety. These include
- psychotherapy
- stress-reduction techniques—meditation, relaxation training, breath therapy, and biofeedback training
- journaling
- bioenergy—working on all of the chakras

with mental/emotional issues associated with your condition

- hypnosis
- body-work therapies

Spiritual and Social Health Recommendations

These are the same as for depression, although meditation is particularly helpful for anxiety.

Addictions

Prevalence

Drug use in the United States has become an epidemic and is especially heavy among men. The incidence of alcoholism among men is five times greater than it is for women. Men use illicit drugs two to three times more than women. The national cost of alcohol and other drug abuse in terms of health care, absenteeism, and lost productivity is approximately $166 billion per year. Over 15 million people are estimated to experience significant health problems as a direct result of their alcohol use.

The diseases most often associated with alcohol abuse are liver disease (cirrhosis), cancer, and heart disease. Among young alcoholics, the death rates from suicide, accidents, and cirrhosis are ten times higher than normal. Alcoholics shorten their life expectancy by about twenty years, and nearly half of the violent deaths from accidents, suicide, and homicide are alcohol-related, as well as half of all automobile fatalities. At least 40 million spouses, children, and close relatives suffer from the destructive energy of alcohol abuse. These factors, combined with the effects of other drug abuse, add up to a significant social plague. Recent data shows that 63 percent of all people arrested have illegal drugs in their urine.

Conventional Medical Treatment

Conventional alcohol and drug-addiction rehabilitation programs usually involve detoxification, drug withdrawal, and counseling in both inpatient and outpatient settings. Through the 1980s many insurance companies were covering the costs of four-week stays at expensive (about $10,000 for one month of treatment) residential alcohol and rehabilitation centers. But with the growth of managed care and studies that show the inpatient programs to be no more effective than outpatient, the majority of the patients with addictions are now being treated as outpatients. In 1995, Kaiser Permanente of Colorado completed a study that revealed about 50 percent of the people who complete their outpatient addiction treatment programs remain clean and sober for at least one year.

Many men are required to enter these programs after early detection of their addiction in their workplace and are successful as a result of their strong motivation to retain their jobs. A man's fear of the loss of his job is often a more powerful motivator than the loss of his health.

Risk Factors and Causes

Physical and Environmental Factors

Genetics are an important factor in determining your predisposition to addictions. In identical (same genetic makeup) twins, if one twin is alcoholic, the chance of the other twin's being alcoholic is four times greater than if one fraternal (different genetic composition) twin is alcoholic. A **genetic study** done at UCLA found that sons of alcoholics run a serious risk at an early age of developing a craving for addictive drugs such as nicotine, marijuana, and alcohol. This suggests that the genetically addictive brain is biochemically altered so that the individual is more susceptible to craving for a range of addictive drugs and even compulsive disorders such as sex, food, and gambling addictions. **The conclusion from hundreds of studies is that alcoholism, and to some extent drug abuse, is more of a disease than a personality disorder.** The findings also confirm that irresistible cravings (alcohol, drug, and food addictions) and compulsive behavior disorders (sex and gambling addictions) are associated with a problem in the functioning of the reward-pleasure centers of the brain involving the neurotransmitters (serotonin, opioids, dopamine) and enzymes that control them. Although the malfunction begins with a gene, it can be made worse by psychological, sociological, and other environmental factors that can either trigger or mitigate genetic predisposition.

Researchers now believe that the root cause of addictive and compulsive diseases may be a **defect in the gene** that regulates the function of a specific receptor called dopamine D2, located in that part of the brain that is the center for feelings of reward. In addition to this genetic theory, some scientists also believe that the alcohol and drug abuse itself may actually cause a disruption in the normal neurotransmitter pathways that mimics the defects that were thought to be purely genetic. For example, habitual use of cocaine can cause these neurotransmitter changes in just a few weeks or months, after which they become difficult to reverse.

Hypoglycemia is a significant risk factor in causing alcoholism—some studies have suggested it may be present in 90 percent of alcoholics. With a drop in blood sugar (hypoglycemia), a number of symptoms can occur—rapid heart rate, hunger, excessive sweating, craving for sweets, headaches, loss of concentration, and anxiety. All of these symptoms can be immediately though temporarily relieved by drinking alcohol, which works powerfully as a sugar. Since marijuana, amphetamines, cocaine, nicotine, and caffeine can all produce these hypoglycemic symptoms, it is not uncommon for users of these drugs to frequently drink alcohol as well. Hypoglycemia can be a significant cause of depression, anxiety, and mental confusion. A weak pancreas and adrenal glands, as well as hypothyroidism and a poorly functioning pituitary gland, may contribute to hypoglycemia. It is part of a vicious cycle that leads to a dependency on alcohol to alleviate its symptoms.

Another factor contributing to the altered neurochemistry of the addictive brain may be **poor nutrition.** Ironically, we live in one of the most affluent nations in the world, yet our diets often fail to provide minimum nutritional benefit and can even be harmful. Our fast-food, high-sugar diets—consisting of synthetic foods heavily laced with pesticides, hormones, and herbicides—routinely deplete our vitality and contribute to a variety of diseases. There is certainly convincing evidence that our modern diet has created the growing problem of hyperactivity. Excessive sugar intake may also predispose children to developing the addictive brain neurochemistry that makes them susceptible to problems with alcohol, psychoactive drugs, and other compulsive disorders.

In addition to contributing to addictions, **nutritional deficiencies** can often result from alcohol and drug abuse. As deficiencies, in turn, create further cravings, the cycle of dependency can eventually alter brain biochemistry. The loss of nutrients can include the minerals zinc, chromium, manganese, magnesium, calcium, copper, and iron and the B vitamins.

Food allergy is also a cause of alcoholism. Some people are allergic to the foods from which alcohol is made, such as wheat, potatoes, or rye. One of the ways the body reacts to foods to which it is allergic is to produce its own addictive opioid endorphins. These create feelings of euphoria, then subsequent withdrawal or hangover, which is then relieved with more alcohol.

By altering brain chemistry, **environmen-tal toxins** such as gasoline, cleaning solvents, and formaldehyde (a common indoor air pollutant found in many building materials) can also contribute to alcoholism.

An excess of sugar and alcohol fuels an overgrowth of yeast *(Candida albicans)* organisms, called **candidiasis.** This condition can weaken the immune system, which even further stimulates the overgrowth of candida. Candidiasis mirrors many of the symptoms of hypoglycemia—especially fatigue and anxiety—which can temporarily be relieved by drugs and alcohol.

Mental and Emotional Factors

Chapters 4 and 5 detail several reasons why men probably experience alcohol and drug abuse to a much greater extent than women. These primarily relate to men's repression of feelings.

- Men do not release their emotional pain as easily as women.
- Men are more doers and tend to act out their pain with alcohol and drugs.
- There is more societal permission for men to drink alcohol and take drugs.
- Men are more out of touch with their spirit than women and use drugs to try to "feel something."
- Men find the machismo of drugs more exciting than do women.

Regardless of your genetic predisposition, emotions and belief systems can have a profound affect on creating addictive behavior. The probable **emotional causes** contributing to **alcohol abuse** can include feelings of guilt, hopelessness, self-rejection, or inadequacy. Emotional causes for **drug abuse** may include fear of taking responsibility or an inability to accept and love oneself. Louise Hay addresses the emotional sources of addictions in her book *You Can Heal Your Life.*

Holistic Medical Treatment and Prevention

The following holistic treatment program for addictions was developed by Gabriel Cousens, M.D.

Physical and Environmental Health Recommendations

Environment. As with the conventional medical approach, begin treating addictions in a somewhat secluded residential setting **away from home** in order to detach yourself from previous addictive behavior patterns. One of the most effective holistic retreat facilities for treatment of addictions is Dr. Cousens's Tree of Life Rejuvenation Center in Patagonia, Arizona. His program focuses on specific **biochemical repair.** Neurotransmitter pathways are maintained with a vegetarian diet, psychological, and spiritual support.

Diet. Reaching optimal blood pH is critical for maximum mental and metabolic functioning. Measuring blood pH in response to diet is an important part of the Tree of Life program. In this way they are able to personalize the vegetarian diet to create optimal acid-base balance. Since hypoglycemia—low blood sugar—plays such a significant role in con-

tributing to alcoholism, a **hypoglycemic diet** is recommended. Healthy snacks (nuts, seeds, fruit, or vegetables) between meals prevents a drop in blood sugar, which may trigger alcohol cravings. The first step in biochemical repair is to avoid all hypoglycemic activators such as sugars, caffeine, and nicotine (including chewing tobacco). These last two substances both produce hypoglycemic symptoms through an overstimulation of the adrenals that can keep the addictive cycle going. The dietary emphasis for treating addictions is to eat whole and organic foods, free of additives, chemicals, and hormones.

Vitamins, minerals, and nutritional supplements. The following nutrients are an integral part of a holistic alcohol and drug addiction program, primarily because they help to relieve and prevent hypoglycemia, which contributes significantly to the cycle of addiction. Combined with an individualized neurotransmitter and endocrine rebuilding program, these nutrients are best administered by a highly skilled holistic practitioner. They include

- chromium picolinate—to rebalance sugar metabolism
- glutamine—to reduce the craving for alcohol, other drugs, and sugar. It also stimulates GABA production (see holistic treatment for anxiety), which helps with sleep and relaxation. Dosage: 1,000 mg, 4 to 6x/day between meals on an empty stomach.
- calcium and magnesium—to aid in detoxification, relax the system in a way

that diminishes irritability, anxiety, unstable emotions, muscle spasm, and insomnia

- pantothenic acid—to strengthen the adrenals for the normal production of all the adrenal hormones, and to diminish sugar cravings
- niacin—to stabilize blood sugar
- vitamin C and B complex—to help relieve adrenal stress
- vitamins B_6, B_3, copper, iron, folic acid, phenylalanine, and tyrosine—to aid in biochemical repair of the dopamine neurotransmitter system

Exercise. Regular aerobic exercise is useful in revitalizing a body debilitated by drug and alcohol addiction.

Candida treatment program. This consists of a strict candida-control diet. Antifungal prescription drugs, such as Nizoral, Diflucan, or Sporonox, can be used with caution (they are potentially toxic to the liver). With alcohol addiction, it is preferable to use a homeopathic remedy to kill the candida, along with an acidophilus/bifidus preparation. A number of books are available on treating candida, which is also covered in detail in *Sinus Survival.*

Acupuncture. Acupuncture has been used successfully to treat addictions by Lincoln Hospital in New York City for over twenty years. Increasingly acupuncture has proven to be effective at treatment centers throughout the country for the detoxification and withdrawal from drugs, alcohol, and nicotine.

Mental and Emotional Health Recommendations

Refer to "Holistic Medical Treatment and Prevention" for depression for an explanation of these therapies. Since addictions typically accompany depression, many of the following therapies are effective for both conditions.

- psychotherapy
- stress-reduction techniques
- journaling
- bioenergy
- hypnosis
- body-work therapies

Spiritual and Social Health Recommendations

A number of twelve-step programs with a spiritual orientation are helpful in overcoming addictions. The most popular perhaps, Alcoholics Anonymous (AA), is quite helpful in treating alcoholism by providing group support for abstinence and behavioral modification. The holistic spiritual and social recommendations for treating drug or alcohol addictions are the same as for treating depression.

The effectiveness of the biochemical aspect of Dr. Cousens's holistic approach, outlined in this chapter, for treating **alcohol addiction** has been validated by an independent study done by Joan Matthews Larson, Ph.D. at the Health Recovery Center in Minneapolis, Minnesota, and a number of other studies. Dr. Larson's study was published in the *International Journal of Biosocial and Medical Research*. The study documented the following results:

- Alcohol cravings from the outset to discharge had dropped from 84 percent to 9 percent.
- Anxiety dropped from 64 to 11 percent.
- Poor memory dropped from 69 to 11 percent.
- Insomnia dropped from 44 to 6 percent.
- Tremors and shakiness dropped from 44 to 2 percent.
- Depression dropped from 61 to 5 percent.

Dr. Cousens's holistic treatment program has been found to be effective in treating drug abuse as well. With the biochemical approach alone, research at the Health Recovery Center showed that 92 percent of the clients were abstinent after six months, and 74 percent remained abstinent three and one-half years later. This compares to an average abstinence rate of 25 percent for clients using other drug treatment programs at one year. This is the same rate as for those who tried to break their drug addiction without using any program.

Dr. Cousens attributes the success of his holistic medical treatment program for alcohol and drug addiction to its emphasis on the repair of the body **as well as** the mind and spirit.

The primary contributors to this chapter are Gabriel Cousens, M.D.; Harriet Ivker, L.C.S.W., a psychotherapist practicing in Littleton, Colorado; Joel Miller, M.D., a psychiatrist in Denver, Colorado; and Scott Shannon, M.D., a psychiatrist in Greeley, Colorado.

C a r d i o v a s c u l a r   D i s e a s e

Coronary Artery Disease (CAD)
(Heart Disease)
Hypertension
(High Blood Pressure)

Prevalence

Arteriosclerosis—"hardening of the arteries"—including heart disease, is of fairly recent origin. Before 1920, heart attacks and strokes due to hardening of the arteries were extremely rare. By 1950, heart attacks had become the leading cause of death in the United States and Europe. Known medically as myocardial infarctions, heart attacks cause 20 percent of all deaths in the United States, and total arteriosclerotic events are by far the leading cause at 30 percent of all deaths. Heart attacks, however, reached their peak in 1968 and since then have steadily declined in both incidence and death rate. By 1994, heart attacks had decreased by 50 percent and the incidence of strokes was down by 60 percent. Although we've made good progress with both preventive and therapeutic measures, heart disease is still the leading killer of men.

Anatomy

The heart is a fist-sized organ located to the left of the midline between the lungs. It is a muscular organ with hollow chambers separated by valves that assist the heart in its function of supplying blood to the organs of the body. The two right chambers drive blood through the lung circuit where carbon dioxide is exchanged for fresh oxygen. The left two chambers, which pump more powerfully, provide the pressure to draw the oxygen into the blood from the lungs and drive it to the farthest reaches of the rest of the body.

The heart supplies blood to itself through a series of *coronary arteries,* the largest of which are located on the heart's outside surface, facing the lungs and other tissues. When these coronary arteries are severely blocked and the blood vessel walls degenerate, the condition is known as *arteriosclerosis* (or atherosclerosis). In the heart, this obstructive process is called coronary artery disease (CAD), or ischemic heart disease (IHD).

Symptoms and Diagnosis

Coronary artery disease most commonly manifests as angina, a pressure-like, squeezing type of pain in the left-center chest and frequently radiated to the left shoulder and left upper arm. The pain can occasionally radiate, also, to the neck, chin or back. Angina usually occurs with physical exertion or marked stress and typically subsides in a few minutes with rest. The pain is often accompanied by sensations of shortness of breath and anxiety, and at times is misdiagnosed as heartburn or indigestion. Angina is usually present when at least one constricted artery approaches 75 percent obstruction.

On investigation, the suspected diagnosis of coronary artery disease can be confirmed by abnormalities of:

1. electrocardiograms taken while walking on a treadmill
2. arteries seen with injections of dye with angiograms
3. heart circulation with radioisotope scans

Some one-third of men experiencing a heart attack have not had these warning signs of angina—or the anginal episodes have been ignored or unrecognized. About 30 to 40 percent of men experiencing a heart attack die before reaching a hospital.

Conventional Medical Treatment and Prevention of Heart Disease

Perhaps because many of its risk factors and causes have been well-identified, conventional medicine now does more to prevent the onset of heart disease than it does for any other chronic disease. The conventional medical prevention of and treatment for CAD begins with taking a **history** to determine any significant **hereditary risk** for arteriosclerosis and to ascertain the presence of any symptoms of exertional chest pain, shortness of breath, or heart rhythm disturbances. **Examination** for early evidence of hardening of the arteries, sometimes ascertainable quite early in the retina of the eyes, is followed by the laboratory assessment of blood **cholesterol** and **triglyceride** levels.

Once arteriosclerotic disease or high levels of cholesterol have been diagnosed, conventional treatment emphasizes physical **exercise** and aerobic activity. Smoking is strongly discouraged, and nicotine addiction is treated with prescriptions for nicotine patches and/or gum. Conventional measures also reduce **cholesterol** by dietary restriction of cholesterol and fat, and by prescribing cholesterol-lowering drugs.

The lowering of the fat content in the diet appears to be helpful and much more effective than the limitation of cholesterol. The fear of egg yolks, which are high in cholesterol, has largely been dispelled by numerous studies showing that reasonable egg consumption bears little if any relationship to blood cholesterol.

Drugs employed to artificially **lower blood cholesterol** levels include colestipol (Colestid), cholestyramine (Questran), clofibrate (Atromid-S), gemfibrozil (Lopid), lovastatin (Mevacor), pravastatin (Pravachol), simvastatin (Zocor), probucol (Lorelco) and niacin (vitamin B_3) derivatives (Nicobid, Nicolar).

Medical science continues to debate the use of cholesterol-lowering drugs. Although many early studies found that administering drugs lowered cholesterol and in some instances lowered the incidence of heart attacks, the gains were generally small. It was found that **total mortality from all causes was greater than in groups in which no drugs were used.**

A 1992 article in *Circulation* found that in eighteen of nineteen studies, aggressive attempts using drugs to lower cholesterol increased the incidence of chronic obstructive pulmonary disease, hemorrhagic stroke, pneumonia, influenza, liver cirrhosis, digestive diseases, alcohol dependence, suicide, and malignancies (including liver and lung cancer, lymphomas, and leukemias). **Significantly increased mortality from all causes appeared in the groups of persons who used drugs to markedly decrease their serum cholesterols.** These alarming associations tended to be present to the greatest extent in persons whose blood cholesterol was below 160 mg/dl; in some studies these associations appeared only in

persons in whom drugs had been used to lower cholesterols. The same study in *Circulation* also warned of significant mortality risks from cancer, cerebral hemorrhage, suicide, and alcoholism when drugs were used to lower cholesterol.

Depression has also been linked to very low blood cholesterol levels, whether resulting from treatment or not. In men over seventy, depression was three times more common in those with low cholesterol compared to those with higher concentrations. In September of 1991, the *Journal of the American Medical Association (JAMA)* reported a study of twelve hundred healthy business executives with risk factors for CAD. The group intensively treated with cholesterol-lowering and blood-pressure-lowering drugs reduced CAD risk factors 46 percent compared to the control group treated in the "usual" fashion. **However, ten years later, there had been 45 percent more deaths from all causes in the aggressively treated intervention group compared to the "usual care" control group.**

Another concern arose with the findings that treatment with Colestid, 30 mg daily for six months, in patients with one subtype of hereditary cholesterol problems resulted in a 30 percent reduction in blood carotene (a critical antioxidant) concentrations. The "statin" cholesterol-lowering drugs—Mevacor, Pravachol, and Zocor—also partially block the body's synthesis of coenzyme Q10, a powerful antioxidant that itself is of value in preventing and treating heart disease. Although initial reports of treatment with statin drugs have demonstrated decreases in both cardiovascular deaths and deaths from all causes, caution may well be advised, since undesirable results of previously used cholesterol-lowering drugs became apparent only after ten years of use.

One British author found a higher mortality in patients treated with Atromid-S or Lopid than those treated with a placebo, and insignificant differences with Questran versus placebo. A Swedish authority reviewed twenty-two cholesterol-lowering trials between 1970 and 1990 and concluded that **lowering serum cholesterol does not reduce mortality and is unlikely to prevent coronary artery disease.**

Conventional **surgical treatment** of advancing coronary artery disease utilizes procedures to dilate constrictions in coronary arteries—**angioplasty** or **balloon dilation**—and **coronary bypass surgery** to fashion new channels around constricted areas. Recent reports are less enthusiastic about balloon catheter procedures because constrictions commonly recur after weeks or months. Although bypass surgery appears to help reestablish circulation temporarily and give relief of anginal pain, a significant portion of bypass grafts are found to be closed off after a few months or years, blocked by the development of plaque in the bypass graft or by clotting. **These procedures do nothing to halt or reverse the insidious progression of the arteriosclerosis.** One year after surgery, arteriosclerosis is found in the grafts of one of every three patients operated on.

At times of acute heart attack, conventional treatment focuses on injection of substances to dissolve the clot that is frequently the terminal event completely sealing off an important artery. The use of heparin, an anti-clotting agent, has also shown promise.

The use of **aspirin, a platelet inhibitor, reduces the risks of second stroke and coronary events** and has been suggested as a preventive in patients with known coronary artery disease and stroke risks.

Risk Factors and Causes of Heart Disease

Most authorities agree that **the initiating event in arteriosclerosis consists of a mild injury to the lining cells of the arteries.** The cause of most of these vessel injuries has so far escaped scientific explanation. These small tears have been observed in autopsy specimens in children as young as eight years of age. The body sends inflammatory chemicals and platelets (a blood-clotting factor) to the site of the injury to begin the healing. Precipitated by free radicals, this inflammatory process is similar to the redness and swelling seen about three to five days after a wound of the skin. Healing progresses to the anti-inflammatory stage, provided that adequate **antioxidant substances** (including vitamins A, C, and E) are present to neutralize any tendency of the free-radical reactions to proliferate out of control. If the free-radical oxidation of fatty acids is not neutralized, a destructive reaction follows that can cause toxic changes in the arterial lining cells that incorporate oxidized "bad" cholesterol (LDL) into a thickening called **plaque.** Made up of a combination of proteins, blood platelets, cholesterol, fibrin (a blood-clotting factor), and inflammatory chemicals, plaque can also attract calcium, creating a hardness that gives rise to the term **hardening of the arteries.**

This hardening and thickening occurs throughout much of the arterial system of the entire body, and its resulting obstructions look like hardened sludge inside a forty-year-old iron water pipe. Arteriosclerosis can progress to cause heart attacks, strokes, and loss of circulation to the kidneys and legs. As more and more plaque is deposited, the walls of the arteries thicken, resulting in symptoms of compromised blood supply when the hollow, blood-carrying space inside the artery is at least 75 percent choked off.

Authorities call heart attacks and strokes **lifestyle diseases.** They are related to the following four factors: (1) From the 1920s to the 1960s, adult smoking increased dramatically, reaching a high of 46 percent of all adults by the late sixties. (2) By the mid-twentieth century, people living in industrialized nations consumed much less complex carbohydrates—starchy vegetables, whole grains, and legumes—and greatly increased their consumption of sugar and fat compared to the late 1800s. (3) As a nation we became much more sedentary, as (4) psychological and social stresses grew enormously.

All of these factors contributed to this rapid rise of heart disease as the number one cause of death. Coronary artery disease, which can lead to heart attacks, can result from a number of these risk factors. The classical risk factors include heredity, diabetes, and lifestyle, including smoking, high cholesterol, and high blood pressure.

Physical and Environmental Factors

Heredity. It is known that severe genetic problems contribute to CAD in a small number of families, in which some males can have heart attacks in their twenties. In a larger group of genetically linked subtypes of heart disease, the hereditary influence is present but not nearly so devastating.

People with **diabetes** run higher risks for development of arteriosclerosis and heart disease. Higher blood insulin levels predispose diabetics to a decrease of fat metabolism, which can speed up the degenerative changes leading to arteriosclerosis. Type II diabetes, related to a moderately strong genetic predisposition, leads to several other biochemical changes including higher compensating levels of corticosteroids, greater biochemical stress, and formation of destructive forms of oxygen called free radicals.

Research in the 1960s and 1970s established **high blood pressure**—hypertension—as a risk factor for the development of coronary heart disease. Not only does elevated blood pressure further damage the lining of arteries, the stress factors that predispose people to develop high blood pressure in the first place also contribute to the biochemical changes producing more free radicals and deterioration of blood vessel walls.

The advent of mass-produced cigarettes and their eventual use by 46 percent of adults in the United States by the 1960s makes **smoking** a significant personal environmental contributor to CAD. The recent reduction in smoking, one of the classical risk factors for heart attacks, has been a contributor to the decline in heart disease.

There is no question about the relationship of **high cholesterol** and the future risk of heart attack and stroke. The causes of high cholesterol in most people are still questioned. Some 80 percent of the cholesterol in the body at any time is synthesized in the liver. The remainder comes from dietary sources. Cholesterol is an essential chemical that in turn produces several major hormones including progesterone, estrogen, testosterone, cortisone, and dehydroepiandrosterone (DHEA). The evidence that high dietary intake of cholesterol can lead to the deposit of cholesterol in arterial walls is not persuasive. There is much more evidence that oxidized fats (rancidified fats) promote free-radical changes in the lipoproteins that carry cholesterol in the bloodstream. These lipoproteins trigger a complicated process in which damaged areas in arterial walls undergo changes in lining cells, which then begin to take in cholesterol and debris from the bloodstream. Over the years, this can lead to the thickening and buildup of cholesterol plaque and the narrowing of the arteries.

Recent careful research, however, has found that classical risk factors do not by any means account for all heart attacks. One analysis showed that 50 percent of men hav-

ing heart attacks had none of the three risk factors that most authorities put at the top of the list: high cholesterol, high blood pressure, and smoking. Another study showed that 46 percent of men with triple-vessel coronary artery disease had excellent levels of "good" cholesterol. A third found that risk for dying from all causes for the 25 percent of men with the highest cholesterol levels was only 21 percent higher than for the 25 percent of men with the lowest levels.

Several **other risk factors** are less accepted by many authorities. However, solid evidence shows that some of these may be more important than the classical risk factors. These additional risk factors include the following:

The presence of a **diagonal earlobe crease** has been recognized as a clinical sign of early arteriosclerotic disease. Not a true risk factor, this early indicator is nonetheless a reliable predictor of increased risk of later cardiac events.

Height can be a mitigating factor for heart disease. Men taller than six feet one inch experience a 35 percent lower risk of heart attack compared to very short men. The reason for the association is unclear.

Homocysteinemia is a hereditary defect in the metabolism of two amino acids, methionine and cysteine. Authorities believe that this defect alone explains up to 20 percent of the total risk for arteriosclerotic cardiovascular disease. This genetic defect can be totally overcome through the use of vitamins. We'll discuss this shortly.

Elevated fibrinogen is in part genetically

determined. It can appear in diabetes, obesity, high blood pressure, kidney disease, excessive blood clotting, elevated bad cholesterol (LDL-C), low levels of good cholesterol (HDL-C), high blood triglycerides (fats), and during stress. Fibrinogen is a critical factor in blood-clot formation and excess levels hasten clot formation. The final insult in most heart attacks is the formation of a clot in a narrowed artery. Fibrinogen may also contribute directly to the formation of plaque in arterial walls. High plasma fibrinogen is a powerful independent risk factor for heart attack.

Nutrition remains a primary causative factor in arteriosclerosis. Since arteriosclerosis is a relatively new disease on the medical scene, it seems reasonable to look at what specific nutritional shifts preceded the rise of heart disease beginning in the 1920s.

Refining of grains became widespread from 1870 to 1920. The removal of the bran and germ, containing scores of vital nutrients, from wheat, rice, and other grains, resulted in refined and bleached flour with an extremely long shelf life as it practically never turned rancid. Unfortunately, refining also removed 25–98 percent of the many vitamins and minerals in these grains—nutrients essential to reducing the incidence of heart attacks.

Consumption of starch and most whole grains, except rice, declined steadily, until by 1970 the per-person intake of total grains was over 50 percent lower than in 1880. The decrease in whole-grain intake, and the resulting depletion of vitamins and minerals, predisposed Americans to an acceleration of arteriosclerotic problems.

As whole-grain consumption declined, the intake of refined sugar increased. In the century between 1880 and 1980, sugar intake jumped from 4 percent to 20 percent of total caloric intake. Like refined carbohydrates, sugar has had the vitamins and minerals removed. The evidence for increased dietary sugar contributing to the increase in heart disease is so strong that in 1992 the *Journal of the Royal Society of Medicine* concluded that there was **more evidence of sugar as a cause of coronary artery disease than there was for dietary fat and cholesterol.**

To compensate for the loss of calories from reduced consumption of whole grains, Americans increased their intake of calories from fats and oils. Average fat intake reached 45 percent of calories by 1980 and has only recently dropped to 35–40 percent. As Americans' intake of protein shifted more and more to animal sources, saturated fat comprised a larger share of those calories. Well-founded evidence shows that the increase in total fat and saturated fat has contributed significantly to the acceleration of heart disease. After World War II, polyunsaturated fats from seed sources were believed to have less heart-disease risk than saturated fats, whose source was mainly animal meats and dairy products. However, it wasn't long before evidence showed that polyunsaturated oils have two hazards: oxidation and hydrogenation. Oxidation (or rancidification) occurs rapidly as unsaturated chemical bonds are saturated with oxygen. Hydrogenation of vegetable oil interferes with omega-3 and omega-6 metabolism and increases deficiencies of these essential fatty acids. A high percentage of unsaturated oils are hydrogenated to margarine, hydrogenated peanut butter, or solidified vegetable cooking fat. Margarines are no better than saturated fats, and many authorities believe they are actually worse. Fats that are oxidized before being consumed increase the free-radical oxidation of low-density lipoprotein cholesterol (bad cholesterol), which can induce arteriosclerotic deterioration. The mild reduction in total fat intake since 1980 has contributed to the decline of heart disease.

Evidence surfacing in the scientific literature in the early 1980s suggested that **excess stores of iron** were also linked with heart disease. Women who had undergone hysterectomies in their twenties tended to have heart attacks in their thirties and forties—much earlier than most women. They were also found to have increased levels of stored iron. Women who continued to menstruate lost blood and iron every month and did not build up excess stores of iron. Though that report did not attract much interest in medical circles, a much larger study of nearly two thousand Scandinavian men, published in 1992, found the same thing: men with high iron stores had over twice the risk for heart attack as low-storage-iron men.

Not only has our increased consumption of refined grains and sugars created nutritional **deficiencies of vitamins, minerals, and essential fatty acids,** but the average intake of fruits and vegetables among Americans has also declined from the 1880s to the 1970s. This has further restricted vitamin and mineral sources.

Magnesium deficiency produces elevated cholesterol, triglycerides, and "bad" cholesterol (LDL) as well as decreased HDL ("good") cholesterol. In a study of 570 healthy men with no initial evidence of coronary artery disease, the initial average daily magnesium intake of those experiencing heart attacks within five years was 275 mg/day compared to 310 mg/day for those who remained free of heart disease. Magnesium intakes were calculated from meticulous seven-day, weighed duplicate food records.

Deficiencies of zinc, chromium, folic acid, and vitamins B_6 and B_{12} promote and accelerate arteriosclerosis and coronary artery disease. **Copper deficiency** increases the risk of weakening of large arterial walls leading to aneurysms, which may rupture and terminate life abruptly.

Greenland Eskimos, with high amounts of **omega-3 (fish) oils** in their diet have a low rate of heart attack in spite of a high-fat diet. In the United States, following heart attacks, men who eat more omega-3-oil-containing fish have a significantly lower complication rate than those who don't eat fish.

Numerous studies have found that **reduced levels of antioxidants** consisting of major nutritional **vitamins C** and **E,** and **beta-carotene** (made by the body into vitamin A), significantly increase the risk of heart attack as well as stroke. One European study concluded that low vitamin E blood levels are a threefold better predictor of death from heart attack than smoking, high cholesterol, or high blood pressure.

Some, but not all, studies have found the

risk for heart attack rises progressively with increased **caffeine** consumption. In one study, one–two cups/day increased risk 40 percent, five–nine cups/day 80 percent, and over ten cups/day 190 percent.

Another factor contributing to the spectacular rise in heart disease from 1920 to 1968 was the increasingly **sedentary lifestyle** of people whose lives were aided by "labor-saving devices." The number of jobs in society requiring great physical exertion has slowed to a trickle. Being physically unfit greatly increases risk of heart attack (see chapter 3). Mortality rates from heart attacks and strokes are 60 percent lower in the most fit compared to the least fit. Men engaging in medium to high physical activity had a 50 percent lower risk of cardiovascular disease than those participating in only mild physical activity.

Increased air pollution in cities and other areas has also contributed to the increased incidence of heart disease. Air pollution with particulate matter and petroleum residues and industrial solvents, heavy metals, nitrous oxides, and sulphur dioxides have all been on the list of causes. Studies of matched pairs of workers have shown a 30 percent greater risk of death from heart attacks in blue-collar workers exposed to petrochemicals and solvents in their working atmosphere than in white-collar workers who were not as exposed. Improvement in pollution problems may also have contributed to the declining incidence of heart disease since 1968.

Biochemical risk factors for heart disease include a **deficiency of coenzyme Q10 and L-carnitine.** Coenzyme Q10 (ubiquinone) is a chemical taken into the body in small amounts in nutritional form but is largely supplied from synthesis within vital organs. It plays a critical role in energy transport systems in the cells of the body. Blood levels and tissue biopsy levels of coenzyme Q10 in patients with heart disease are significantly lower than in normal persons with healthy hearts. It is deficient in persons with congestive heart failure.

L-carnitine is a nonessential amino acid synthesized from betaine in the liver and kidney. It is present in high concentrations in heart and skeletal muscle. It facilitates movement of chemicals across the membrane of tiny energy units within the cells called mitochondria. Carnitine is essential in energy production and utilization within all body cells, including arterial wall lining cells and heart muscle cells. In coronary artery disease it is easily displaced and lost from heart muscle cells. It is also deficient in persons with heart failure.

Significantly lower levels of dehydroepiandrosterone (DHEA) and **testosterone** are commonly found in men over fifty with heart disease. Over a twelve-year period, men with low DHEA were three times more likely to die from arteriosclerosis and one and a half times more likely to die from all causes than those whose levels were high. The lower the level of DHEA, the higher the rate of death from all causes and death from cardiovascular disease in men over fifty. Low testosterone levels are also found in men who later develop coronary heart problems.

Mental and Emotional
Risk Factors

That nine o'clock on Monday morning is the peak hour of the week for heart attacks is testimony to the devastating effect of **work stress.** From 9–11 A.M. on Mondays is the peak two-hour period of the week for strokes. In primate research, monkeys placed under stress developed significantly more hardening of the arteries than unstressed monkeys whether they were on either high- or low-fat diets. Clearly stress had proven even more important than nutrition.

The risk of heart attack in the first twenty-four hours after the **loss of a spouse or loved one** is fourteen times greater than normal. In the second twenty-four hours, that rate is eight times higher. In the third twenty-four hours, the rate is six times greater, and over the ensuing month, the risk of heart attack remains two to four times the rate of persons who have not experienced this type of loss. **Depression** is the best predictor of serious cardiovascular events such as heart attacks, more so than any other risk factor. Depressed patients after heart attack are six times more likely to die within eighteen months compared to patients who are not depressed.

Type A behavior—typified by an attitude of hostility with resulting high levels of anxiety and accompanying anger—is also an established contributor to heart attacks. Medical students exhibiting high levels of hostility were found in the next twenty-five years as physicians to have four and one-half times the incidence of heart attacks compared to low-hostility medical students/physicians. The risk of having a heart attack increases two and one-half times within two hours after intense anger.

The risk of heart attack has been shown to be significantly higher in men with **control issues**—a fear of losing control—and in those men with **insomnia,** or sleep problems.

Spiritual and Social
Risk Factors

The stress of **social isolation and loneliness** increases the risk of heart disease. Divorced, separated, and widowed men living alone share this risk. More specifically, coronary artery disease is significantly more common in those who are not intimate in relationships. **Fourth chakra** energy is connected to feelings of compassion and the experiences of unconditional love. Heart disease is related to vulnerability and **the predisposition to be critical and judgmental of ourselves.** Blocked energy at this level manifests as a deficiency in giving and receiving love, excessive fear, guilt over acts of neglect, and bitterness deriving from the belief that one cannot forgive—**the hardened heart.**

Holistic Medical Treatment
of Heart Disease

Physical and Environmental
Health Recommendations

The holistic approach to treatment of coronary artery disease and arteriosclerosis in general begins with **prevention.** Nothing can be done to change the hereditary risk in those few persons with genetically determined, inexorably progressive cholesterol deposition. It is important for all people, however, whether burdened with bad heredity or not, to realize that lifestyle factors play an extraordinarily large role.

Diet. **Prevention** of heart disease begins, as does the prevention of most degenerative disease, by increasing the sources of **whole foods,** particularly fruits, vegetables, whole unrefined grains, fiber, vitamins, and minerals. As recommended in the *Thriving* diet (chapter 3), increase your intake of fruits plus vegetables per day to five or more servings—only 8 percent of Americans meet that standard. Increase daily fiber to at least fifteen grams. Whole grains, fruit and fibrous vegetables, legumes, and members of the bean families supply a surprising amount of fiber. Olive oil appears to be the best vegetable lipid source for use in salads and for sautéing. Increased consumption of fish and fish oil supplies more omega-3 oils, which bring many benefits. Garlic and onions both have active ingredients that reduce blood pressure and improve cholesterol ratios.

Avoid saturated fat (meats and whole-milk dairy products), margarine and other hydrogenated vegetable oils, refined flour products, sugar, and foods lacking fiber. The vast majority of bakery products are still made with refined and bleached white flour, and white-rice consumption far outstrips brown-rice intake. **Reduction of total fat**

and oxidized fat in the diet is important in the treatment of heart disease. Simply following the **Thriving Food Pyramid** (page 70) will reduce fat to 20–30 percent of caloric intake, the desirable range. Remember that margarines and hydrogenated cooking fats should also be minimized; they are probably worse than butter.

Reducing dietary cholesterol from eggs does not consistently affect serum cholesterol. Its effects are probably essentially neutral. **You needn't restrict egg consumption to a significant degree.**

Sucrose (table sugar) in large amounts has repeatedly been shown to decrease HDL (good cholesterol) and increase triglycerides. Persons with sugar cravings and a sweet tooth are particularly at risk.

High fiber diets consistently reduce total cholesterol, LDL, and HDL levels; the latter is affected less, however.

Minimizing coffee and caffeine intake is a wise preventive measure.

Essential fatty acids, including those found in olive oil, are more resistant to oxidation. Eicosapentaenoic and docosahexaenoic acid (omega-3 oils), found primarily in fish and certain plants, given in large amounts (6–12 gm/day), neutralize part of the inflammatory process leading to plaque in arterial walls and are thus helpful in treatment. Flaxseed oil, one to two tablespoonfuls daily, is an acceptable alternative.

In persons with known coronary or cerebral arteriosclerosis, **antiplatelet factors** can reduce clotting tendencies in the same way aspirin does. Nutrients including adequate amounts of vitamins B_6, choline, C, and E, omega-3 oils, magnesium, garlic, and onions in the diet can be very effective in this regard. Some studies have shown vitamin E to be 20–45 percent better than aspirin for this purpose. Bromelain, a proteolytic enzyme of the pineapple plant, also inhibits the platelet aggregation (stickiness), which leads to clot formation.

Alfalfa in animal studies tends to break down cholesterol plaques and helps the rebuilding of arterial walls.

More important than reducing cholesterol is **achievement of a better balance of antioxidants to free radicals,** which leads to both improvement in cholesterol ratios and reduction of coronary plaque. The reasonable reduction of cholesterol is a worthy goal, but can often be accomplished by decreasing free radicals through lifestyle change and the addition of nutritional antioxidants.

Vitamins, minerals, and nutritional supplements. To prevent deficiencies that accelerate arteriosclerosis, take adequate daily amounts of the following **vitamins:**

- C—1 gram or more
- beta-carotene—15,000–25,000 IU
- B_1—25 mg or more
- B_2—10–25 mg
- B_6—25–100 mg
- B_{12}—100–200 mcg
- folic acid—400 mcg
- E—400 IU

Niacin (vitamin B_3) decreases serum cholesterol up to 20 percent and triglycerides up to 40 percent when taken in 500–1,500 mg amounts daily. Many people will have marked flushing of the skin when taking niacin. The flushing of the skin is a nuisance and not a medical problem and is often greatly reduced by taking niacin with food. There is also a "flush free" brand of niacin found in some health food stores called Niacitol. The usual dosage is 500 mg 2x/day. "Good" cholesterol (HDL) frequently increases with niacin.

Pantethine (vitamin B_5), 300 mg three times daily, also increases HDL while lowering total cholesterol and triglycerides. It is rapidly depleted in hearts with deficient oxygen supply. It is inexpensive.

Vitamin C lowers cholesterol and triglycerides, beginning at 0.5–1 gm/day. Vitamin C given intravenously decreases vascular resistance in smokers, and given during a heart attack significantly improves survival (1–3 gm/day).

The acceleration of coronary arteriosclerosis in homocysteinemia, the hereditary risk factor mentioned above, is prevented by treatment with **folic acid,** 400–800 mcg/day; **vitamin B_6,** 100 mg/day; and **vitamin B_{12},** 1 mg daily. Continued intake is lifelong and wholly preventive. Expensive diagnostic tests to show the defect are usually not necessary. Most good megadose vitamins will have these amounts of nutrients except for B_{12}.

Suggested daily **minerals** include

- calcium—800 mg
- magnesium—400 mg
- zinc—at least 15 mg
- copper—2 mg
- chromium—200 mcg
- manganese—15 mg

- selenium—200 mcg
- silicon—2 mg

Chromium supplements of 200 mcg/day have been shown to increase HDL levels 16 percent in as little as two months.

Magnesium in dosages of 400 mg/day has raised HDL 33 percent and reduced total cholesterol 14 percent. Magnesium given intravenously early after onset of symptoms of heart attack improves survival 25 percent and helps maintain a normal blood pressure. Magnesium given before analgesics reduces pain during a heart attack.

Increased intake of **antioxidants** in food and supplements lowers the incidence and slows the progression of coronary arteriosclerosis. They can also help in reducing existing disease. The free-radical oxidation of fatty acids begins in fats before consumption and continues within the bloodstream following digestion. For this reason, eating less saturated fat and unsaturated fat, which is especially subject to rancidification, reduces heart disease. Higher **vitamin E** levels in blood tests and higher intakes of vitamin E from food and supplements are consistently correlated with lesser amounts of arterial plaque, and a lower incidence of coronary artery disease and heart attacks. In reducing free-radical damage to blood vessels, all aspects of the antioxidant defense system are important. They include previously mentioned physical exercise, more appropriate management of stress, the avoidance of environmental toxins, and the adequate intake in food and supplements of vitamins and minerals mentioned above.

The twenty-year mortality rate of men consuming at least one ounce of fish/day is 50 percent lower than that of non-fish-eating men. The effect is probably due to **omega-3 oils** in fish. Four grams daily is desirable. Greenland Eskimos have an extremely low incidence of heart disease in spite of a very high fat intake from mammal blubber. What is believed to be protecting them is a high intake of omega-3 oils from fish. It can also be obtained from flaxseed oil.

As mentioned earlier, **excess amounts of iron contribute to the chemical promotion of arteriosclerosis.** Donating blood and taking supplements without iron reduce excess iron stores and aid in preventing heart disease.

L-carnitine is a nonessential amino acid that has a marked effect on improving lipid values. One-year survival after heart attack in patients taking four grams of L-carnitine per day showed a tenfold improvement over those treated with placebo. L-carnitine normalized cholesterol in 90 percent of subjects of one subtype of hereditary cholesterol problem and reduced triglycerides to normal in 100 percent of another type. One hundred percent of all these patients reduced total cholesterol to near normal levels. Carnitine significantly decreases triglycerides and LDL while increasing HDL. Rapidly depleted in hearts that have a compromised blood supply, carnitine should be taken in doses of one to three grams per day.

Angina and treadmill test performance significantly improve on treatment with L-carnitine compared to placebo treatment.

After intravenous injection of a form of L-carnitine, various measures of heart function in patients with moderately advanced coronary artery disease improved 10 percent to 45 percent.

Phenols, contained in wine, even in solutions diluted a thousandfold, inhibited LDL free-radical oxidation much more significantly than vitamin E.

An outstanding free-radical scavenger, **coenzyme Q10** has significantly improved angina and treadmill performance of patients with heart disease, while also lowering free-radical levels. Co-Q10 is a powerful antioxidant, more powerful even than vitamins A, C, and E. It also improves circulation by facilitating movement of red blood cells through the tiniest arteries. In animals, pretreatment with coenzyme Q10 significantly protected against reperfusion injury, in which blood is released into an organ that has been blood deficient, following cardiac surgery for example. The percentage of vessels open was nearly three times greater than with placebo treatment. In a study of patients with symptomatic mitral valve prolapse who recorded isometric handgrip test baseline scores, those patients treated with Co-Q10 (140 mg/day for eight weeks) became normal in seven of eight cases, whereas none of those patients given placebo showed normal scores.

Glycosaminoglycans are a group of body-biosynthesized (produced in the body) compounds important to the structure of a common connective-tissue protein called **collagen.** Mesoglycan, a derivative of glycosaminoglycans, can be obtained from al-falfa or by itself. It lowers total cholesterol and raises good cholesterol, preventing damage to arterial linings and maintaining their structure and preventing clot formation. One hundred mg daily impressively improves arterial integrity, function, and structure.

Available in most health food stores, the **hormone DHEA** when administered to men with heart disease appears to improve survival, although experience is not extensive. Men with normal cholesterols who had heart attacks showed decreased levels of testosterone and DHEA, compared to healthy men. Reasonable doses should not exceed 25 mg per day.

Biomolecular therapy. **Chelation,** a procedure used to remove heavy metals from the body in acute and chronic poisoning, has often been used as an alternative treatment for advanced coronary arterial disease. Many patients choosing chelation have advanced disease, including some who have had one or more coronary artery bypass operations. Numerous stories of significant improvement have been reported. I am not aware of a well-done, well-controlled study that has settled this controversial issue. One of the great criticisms of chelation—that it destroys kidney function—has been thoroughly disproven. It appears to pose no significant complications. Although not yet approved by the FDA, chelation is currently legal in most states.

Herbs. A number of herbs can enhance blood chemistry to reduce the danger of heart disease. These include:

- **Diosgenin,** a plant-derived sapogenin that inhibits cholesterol absorption, decreases LDL (bad) cholesterol, and increases HDL (good) cholesterol in rats.
- **Indian gooseberry** (amla, an Ayurvedic herb). Fifty mg daily has been shown to reduce cholesterol levels 12 percent in four weeks.
- **Commiphora mukul** (gum guggulu), another Ayurvedic herb, reduces platelet adhesiveness and increases clot-dissolving actions in the body. Cholesterol decreased 22 percent, triglycerides decreased 27 percent, and HDL increased 36 percent at sixteen weeks with doses of 2.25 grams twice daily.
- **Garlic.** Twelve gm/day of garlic pearls was shown to reduce cholesterol 12 percent and triglycerides 17 percent and increase HDL 13 percent in three weeks. Eight hundred mg daily of concentrated garlic powder reduced cholesterol 12 percent in three months.
- **Ginger** lowers cholesterol and decreases platelet aggregation more than onions or garlic (1 gm of powdered ginger daily). *Crataegus oxycantha* **(Hawthorn berry)** extract, $\frac{1}{4}-\frac{1}{2}$ tsp twice daily, has a protective effect on arterial walls. **Catechin,** 400 mg twice daily, and 40 mg of **Ginkgo biloba** twice daily have beneficial arterial effects as well.

Exercise. If you were raised in a family that valued physical activity and exercise, consider yourself lucky, because exercise is a significant factor in prevention of heart disease. If you weren't so lucky, it's not too late, but you must start gradually. Physical activity, including aerobic exercise, is probably the most reliable way of increasing "good" cholesterol. **Long periods of consistent exercise have been shown to reduce cholesterol/HDL ratios 15 percent and increase HDL 10 percent.** In men who exercise, fibrinogen, the clotting factor significantly correlated with coronary heart disease, is a highly significant 11 percent lower than in sedentary men.

One caution should be noted, however. **For those sedentary people with known heart disease, the risk of heart attack can increase a hundredfold with sudden, unaccustomed heavy exercise,** compared to moderate-mild exercise! The sedentary, unfit, overweight male who suffers a heart attack shortly after an hour of vigorous snow shoveling is the classic example.

For those with advanced heart disease, the **aerobic exercise prescription must begin very gradually.** Just a little activity becomes aerobic for those with severe cardiac limitations. Exercise helps in quitting smoking. Exercise decreases synthesis of adrenaline-like chemicals in the body, which reduces blood pressure and excessive clotting tendencies.

In normal volunteers who regularly practice **yoga,** the measure of fibrinolysis (the ability of blood to dissolve clots), a valuable asset in destroying the clots that shut off circulation, has been shown to be significantly increased.

Acupuncture has been shown to be quite effective in helping to quit **smoking.** It is so successful that some industries now pay for this special acupuncture service for insured employees.

Blood Tests. With a strong family history of heart disease or elevated cholesterol, you should obtain the following blood tests:
• total cholesterol, HDL, LDL, and triglycerides; the total chol/HDL ratio is important—it should be 4.0 or less
• homocysteine
• DHEA-S (sulfated)
• testosterone
• red blood cell magnesium

Mental and Emotional Health Recommendations

Heart disease is related to the **fourth chakra.** According to Carolyn Myss in *Anatomy of the Spirit,* mental and emotional issues related to this chakra include
• love and hatred
• resentment and bitterness
• grief and anger
• self-centeredness
• loneliness and commitment
• forgiveness and compassion
• hope and trust
Emotionally, heart disease represents a hardening of the heart. According to Louise Hay, heart attacks are triggered by "squeezing all the joy out of the heart, in favor of money or position." Her affirmations for heart disease include "I lovingly allow joy to flow through my mind and body and experience" and "I bring joy back to the center of my heart. I express love to all."

Since emotional stress contributes to heart disease, stress management in the form of regular practice of **meditation** or **relaxation techniques** should be a part of your specific program. Attitudes, too, are important. Hostility, the prototype of negative attitudes and the key factor in type A behavior, promotes heart disease. Modification of hostility, anger, and depression through **counseling** can also be an important preventive measure. Reshaping attitudes and beliefs around the experience of unconditional love is as important as all the other factors I could mention.

In 1991, Dr. Dean Ornish published his work documenting striking reversal of arteriosclerosis in people without drugs and surgery. In addition to a strict vegetarian diet and three hours of brisk exercise per week, his program for reversing advanced heart disease includes
• meditation, practiced daily
• mental imagery, picturing the arteries dilating with improved circulation
• group counseling sessions for an hour and a half twice weekly to learn stress management and to resolve past stressful issues

Social and Spiritual Health Recommendations

The presence of supportive family and friends during and after a heart attack greatly increases survival and shortens hospitalization.

Randolph Byrd, M.D., conducted a well-known study of patients admitted to a hospital with heart attacks. Unbeknownst to any of these patients, one group was made the object of daily organized prayer and the other was not. Byrd found that the death rate, complications, use of antibiotics and diuretics, requirement for resuscitation, need for mechanical respiration, and incidence of congestive heart failure were all significantly reduced in those for whom prayers were offered compared to the group that had received no prayers.

Congestive heart failure is an aspect of heart disease encountered in aging men, usually over sixty-five. It responds to many of the same holistic medical therapies included in the treatment of coronary heart disease. Coenzyme Q10 and L-carnitine are highly effective in treating this condition.

Heart rhythm disturbances (arrhythmias) likewise respond to many of these same options. Magnesium and coenzyme Q10 are most notable in this regard.

Hypertension (High Blood Pressure)

Prevalence

Hypertension, or high blood pressure, is common in the United States. Among adults, an estimated 20 percent of the white population and 30 percent of the black population have blood pressures about 165/95 mmHg (millimeters of mercury). Hypertension contributes significantly to arteriosclerosis. The greatest damage occurs from elevated blood pressure sustained over long periods, which can lead to significant increases in risk of stroke, heart attack, congestive heart failure, and kidney damage.

Hypertension is a result of the narrowing of arteries throughout the body. **Arteriosclerosis** (hardening of the arteries) contributes modestly to this change, but the major factor is the constriction of the muscular layer around the smallest arteries (arterioles). This constriction occurs in vast areas of the body when the fight-or-flight reflex is triggered, in order to shunt blood away from the intestines, skin, and core organs to the muscles to be used in physical combat or flight. As constriction occurs, the blood vessels increase their resistance to the flow of blood and the heart works harder to sustain a higher blood pressure to force more oxygen-containing blood into the tissues supplied through constricted arteries. High blood pressure, then, takes a gradually increasing toll in malfunction of the heart and begins to damage the blood vessels of a variety of organs, including the brain, kidney, and the heart itself.

The top number of a blood pressure reading, called the systolic pressure, measures arterial pressure as the heart muscle contracts; while the bottom number, or diastolic pressure, is the measurement during the relaxed phase of the heart's pumping cycle—the pressure between heart beats.

Symptoms and Diagnosis

Verifying the presence of hypertension is not easy. At least three random elevated blood-pressure readings are required to diagnose hypertension. Some people elevate their blood pressure only in the presence of a doctor or nurse—the so-called white-coat effect. Careful documentation in hospitalized patients has shown a rise of as much as 25 mmHg in the blood pressure as the doctor enters a room to check a patient. Repeated blood pressure readings taken at home by the patient himself or by family members will usually bring to light this discrepancy. A blood pressure that is elevated only in the doctor's office should not be treated by drugs. Most often hypertension presents no obvious symptoms. However, recurring **headaches** in some people may indicate elevated blood pressure. Another common symptom is **tinnitus,** characterized by a faint ringing or buzzing in the ears.

Conventional Medical Treatment

The most common blood pressure levels that trigger a physician's decision to use drug treatment for hypertension are a sustained elevation of 140/90 mmHg or higher. Some experts cite large studies that confirm that drug treatment in mild and moderate hypertension lessens heart disease risks but often does not bring greater longevity due to the serious side effects of the drugs. Diuretics have long been known to have serious effects in removing essential minerals from the body (potassium and magnesium), and recently calcium channel blockers have been linked with a higher death rate and higher complications of clotting due to an increase in a body

chemical called thromboglobulin. Other side effects affecting quality of life reported in the use of nearly all classes of the drugs mentioned below are impotence and decreased libido.

Although most physicians begin treatment of hypertension with suggestions to **reduce dietary salt, lose weight, and begin or continue exercise,** the most common approach in conventional treatment is the prescribing of medications. The classes of drugs used, with a few of the commonly used drugs in each category, include alpha adrenoreceptor blockers (prazosin [Minipress]); alpha adrenoreceptor central inhibitory stimulants (methyldopa [Aldomet], clonidine [Catapres]); beta adrenergic blockers (nadolol [Corgard], propanolol [Inderal], atenolol [Tenormim]); angiotensin converting enzyme inhibitors (lisinopril [Zestril, Capoten, Vasotec]); diuretics (hydrochlorothiazide [Hydrodiuril], hydrochlorothiazide-triamterene [Dyazide], and furosemide [Lasix]); calcium channel blockers (verapamil [Calan], diltiazem [Cardizem], and nifedipine [Procardia]); rauwolfia derivatives; and vasodilators.

Advertising by the American Heart Association insists that an antihypertensive drug, once started, must be continued for life. This is not true. Many persons on drugs, having made important lifestyle changes as outlined below, can safely go off their medications.

Risk Factors and Causes

Ninety-five percent of cases of high blood pressure are "primary," meaning they occur with no other identified predisposing cause.

Nearly all of these are arbitrarily called "essential" hypertension with conventional wisdom teaching that there is no discernible cause. A number of factors, however, are quite obviously related.

Physical and Environmental Factors

Genetic factors can make offspring significantly more vulnerable to influences of excess sodium and loss of potassium. The genetic factor is probably not large compared to conditioning experiences and other lifestyle factors.

Environmental risk factors include exposure to **toxic substances** that increase blood pressure. These include lead (gasoline, paint, drinking water) and cadmium (batteries and cigarettes). Hypertensive patients have higher blood levels of lead and three to four times higher amounts of cadmium than nonhypertensive persons. Toxins provoke increased levels of oxygen free radicals in the body, and hypertension is on the long list of diseases linked to this problem.

Potential environmental **inhalant sensitizing agents** include chemical odors (natural gas, gasoline fumes, chlorine), air pollution, auto exhaust, soft plastic, cleaning chemicals (Lysol, phenol), perfume, polyurethane, tobacco smoke, polyesters, fiberglass, Naugahyde, new carpeting, formaldehyde, pesticides, pest strips, and foam rubber.

When other measures do not yield improvement and control of blood pressure, consider possible **environmental** and **food sensitizers.** The probability that inhalant and food sensitivities will play a role in hypertension is greater in persons with a personal or family history of allergies, in those with food cravings or habitual ingestion of a great amount of a few foods, and in those whose hypertension seems to come and go. Careful history taking and food elimination and reexposure trials can identify offending sensitizing agents. The most common food offenders include chocolate, corn, nuts (especially peanuts), pork, coffee, milk, wheat, rice, beef, shrimp, seafood, chicken, and apples.

Nutritional factors for hypertension can include **mineral deficiencies.** Deficiency in calcium, magnesium, potassium, or zinc from the diet is known, also, to contribute to high blood pressure. Excess sodium, chiefly from salt, raises blood pressure in the one out of six persons who is sodium sensitive.

In laboratory rats, groups consuming 10, 15, and 20 percent of total calories as **sucrose** (sugar) for fourteen weeks had significantly higher systolic BP than rats consuming no sucrose. Sucrose in Western diets averages more than 20 percent of calories. Studies in humans also suggest increased salt retention and elevated BP occurs with higher intake of most sugars.

Alcohol in modest or great amounts increases the risk for high blood pressure, and **coffee** and **caffeine** in some but not all studies lead to mild elevations. Smoking and tobacco use increase the risk of high blood pressure (especially the malignant variety).

Overweight persons have a higher risk of developing hypertension. **Obesity** places increased demands on the heart, and changes in hormone chemistry are thought to explain this risk.

Sedentary lifestyles are also a risk factor. Since the tension from stressful experiences is dissipated during physical exercise, sedentary persons may simply miss the opportunity to wind down. The elevated blood pressure that occurs with athletic or vigorous physical exertion is much less damaging because it does not remain sustained after the exertion is terminated. In fact, the slow rise in blood pressures that accompanies aging in most people occurs least often in people who remain physically fit. The risk of hypertension is 50 percent greater in those in poor shape than in those who are highly fit.

Mental and Emotional Risk Factors

The fight-or-flight (arousal) response is triggered by all phenomena perceived to be threatening and by events that require adaptation. Documented types of **stress** that can lead to elevated blood pressure include public speaking, performance tasks, work-site pressures, and ongoing family conflicts. Other research-confirmed factors contributing to hypertension include increased life dissatisfactions, impatience, and type A behavior including increased hostility and anger. Imagined stresses can also raise blood pressure equivalent to that from real stresses. Elevated blood pressure also develops in subjects who suppress or repress emotions while maintaining a calm exterior.

In the October 1996 issue of the *American Journal of Public Health,* researchers from the Harvard School of Public Health in Boston and the Kaiser Foundation Research Institute of Oakland, California, reported on their study of high blood pressure within the black community. They found that the risk of hypertension among blacks seems related to experiences of racial discrimination and whether victims challenge unfair treatment. In general, black professionals who are conscious of discrimination and who challenge unjust or unequal treatment appear to be at lower risk of elevated blood pressure than black working-class men and women who may be less aware of discriminatory acts and less likely to challenge them.

Psychological research of the 1950s and 1960s identified two types of elevated blood pressure reactions. The first pattern of hypertension, called the exercise type (probably the same as the "hot reactor" type popularized by cardiologist Robert Eliot, M.D., in the 1980s), occurs when the sympathetic nervous system overreacts to stressful stimuli, with overt and visible emotional disturbance. The second type—high resistance—is encountered when suppression or repression of emotions is accompanied by a calm exterior appearance. Hypertension is seen in energy terms as related to frustration and anger, often linked with inflexibility.

Holistic Medical Treatment and Prevention

Some conventional medical authorities have concluded that 40 percent of the time careful attention to lifestyle changes can control blood pressure to the point that medications can be eliminated. The holistic perspective is much more enthusiastic. Our experience has shown that optimizing lifestyle factors, including many options not used by conventional practitioners, can achieve normalization of blood pressure, while eliminating drugs, 80–85 percent of the time.

Physical and Environmental Health Recommendations

Blood pressures respond to moderate and strenuous **physical activity** including walking, running, gardening, and other steady, vigorous activities. Patients who start exercising can usually reduce or eliminate their medications. Exercise is especially effective in patients with mild to moderate hypertension. Low- and moderate-intensity exercise are as good as high-intensity exercise in normalizing blood pressure in mild to moderate hypertension. In severe hypertension, high-intensity exercise is required. Results are seen within a few weeks of starting exercise.

Diet. **Stabilizing weight** to within 5–10 percent of ideal is helpful in persons with hypertension. Blood pressures usually drop promptly as weight loss occurs.

Fiber intake of more than twenty-four grams per day (high in fruits and vegetables), compared to less than twelve grams per day, decreased the incidence of high blood pressure 57 percent in a study of thirty thousand men.

Limit alcohol to one drink or less per day.

Once you have identified offensive foods, strictly **avoid the most sensitizing foods.** To permit mildly or moderately sensitizing foods, use a rotation diet to introduce them independently every three or four days.

Vegetarians have lower blood pressures than consumers of both animal and vegetarian foods (omnivores). Much of the benefit may come from higher amounts of minerals and lower consumption of foods preserved and laced with salt.

Vitamins, minerals, and nutritional supplements. Blood levels of **vitamin C** and other antioxidants are inversely related to systolic and diastolic pressures. In a number of research studies, average pressure decrease with vitamin C intake of over 250 mg/day was 7 percent. Vitamin C acts to oppose the arterial constriction caused by smoking.

Omega-3 oils. Nine grams of fish oil daily for six weeks has been shown to reduce diastolic BP an average of 5 mmHg.

Including adequate daily amounts of calcium, magnesium, and potassium from food and supplements has been shown to reduce blood pressure. Men consuming more than one gram of **calcium** daily compared to those ingesting less than half a gram have a 20 percent lower incidence of hypertension. Men consuming more than 400 mg/day of **magnesium** compared to those taking in less than 250 mg/day have a 50 percent lower incidence, and those consuming more than 3.5 grams/day of **potassium** compared to those ingesting less than 2.5 grams/day have a 55 percent lower incidence. Avoiding excess amounts of **sodium** (salt) is also important. Men need only 1.5 gm of sodium daily, which can be achieved without salting of most foods and by avoiding many commercially prepared foods including pickles, canned foods, preserved meats, and fast foods. **Zinc** reverses the hypertension caused by cadmium exposure in experimental animals. Dosage: 15–30 mg/day.

In hypertension there tends to be a deficiency of **taurine,** a nonessential amino acid obtained in small amounts in food and also synthesized in the body. Adding supplements of taurine lowers blood pressures. Six grams per day has been shown to lower systolic pressure 10 mmHg and diastolic 5 mmHg in seven days, with no effects seen in subjects with normal blood pressures. Taurine indirectly decreases sympathetic constriction, the primary cause of hypertension. Reasonable doses are 1–1.5 gm/day.

Coenzyme Q10 in 100-mg-per-day doses in one group of men reduced average blood systolic blood pressure 10 mmHg and diastolic pressure 8 mmHg.

Herbs. In hypertensive patients with pressures 190–240/70–150 mmHg treated with *Crataegus oxacantha* **(hawthorn berry),** blood pressure decreased in all cases, resulting in pressures ranging from 110 to 175 systolic and 55 to 100 diastolic. In the 1:5 tincture form, 1–1.5 tsp is taken daily.

Garlic and **onion** both have blood-pressure-lowering properties. In some stud-

ies, liberal use of garlic has lowered systolic blood pressure by 20–30 mmHg and diastolic pressure by 10–20 mmHg.

Mistletoe *(Viscum album),* as a whole-plant 1:1 fluid extract, lowers blood pressure in 0.5-ml doses.

Environmental toxins. Reduction in exposure to sources of **lead** and **cadmium** is imperative, including the filtering of drinking and cooking water. Exercising careful environmental controls of *inhalant substances* can yield impressive improvement.

Reduction and **elimination of smoking** is an obvious element in successful treatment. Nicotine is a vasoconstrictive agent, significantly contributing to the blood vessel constriction that occurs in hypertension.

Mental and Emotional Health Recommendations

Relaxation. Significant reduction in systolic and diastolic blood pressures results from biofeedback training, with improvements still present after three years in follow-up. Systolic (top number) measures typically fall 15–20 mmHg from baseline readings and diastolic (bottom number) measures fall 8–12 mmHg. Cortisone levels also fall significantly, as much as 20–25 percent, providing the additional benefit of postponing degenerative disease. Biofeedback does not lower blood pressures in persons with normal readings.

Hypnosis has been found to substantially lower blood pressures an average of 16–20 percent, equivalent to the effect of most medications. Results last through months and years of follow-up.

Practicing **meditation** also consistently decreases systolic and diastolic blood pressures compared to control subjects. Hypertensive African-American patients randomly assigned to three months of Transcendental Meditation have been shown to achieve significantly greater reductions in blood pressures than a group practicing progressive muscle relaxation and very significantly greater blood pressure reductions compared to a lifestyle-modification education group. In long-term follow-up, some meditation studies show twice the benefits of drug treatment. Regular practice of *qi gong,* a Chinese gentle martial art and a moving meditation, has been shown to lower blood pressure and prevent stroke.

Placebo effects depend on **beliefs** that tend to evoke images to which the nervous system responds. What we believe and expect engages the brain and nervous system to act consistently with what we believe. If our beliefs and images are positive, decreased arousal-fight-flight responses drive the nervous and adrenal systems at a lower baseline, lowering blood pressure. In 1982, an Australian study reported on the experience of 1,100 patients acting as placebo controls for a larger number of patients being treated with drugs. Their average initial blood pressure was 158/102. Receiving a daily placebo, the group reduced its average pressure to 144/91 at the end of three years. Forty-eight percent

fell to normal with diastolic pressure below 80 mmHg. Drug-treated patients were only slightly better off than placebo subjects. The profound placebo effect persisted for the three years of the study.

The placebo effect can be greatly enhanced by the use of **affirmations** and **visualization.** These are particularly effective in soothing the nervous system and relaxing the tiny constricted muscles lining the arterial walls. Either picture yourself in a serene vacation setting or imagine the arterial walls letting go of their constriction, becoming softer and more supple (refer to chapter 2 for other techniques). Repeat the affirmation "My blood courses through my arteries like a gentle, freely flowing stream."

The mental and emotional issues associated with hypertension are the same as those contributing to heart disease—**fourth chakra issues** (see heart disease).

Spiritual and Social Health Recommendations

Systolic and diastolic blood pressures recorded in children who are reading aloud are significantly lower if they are reading in the presence of a friendly dog. Similar reductions occur in the elderly with **pets** present.

Ninety-six hypertensive patients age sixteen to sixty were exposed to a series of long-distance bioenergetic treatments by a healer. Forty-eight were randomly selected to receive the treatments and the remainder acted as an untreated control group, all continuing their usual drug treatment. Neither patients nor attending physicians knew who received the treatment and who did not. Each healer engaged in relaxation, followed by attunement with a higher power or infinite being, followed by visualization of the patient in a perfect state of health, followed by an expression of thanks to the Source of all power and energy. The systolic blood pressure improved significantly in 92 percent of the treated group versus 74 percent of the control group.

The primary contributor to this chapter is Robert A. Anderson, M.D., practicing holistic family medicine in Mukilteo, Washington.

E n d o c r i n o l o g i c a l   D i s e a s e

Diabetes Mellitus (Diabetes)

Prevalence

Diabetes is a chronic disease that adversely affects the way your body turns food into energy. This chronic disorder of carbohydrate, protein, and fat metabolism does not occur to any extent in primitive peoples, but is a phenomenon of industrialized societies. The incidence of diabetes in the United States is about 5 percent of the population, affecting 15 million Americans. It is the seventh leading cause of death and can contribute significantly to kidney failure, heart attacks, blindness, and strokes.

Symptoms and Diagnosis

The diagnosis of diabetes depends on the finding of a morning fasting blood sugar level (glucose) of 140 mg/dl or greater on at least two occasions; blood sugar concentration of 200 mg/dl or more at two hours after the ingestion of 75 gm of sugar; and classical signs of **excessive thirst** and **appetite, frequent urination,** and **weight loss.** Other symptoms include fatigue, blurry vision, tingling or coolness of the hands and feet, and frequent infections.

When food is digested, it is turned into glucose, a form of sugar that fuels the body and all its tissues and organs. **Insulin** is a hormone produced in the pancreas that allows glucose to enter the cells of all tissues. Insulin is attracted to insulin-receptor sites on the surfaces of the cells in the body, where it facilitates the passage of molecules of sugar through the membrane surface into the body of each cell. The cells utilize the molecules of sugar as their major source of fuel.

Diabetes results either from (1) a **lack of insulin production** in specialized cells of the pancreas or from (2) inability to properly utilize insulin at the receptor sites on the cell surfaces. When insulin is deficient or cannot be utilized by the cells, they become fuel-depleted, while sugar in the bloodstream rises to high levels. In uncontrolled cases of **juvenile diabetes,** extreme deprivation of sugar in the cells of the brain can cause unconsciousness (diabetic coma), and the excess burning of fat for fuel creates a serious condition called diabetic ketoacidosis.

In adult-onset diabetics, **stress** combined with **dehydration** can lead to a life-threatening condition called hyperosmolar nonketogenic coma. This and ketoacidosis are life-threatening emergency situations requiring urgent hospitalization.

Long-term complications of diabetes include damage to the retina of the eye, kidneys, peripheral nerves, and blood vessels. Diabetics tend to have premature onset of arteriosclerosis, heart attacks and strokes, and poor circulation. Thyroid function is impaired in uncontrolled diabetics.

Conventional Medical Treatment

Upon proper diagnosis, management of diabetes begins with proper **nutritional control:** eliminating simple sugars, increasing carbohydrates to 60–70 percent of caloric intake, and decreasing fat. In juvenile diabetics, **insulin** becomes required, sometimes after a "honeymoon" period when sugar levels are temporarily easier to control. Proper insulin adjustment, based on blood sugar readings, is imperative. In "brittle" diabetics (whose blood sugar levels rapidly fluctuate), a device known as an insulin pump may be used.

In adult-onset diabetics, nutritional considerations are equally important as in Type I treatment. Appropriate exercise is prescribed. Ninety percent of Type II diabetics are overweight, and **weight loss** for these obese persons is important. Prescription of **oral antidiabetic agents** is common. Fre-

quently prescribed drugs include the sulfonylureas (Diabeta, Diabinese, Glucotrol, Glynase, and Amaryl). Other new oral antidiabetic medications are Glucophage and Precose.

Many physicians recommend that their diabetic patients obtain a glucometer, a device that measures blood sugar with a simple poke of the finger. Although it is important to obtain periodic fasting blood sugars, a blood test called glycohemoglobin will tell you how effective your blood sugar management has been for the previous six weeks.

Conventional treatment includes careful attention to the **complications of diabetes,** which include neuropathy (nerve pain and numbness), accelerated arteriosclerosis, retinopathy (eye damage), sexual dysfunction, and neurogenic loss of bladder control.

Risk Factors and Causes

Diabetes occurs in two forms. **Juvenile diabetes (Type I)** has its onset in infancy, childhood, and young adulthood up to about age thirty-five. It results from total destruction of beta cells in the pancreas, the site of insulin production. Juvenile diabetics are inevitably **insulin-dependent,** and they take injections of insulin. Recent research links onset of juvenile diabetes to exposure to cow's milk early in life (see below). Recent studies have also shown nitrate concentrations in drinking water to be significantly linked with increased risk of juvenile diabetes. It is believed that one of the concentrates produced from the breakdown of nitrates—N-nitroso compounds—can produce beta-cell damage.

Adult onset-diabetes (Type II) can occur at any time in adulthood, and these types of diabetics may or may not require treatment with insulin. Although adult diabetics have sufficient insulin, its utilization at the cell membrane site is compromised. Increased sugar intake and lack of exercise can aggravate this risk. In adult-onset diabetes, **hereditary factors** play a major role. **Other causative factors are obesity, smoking, lack of antioxidant nutrients, and insufficiency of vitamins B$_6$ and biotin and magnesium.** The risk of developing Type II diabetes for those smoking more than twenty-five cigarettes per day is twice that of non-smokers.

Use of certain **drugs** increases risks for induction of diabetes. These include corticosteroids (cortisone, prednisone); estrogens, including oral contraceptive agents; thyroid medications; catecholamines (adrenaline-like drugs); diuretics; antidepressants and other psychotropic medications; chemotherapy drugs; and isoniazid (a tuberculosis drug).

Stress is unequivocally related to both causing and controlling diabetes. The stress of marital or personal separation is associated with onset of diabetic symptoms. In children five to nine, a history of loss or threatened loss increased the risk of developing Type I diabetes 80 percent, compared to a group with low levels of loss or threat of loss. Stress increases cortisone, which opposes insulin. Stress is likewise a significant contributor to the onset of Type II diabetes. In experimental situations where dietary intake and muscular activity are held constant, episodes of elevated blood sugar, diabetic acidosis, and near-coma have been induced by intentional exposure to stress-evoking circumstances. Insulin requirements are invariably increased during times of increased stress when the stress is not managed well.

Energy diagnosticians and medical intuitives who are aware of energy fields sense diabetes as a disorder related to the **third chakra.** Blocked third chakra energies (related to the solar plexus and the adrenal and pancreatic glands) manifest **in issues of responsibility** and often include

- resentment or fear of having to take responsibility for another person or for oneself
- resentment in children when their parents—out of ineptitude, immaturity, or alcoholism—require parenting by their children
- codependent excuse-making for the irresponsible behavior or attitudes of others
- efforts to prevent others from maturing into self-responsibility because of loss of control over those others
- anger resulting from being neglected or ignored while constantly giving to others

Studies also suggest that **suppressed anger** plays some role in diabetes onset.

Holistic Medical Treatment and Prevention

Physical and Environmental Health Recommendations

Diet. The **best standard diet** omits simple sugars and processed grains and favors high complex-carbohydrates, fiber, fruit, and vegetable intake with modest protein and low fat consumption.

Starchy foods vary significantly in the degree to which they raise blood sugar levels. They are also digested at varied rates. **Potentially useful foods** that tend to raise blood sugar less (having a low glycemic index) include legumes (beans, peas, peanuts, soybeans), pasta, grains (including parboiled rice and bulgur or cracked wheat), fruit (apples, oranges), fructose, dairy milks, and whole-grain breads such as pumpernickel. All these foods have a significantly lower glycemic index than white bread.

Vegetarian diets that include little or no sucrose are known to control blood sugars well. Nerve pain, or diabetic neuropathy, was completely alleviated or partially relieved in diabetics who adhered to a program of exercise and a vegetarian diet of unrefined foods. Although numbness persisted, it was noticeably improved within twenty-five days. Studies have shown that vegetarians eating a diet of meat or poultry less than once per week have a 38 percent lower risk of diabetes than nonvegetarians.

In Type I patients with compromised kidney function who were treated with a **low-protein, low-phosphorus diet** for three years, kidney function deteriorated 67 percent more slowly compared to patients on a standard American Diabetic Association diet. (Their protein consisted of one ounce per kilogram of ideal body weight/day. Phosphorus intake was less than one gram/day.)

High-fiber foods—whole grains, vegetables, and fruits—lower blood sugar and insulin levels and decrease insulin requirements.

Cow's milk. Children exclusively breast-fed for their first ninety days have a 35 percent lower risk of developing juvenile insulin-dependent diabetes compared to those not breast-fed. Those given cow's milk formula in their first ninety days of life are 52 percent more likely to develop diabetes than those not given cow's milk. Cow's milk contains a protein closely resembling a surface molecule in insulin-producing pancreatic beta cells. Immune cells reacting to the milk also attack the beta cells, gradually destroying them. Antibodies to this unique seventeen-amino-acid protein found in cow's milk were present in 100 percent of newly diagnosed Finnish diabetic children. This antibody was not present in nondiabetic healthy children or adults. The link between cow's milk and diabetes in susceptible populations is clear. Studies have also shown an 88 percent correlation between the amount of milk drunk by children and the risk of diabetes. Preventing juvenile diabetes begins with the promotion of **exclusive breast-feeding** for infants for at least three to six months and the sparing use of cow's milk in early childhood.

Obesity is a highly significant predictor of adult-onset diabetes, particularly in those with a genetic predisposition. In one review, obesity increased the likelihood of Type II diabetes 400 percent compared to normal weight persons. Obesity is a more specific predictor of diabetes than lack of exercise.

Free radicals have been implicated in the immunological process that leads to juvenile diabetes. Persons on diets higher in **antioxidants,** such as those found in the Orient, have less Type II diabetes.

Vitamins, minerals, and nutritional supplements. **Vitamins C, E.** Diabetics given vitamin C, 1 gm/day for three months, had an 18 percent improvement in blood sugar control. Elderly diabetics significantly improved glucose control after receiving 900 mg of vitamin E each day for four months.

In diabetics whose **vitamin B$_6$** status is normal, double-blind studies show that the addition of 50 mg/day of B$_6$ as a vitamin supplement improves long-term blood sugar control 6 percent. A form of Vitamin B$_6$ called pyridoxine alphaglutarate, given 600 mg three times daily for four weeks to insulin-dependent juvenile (Type I) diabetics, decreased fasting blood sugars by 30 percent and improved long-term blood sugar control 32 percent. Using the same treatment, Type II diabetics experienced a 24 percent decrease in fasting blood sugars and a 24 percent improvement in long-term blood sugar control. After stopping the pyridoxine al-

phaglutarate, all values returned to previous levels within three weeks.

Average **blood biotin** (a B vitamin) levels are significantly lower in Type II diabetic patients compared to healthy controls. Raising blood biotin decreases fasting blood sugar levels in diabetics. The blood sugars of Type II diabetics taken off insulin and treated with 16 mg/day of biotin for one week decreased significantly.

Inositol, given 500 mg twice daily to diabetics with peripheral neuropathy, has been reported to significantly improve nerve sensation.

Chromium aids insulin action and assists in losing weight. A therapeutic dose may range from 200 mcg to 1,000 mcg/day.

Zinc tends to be utilized in higher amounts in diabetics and zinc supplementation is a wise precaution (30 mg/day).

Magnesium levels in diabetic patients are lower than in healthy people. Levels in diabetics with heart complications were significantly lower than those without heart involvement. Magnesium levels in elderly persons are significantly lower than those of younger persons. Blood tests typically understate tissue levels of magnesium. Therefore, it's much better to use the *red blood cell* magnesium test. Insulin production and insulin utilization improve greatly in magnesium-supplemented Type II diabetics (400–800 mg/day).

In adults with Type I diabetes compared to age-matched nondiabetic controls, the average concentration of white blood cell **vitamin C** was 33 percent lower; there was no significant difference in vitamin C intake between these two groups, whose intakes were both above the RDA. It is not totally clear whether these deficiencies exist before onset of the diabetes or result from it. The implication for increasing vitamin C intake to remedy this deficiency, however, is quite apparent.

Manganese levels are also low in diabetics. Manganese should be taken in dosages of 5–15 mg per day as a supplement.

Iron levels are elevated in 50 percent of poorly controlled Type II diabetics. The most accurate index of iron stores is a blood ferritin test. Patients with elevated ferritin have been treated with an iron-chelating agent (intravenous desferrioxamine)—10 mg/kg twice weekly for five to thirteen weeks— which removes iron. In 90 percent of those treated, in spite of the discontinuance of oral antidiabetic drugs, significant improvement occurred in blood sugars and triglycerides. Iron stores can be decreased by blood donations and avoiding iron in supplements.

Supplementation with **omega-3 fatty acids** such as flaxseed oil, omega-6 fatty acids such as primrose oil, and sardine and marine oils can (1) enhance insulin-binding to cells, (2) improve the pain and numbness of diabetic neuropathy, and (3) improve circulation.

Levels of dehydroepiandrosterone **(DHEA),** an adrenal hormone, are consistently and significantly lower in diabetics than in healthy persons. In animals, DHEA improves diabetic control. Present research will shed light on the possibilities for human use.

Herbs. Two **bioflavonoids,** catechin (1 gm daily) and quercetin (400 mg twice daily), have been shown to stimulate the action of insulin and to scavenge free radicals. They are frequently helpful in controlling symptoms of diabetic neuropathy.

Aloe, one-half teaspoonful daily for four to fourteen weeks in Type II patients, has been shown to reduce fasting blood glucose from levels in the high 200s to 150 mg/dl.

Type II patients given 100 or 200 mg/day of **ginseng** for eight weeks improved fasting glucose levels and had a weight loss. Those receiving 200 mg/day demonstrated improvement in long-term sugar control. Ginseng was four times as effective as a placebo in normalizing blood sugar levels.

Compared to baseline control values, non-insulin-dependent patients given 100 gm/day of defatted **fenugreek seed powder** for ten days decreased their fasting blood sugars 30–65 percent.

Momordica charantia **(bitter melon),** prepared as a juice of the unripe tropical Asian fruit, lowers blood sugar (25–50 gm three times a day).

Gymnema sylvestre is an Ayurvedic blood-sugar-lowering botanical contained in a product called Bio Gymnema taken up to three capsules three times daily.

Onion and **garlic** have both been shown to have blood-sugar-lowering effects and can be used liberally with benefit.

In patients with Type II disease due to liver cirrhosis, 600 mg of **milk thistle** (silymarin) daily significantly reduces average fasting blood sugar, daily insulin need, fasting insulin levels, and blood free-radical levels.

Exercise. **Aerobic exercise** more than once a week reduced the risk of developing adult-onset diabetes 36 percent in a study of 21,300 male physicians. Those exercising five or more times a week reduced the risk of developing diabetes 48 percent. A thirty-five-year study placed the risk reduction at 42 percent. Regular aerobic exercise postpones by ten to twelve years the onset of diabetes in those with a family diabetic history.

In 550 Type I diabetics, the six-year mortality rate in those exercising moderately to strenuously was 6 percent compared to 19 percent for those exercising mildly to not at all. The mortality rate decreased 71 percent in the high-exercise group over six years.

Men with Type II diabetes exercised on a treadmill sixty minutes daily at 60 percent of maximal heart rate. Their average blood sugar two hours after a sugar load dropped from 227 to 170 mcg/dl after only one week; blood insulin fell from 172 to 106 mcg/ml; and 80 percent had normal glucose and insulin tolerance tests at the end of the week. **Exercise increases availability of insulin receptor sites.**

Weight training programs of three sessions per week for ten weeks also improve blood sugar readings.

Smoking. In persons who have quit smoking, the risk for developing Type II diabetes drops 20 percent in only two years. Smoking appears to hasten onset of Type II diabetes.

Kidney damage, a consequence of chronic diabetes, progresses four and one-half times as rapidly in smokers as nonsmokers.

Mental and Emotional Health Recommendations

Stress. Diabetics who learn to incorporate **stress management techniques** have far better blood sugar control. Relaxation practices, exercise, and changing belief systems and attitudes are all helpful in managing stress.

Biofeedback, relaxation, and yoga. Learning these practices is a major part of managing stress while reducing its damaging effects. Three diabetic subjects with non-healing diabetic ulcers of the toe, ankle, and leg participated in twenty sessions of biofeedback training in fifteen weeks. Two of the three showed significant healing. Practicing biofeedback, meditation, and autogenic training all decrease circulating-cortisone levels, improving diabetic control.

Type II patients engaged in **yoga therapy** that included visceral-cleansing procedures, body postures, and breathing exercises for ninety minutes in the morning and sixty minutes in the evening. After forty days of practice there were significant improvements in oral glucose tolerance and in the amount of oral hypoglycemic agents taken. Average fasting blood sugar decreased from 135 to 100 mg/dl. Seventy percent showed good to fair response to therapy.

Responsibility issues. Based on energy diagnosis linking diabetes with issues of responsibility, conflicts over this issue may require professional counseling for resolution.

Proactive education. Diabetic subjects participating in a forty-five-minute educational and medical decision-making program with home follow-up showed significant improvement in their condition. This included fewer physical limitations in daily living and better sugar control than those of a control group not participating in the program. The results persisted four months later. In every disease, a patient's informed awareness and participation in decisions insures a better outcome.

The primary contributor to this chapter is Robert A. Anderson, M.D., practicing holistic family medicine in Mukilteo, Washington.

Chapter 15

Gastrointestinal Disease

Irritable Bowel Syndrome (IBS)
Constipation
Peptic Ulcer
(Gastric or Duodenal Ulcer)

Prevalence

Although none of the chronic diseases of the gastrointestinal tract ranks among the top ten most common diseases afflicting men, an estimated 95 million Americans suffer gastrointestinal upsets from time to time. Irritable bowel syndrome (IBS), sometimes described as frequent indigestion, affects about 15 percent of the population and is high on the list of physical discomforts for men under forty-five years of age. An estimated 4 million Americans suffer from chronic constipation every year, and about $725 million a year is spent on laxatives. It is most common in men over the age of sixty-five. Antiulcer drugs, led by Zantac and Tagamet, are the most commonly purchased prescription drugs in America—mostly by men.

IRRITABLE BOWEL SYNDROME (IBS)

Anatomy

The gastrointestinal tract, beginning in the mouth and ending at the anus, is a thirty-plus-foot processing tract for the digestion of food. This digestive process is described in more detail in chapter 3, beginning on page 70.

Symptoms and Diagnosis

A healthy digestive tract produces well-formed, loglike, light brown, easily passed stools that are about two finger widths in diameter, and with no accompanying mucus. Ideally, you should never "feel" your GI tract. Belching or burping, bloating, passing gas, diarrhea, dry or hard stools, days of skipped bowel movements are all variations of normal GI function. Irritable bowel syndrome has also been called spastic colon, mucous colitis, colitis, or functional bowel disease. The so-called irritated bowel is characterized by *intermittent bouts of diarrhea and constipation usually occurring in the morning.* Symptoms of this condition are usually precipitated by eating. Other symptoms might include

- abdominal pain
- distension and bloating
- painful bowel movements
- excess production of mucus in the colon (large bowel)
- nausea
- loss of appetite
- anxiety and/or depression

Because of both the variety of related symptoms and the number of possible inter-related causes, diagnosis can be difficult. Usually the diagnosis is made through a process of elimination (no pun intended), re-lying heavily upon a detailed medical history and physical examination. Given the multiple causes of this condition, a number of tests may be performed to determine the diagnosis. These might include

- comprehensive stool analysis with parasitology
- lactose breath test
- hydrogen breath test
- food sensitivity test
- food allergy test—elimination diet
- intestinal permeability screening for "leaky gut" syndrome

Conventional Medical Treatment

Most people with IBS are treated with **anti-spasmodic medications,** such as Bentyl, Donnatal, Levsin, or Lomotil. They are usu-ally advised to add fiber to their diet and avoid caffeine.

Risk Factors and Causes

Physical and Environmental Factors

Food allergies and sensitivities. Two-thirds of the people with IBS have at least one **food intolerance** and many have multiple sensitivities. This is considered the most common cause of IBS. The most common foods that cause difficulty for the bowel are milk and **dairy products, wheat, coffee, chocolate,** citrus, corn, eggs, nuts, rye, potatoes, and barley oats. The first four are the most common.

Lactose intolerance. **Lactose is a sugar in all milk products,** and many people with IBS are deficient in the enzyme that breaks down lactose in the intestine. This results in fermentation of lactose by bacteria and bloat-ing and inflammation.

Sugar intolerance. A high percentage of IBS sufferers have difficulty breaking down **disaccharide sugars**—mannitol, sucrose, sorbitol, fructose, etc. The result is gas, bloat-ing, and possible diarrhea. People with IBS who react to sugar can even react to sugars in fruit, especially citrus. Often people with can-didiasis, or yeast overgrowth, are much more sensitive and react strongly to both sugar and fruits. A hydrogen test can detect sugar fer-mentation.

Excess antibiotics and medications. Antibiotics often cause temporary bouts of diarrhea and GI distress because they kill healthy bacteria in the intestine. This allows **yeast (candida) organisms,** to overgrow and cause symptoms. This condition, which most often follows repeated courses of antibiotics, is called dysbiosis or **candidiasis.** It can render the colon defenseless in the face of other opportunistic infections caused by bacteria or parasites. Dysbiosis can also lead to **leaky gut syndrome.** This occurs when candida organisms eat through the mucosal lining of the small intestine allowing larger-than-normal food particles to be absorbed into the bloodstream. Failing to recognize these particles as nutrients, the immune system attacks them as allergens or foreign substances, which is often the cause of severe food allergies. Studies have revealed leaky gut to be quite common in people with IBS. Steroid medications, such as prednisone, and NSAIDS (nonsteroidal anti-inflammatory drugs), such as ibuprofen, can also affect the normal balance of gut bacteria and cause thinning of the intestinal lining.

Environmental toxins. **Chemical contaminants from air, food, and water** can all contribute to IBS symptoms. Pesticides, herbicides, flavorings, preservatives, food coloring, and other toxins can all contribute to gut inflammatory disorders as well as dysbiosis, acid/alkaline imbalances, and leaky gut.

Infection. Both high- and low-grade infections may contribute to IBS directly or through a constant state of dysbiosis. The **toxins released by disease-causing microbes** can cause or contribute to any or all IBS symptoms. Leo Galland, M.D., a noted researcher and author of *Superimmunity for Kids,* finds the parasite *Giardia* in almost 50 percent of his patients.

Low-fiber/high-saturated-fat diet. It is well known that **insufficient fiber in the diet** can cause IBS symptoms. Foods high in saturated fat, which tend to move more slowly through the bowel, can also disrupt the balance of **bowel flora** and increase inflammatory responses in the bowel lining.

Mental and Emotional Factors

Marshall Friedman, M.D., was the gastroenterologist who first taught me about irritable bowel syndrome, during my family practice residency nearly twenty-five years ago. With regard to the causes of IBS, he used to say, "It's not what you eat, it's what's eating you!" I now realize that in many cases it does matter what you eat, but I've also confirmed that there is almost always a significant emotional component to creating this uncomfortable physical condition.

Nearly every patient with IBS complains of anxiety, depression, feelings of hostility, fatigue, and sleep problems. Some studies have shown higher levels of anxiety and depression in IBS patients once the illness is present, rather than before its onset. The IBS itself may contribute to the anxiety and/or depression. Most people with IBS tend to be excessively **controlling** of themselves, **self-critical,** and **fearful.** They tend to be meticulous, detail-oriented, and want to appear as if in control. This leads to the physical pattern of diarrhea (release of control, eruption) and constipation (withholding feelings and honest, vulnerable expression of personal needs).

The small bowel is associated with the **third, or solar plexus, chakra.** The mental/emotional issues associated with this chakra that are most related to IBS are gut-level fear and intimidation, trust, self-confidence, care of oneself and others, and personal honor.

Holistic Medical Treatment and Prevention

Physical and Environmental Health Recommendations

The basic strategy for this aspect of the holistic treatment is to **reduce toxic irritants,** inflammation, and spasm; **repair damaged mucosal lining** of the intestine and overcome leaky gut syndrome; **enhance digestive enzymes; increase fiber; promote healthy bacteria; stabilize sugar metabolism, stool consistency, and regularity.**

Diet
- Increase **fiber** with high-fiber vegetables, such as beans, beginning with two to three servings daily, lightly steamed, for two to three weeks. Then begin adding new vegetables in salads gradually and note how well you tolerate them. Add one to two rounded teaspoons (five grams) of psyllium

to eight ounces of water in the morning and evening.
- Follow an anti-candida, **hypoallergenic diet** for three months. Cut out most common allergens for two to three weeks (dairy, wheat, corn, etc.). Then reintroduce them one at a time and rotate every four days and note your reactions.
- **Avoid known allergens** and food sensitivities as determined by lab testing.
- **Drink** at least your minimum daily requirement ($\frac{1}{2}$ oz/lb of body weight) of bottled or filtered water.
- Make eating an excuse to relax! **Eat slowly,** don't overstuff, and **chew thoroughly.**
- Eat only **organic, unprocessed whole foods.**
- Minimize animal-protein foods.
- Try **avoiding fruit and sugars** for three weeks. Gradually reintroduce and be aware of any reactions.

Nutritional supplements. In addition to a **high-fiber** diet, take five or more grams of psyllium or a professional product called Ultrafiber (made by HealthComm) containing both soluble and insoluble fibers.

Take eight grams of **L-glutamine** daily before meals for four weeks; then maintain at 500 to 1,000 mg before meals. L-glutamine is the most abundant amino acid in the body. It is used by the intestinal mucosa for fuel and repair. It is also effective in lowering sugar and alcohol cravings.

Available only through physicians, **Ultra-Clear Sustain** is a specific therapeutic food product developed by Jeffrey Bland, Ph.D., at HealthComm in Gig Harbor, Washington, for healing the intestinal mucosa.

Herbs. Take one to three enteric-coated **peppermint oil** capsules between meals. According to a double-blind crossover study, enteric-coated peppermint oil can significantly reduce abdominal symptoms of IBS.

Antispasmodic herbs can help relax the intestinal mucosal lining while promoting the relief of gas. All of them can be taken alone or in combination, and as a tea. They include chamomile, valerian, rosemary, peppermint, fennel, and lobelia.

Taken fresh or as a powder, **ginger** can be added to food or taken as a tea. It is effective in relieving gas and bloating and promoting digestion.

Mental and Emotional Health Recommendations

Psychotherapy. Counseling is sometimes effective in treating IBS. When you are able to relax, your digestion can dramatically improve. When the physical factors contributing to IBS are treated first, many people seem to experience less anxiety and have an increased capacity for self-expression and improved sleep. The psychotherapy most effective for IBS is **body-centered therapy,** such as integrated-body psychotherapy (IBP), Hakomi, or a breath therapy. These allow you to more easily identify and express painful emotions while simultaneously feeling in control.

Affirmations and visualization. Louise Hay's affirmation for indigestion is "I digest and assimilate all new experiences peacefully and joyfully." For diarrhea, "My intake, assimilation, and elimination are in perfect order. I am at peace with life."

You can be very direct with your affirmations relating to IBS. For example: "My bowel is relaxing and is at peace." "My intestinal mucosa is healing and getting stronger every day." "I am eating only foods that nurture and heal the lining of my bowel." While affirming these healing beliefs, visualize an image that represents to you a healthy intestinal lining.

Dr. Todd Nelson's recommended affirmation for IBS is "I now allow the beautiful and perfect unfolding of all the knowns and unknowns of this situation. I trust myself to offer what I can to this situation, and as I relax and breathe, I will be shown the right path. I have no attachment to the outcome."

Biofeedback. This method of learning to control muscle relaxation, in this case the involuntary muscles lining the intestine, was discussed in chapter 12, page 270. It can be helpful in treating IBS.

Bioenergy. The **third, or solar plexus, chakra** is most closely associated with dysfunction of the small intestine. There is some overlap with the second, lower belly or sex, chakra. Any energy medicine therapy, such as **healing touch** or *reiki,* directed toward these chakras can be healing to the bowel. The regular practice of **yoga, *qi gong,*** or **tai chi,** are also extremely beneficial.

Stephen Chang, M.D., an expert in Chinese medicine, describes the following exercise for treating IBS: Begin by lying flat on your back and relaxing. Put the palm of your right hand (if you're right-handed) on your navel and then simply rub gently. Then start to rub clockwise from the center, that is from right to left, first in small circles and then gradually expanding until the upper and lower limits of the stomach and abdomen are being rubbed. When you have completed this first movement, reverse it, rubbing counterclockwise in smaller and smaller circles until you are back at the center of the navel. You need not press down with any force. Rub slowly with gentle pressure. Repeat this clockwise and counterclockwise motion as long as it feels comfortable. While doing this, visualize heat, light, or energy warming and illuminating your entire abdomen. Try to see the blockages and constrictions in your intestines as they release and pass out through your body. Try to picture the damaged cells of the intestinal lining melting away.

This exercise can be performed for as little as two minutes and still have some beneficial effects. The clockwise direction in gradually widening circles can usually help relieve problems with constipation, and the counterclockwise motion can aid in the relief of diarrhea.

Spiritual and Social Health Recommendations

Since IBS sufferers tend to be hyper-responsible and fear the loss of control, they need to learn to **let go**—to trust and surrender in faith to the realization that everything will work out with or without them, just as it was meant to. Any and all of the spiritual practices presented in chapter 5 can help diminish fear and allow for letting go.

The social health recommendations in chapter 6 can help an IBS individual release control in relationships and risk revealing more of himself—to experience greater intimacy.

CONSTIPATION

Symptoms and Diagnosis

The main function of the colon (large bowel) is the reabsorption of nutrients and water and the elimination of toxic waste. The colon requires large amounts of water, high-fiber foods, beneficial bacteria, proper food combinations, and low-stress eating (slow and relaxed) to function properly. Normal colon function results in one to two bowel movements (BM) a day with a light brown, uniform stool that is easily passed. Ideally you should feel only the urge to have a bowel movement and no other physical sensations related to digestion.

Optimal health requires a highly functional digestive tract. Chronic constipation can contribute to and/or aggravate any chronic illness through the accumulation of toxins in the colon, which then find their way through the bloodstream to the rest of the body. This general toxic burden then contributes to lowered immunity, increased inflammation, potential tissue destruction, and fatigue. **Thriving can only occur when the body is fully absorbing nutrients and eliminating as much waste as it is accumulating and manufacturing.** Whatever chronic ailment you're treating, to heal it you must overcome constipation.

Transit time is the length of time it takes for food to travel from the mouth through the digestive tract and out through the stool. This usually takes twelve to eighteen hours. Recently the National Institutes of Health (NIH) suggested the normal frequency of BMs is three to twenty-one per week. While this number may reflect the average American, to have three BMs a week is not "normal." A truly normal, optimally functioning GI tract allows you to have one to three easy, soft, well-formed stools per day. If you're having only three BMs per week, then the transit time is fifty-six hours. This slow transit time can significantly increase colon disease as well as contribute to greater toxicity throughout the body as a result of chronic malabsorption. The NIH may call three BMs per week normal, but if you're training to thrive, I'd call it constipation.

The **primary symptoms** of constipation are
- straining to have a bowel movement (BM)
- infrequent BMs (less than one per day)
- hard and incomplete BMs, usually with associated discomfort or continued sense of fullness
- abdominal distension and bloating
- fatigue
- headaches, achiness
- mental fog
- hemorrhoids or anal fissures

Conventional Medical Treatment

Conventional medicine treats constipation almost entirely with **laxatives,** of which there are three types: bulking agents, stimulant laxatives, and stool softeners.

Bulking agents are fibers and are the usual first line of treatment since increased fiber naturally enhances proper colon function. A number of natural plant fibers are used as bulking agents. Increasing fiber without any other intervention can usually cure **mild** constipation. Psyllium-containing bulking agents are the most popular and often the most effective laxatives.

Stimulant laxatives increase peristalsis, the muscular action of the colon. Most of these products are derived from the herbs senna or cascara. Stimulant laxatives are effective at promoting BMs, but they should only be used for short periods—one to two weeks. Long-term use can cause the colon to atrophy and create dependency and other types of colon dysfunction. Other potential side effects include severe cramping, dehydration and electrolyte imbalance, irritation, and inflammation.

Stool softeners moisten the stools and help to combat the hard, dry stools associated with constipation. Docusate calcium and docusate potassium are the most popular stool softeners. Docusate softens by mixing water and fatty materials in the stool. Stool softeners are usually combined with stimulant laxatives. Both should be used only for short periods while the underlying causes are identified and corrected.

Risk Factors and Causes

Constipation is primarily related to lifestyle choices and is, therefore, very correctable even in the most severe cases.

Physical Factors

Diet. **Foods low in fiber,** high in saturated fats, prepackaged and overly cooked, can decrease normal colon function and stool mobility. Meat, cheese, fried foods, sugar, and white-flour-based foods can all contribute to constipation.

Inadequate water intake can lead to dehydration and cause constipation.

Excess coffee, alcohol, and soda pop can dehydrate the stool and irritate the colon lining. Many people use coffee in the morning to stimulate a BM, but eventually the colon becomes dependent and an addiction is created.

Physical inactivity slows transit time of stools through the large intestine.

The majority of **prescription drugs, antacids, and even the chronic use of laxatives** can all contribute to constipation.

Mental and Emotional Factors

Mental and emotional issues contributing to constipation are those associated with the **third** or **solar plexus chakra.** (See "Risk Factors and Causes" of IBS.) Louise Hay attributes constipation to refusing to release old ideas, remaining stuck in the past, and being stingy.

Other commonly seen emotional factors are **depression,** withholding feelings, an excessive need for control, sensitivity to criticism, unrealized creative potential, and obsessive/compulsive tendencies. Many people suffering from constipation need to overcome the fear of making mistakes and the need for perfection. Some psychotherapists speculate that early toilet training may be an emotional contributor to constipation.

Holistic Medical Treatment and Prevention

Physical Health Recommendations

Diet
- Increase **fiber**—eat more fruits and vegetables at every lunch and dinner; at least double your current intake. Beans, legumes, and ground flax seeds are especially high in fiber.
- Increase **whole grains,** instead of eating flour-based products such as bread and pastry.
- Increase **water** intake to at least the minimum daily requirement ($\frac{1}{2}$ oz/lb of body weight), and drink most of it between meals to avoid diluting digestive enzymes.
- Reduce or eliminate sugar, milk, coffee, alcohol, meat, and processed food.

Healthy habits to reestablish bowel regularity
- Identify and eliminate the causes of your constipation.
- Always answer nature's call and don't repress your natural urge to have a BM.
- Follow the dietary recommendations.
- Sit on the toilet at the same time every day,

preferably in the morning, even if you don't feel like going.

- Do regular aerobic exercise for thirty minutes three to five times per week.
- Stop using laxatives as soon as possible.
- To reestablish regularity you might need to take an herbal laxative containing either cascara or senna at night before bed for two weeks. This may need to be done under a physician's supervision. If loose stools or diarrhea occur, then the dose of the laxative needs to be reduced until a normally formed stool is established.

Vitamins, minerals, and nutritional supplements. In addition to dietary fiber, you may need **fiber supplements.** Most come in powder form, some in tablets or capsules. Fiber in a powder added to water or diluted juice is most effective. It is best to use a fiber supplement that has a balance of soluble and insoluble fibers, such as Metamucil, Ultra fiber, or Jarrow Gentle Fiber. Add supplementary fiber slowly—one to two grams daily until you reach five grams per day. Listen to your body and watch your elimination to adjust your fiber dosage. In addition to restoring regular bowel movements, supplementary fiber can

- hydrate and keep the stool formed
- feed the beneficial bacteria and promote eubiosis—a positive bacterial balance in the gut that strengthens immunity
- help prevent toxins from being absorbed into the body
- reduce fat uptake, thus reducing cholesterol

- reduce the risk of heart disease and hypertension
- reduce the risk of colon and rectal cancer

In reestablishing normal bowel function, it is essential to create the proper bacterial balance using substances called **probiotics.** In all cases of constipation there is an underlying bowel bacteria imbalance—**dysbiosis**—which occurs when there is more of the bad bacteria than good. The beneficial bacteria are acidophilus and bifidobacteria. It is best to take a high-potency probiotic formula containing acidophilus and bifidus in a powder form. The dosage is one-half to one teaspoon in water A.M. and P.M. Bifidobacteria can promote peristalsis.

Magnesium is essential to peristaltic function. It is estimated that 40 percent of Americans do not get the required daily allowance (RDA) of magnesium. The recommended dosage is 400–500 mg/day in a citrate or aspartate form. If too much is taken, it can cause diarrhea.

Vitamin C can usually soften the stool at higher dosages such as 5,000–10,000 mg/day. Take it as ascorbic acid with bioflavanoids in gradually increasing doses until constipation subsides.

Chinese herbs can act as excellent stool softeners, but you would have to consult with a skilled practitioner to use them.

Mental and Emotional Health Recommendations

Psychotherapy and **biofeedback** are both effective in treating constipation. Because depression is a significant cause of constipation, please refer to the "Mental and Emotional Health Recommendations" for treating depression in chapter 12.

Use eating as an excuse to relax. Slowing down and relaxing promotes digestive secretions and peristalsis. With each meal, stop to take a moment to feel gratitude, breathe freely and deeply, chew your food thoroughly, and visualize excellent digestion and elimination.

PEPTIC ULCER (GASTRIC OR DUODENAL ULCER)

Symptoms and Diagnosis

A peptic ulcer is a sharply defined crater in the mucosa lining the stomach or duodenum (first or upper part of the small intestine). The stomach contains hydrochloric acid and the digestive enzyme pepsin to digest the protein in our food and to help convert the minerals in food into a more digestible form. Normally the stomach and duodenum produce a protective mucous shield against the potentially damaging effects of stomach acid and pepsin. They also secrete substances such as bicarbonates that neutralize the acid when it comes in contact with the stomach and intestinal linings. When this protection breaks down, an ulcer can occur.

Men tend to suffer peptic ulcers more than women. These usually have a chronic or recurrent medical history. Symptoms vary according to the age and location of the ulcer. Pain is frequently described as **burning,** gnawing, or aching. Symptoms can radiate into the back or behind the sternum (breastbone) and are often described as "heartburn." There can be nausea, vomiting, an "empty" feeling in the gut, or pronounced hunger an hour or two after eating. Pain can range from mild to severe and is usually in the upper abdominal area of the solar plexus. Pain occurring with an empty stomach—during the night or between meals—could be the result of a gastric or stomach ulcer; pain shortly after a meal (forty-five to sixty minutes) can be a duodenal ulcer. Most of these same symptoms can occur with **hyperacidity,** a condition that simulates an ulcer but without the actual formation of a crater in the mucosa. This could be considered a "pre-ulcerous" condition—a warning that it's time to respond, before an ulcer becomes inevitable.

Symptoms requiring emergency attention include
- black, tarry stools
- vomiting blood or gastric contents resembling coffee grounds
- searing abdominal pain

The definitive diagnosis of peptic ulcer is usually made through an X-ray study called up **upper GI** or through a gastroscopic examination. The gastroscope is a long tubelike telescope that is passed down the throat through the esophagus for direct viewing of the lining of the stomach and duodenum. If you have been diagnosed with a peptic ulcer, you should be under the care of a physician.

Conventional Medical Treatment

The focus of conventional medical treatment is on reducing gastric acidity with **antacids** and **drugs that block stomach acid secretion.** Current treatment also usually includes an **antibiotic** to eliminate the unfriendly bacteria **helicobacter pylori (HP).** The following treatment is also used to mitigate hyperacidity, but the prescription drugs do not have to be taken for as long as they do when treating a diagnosed ulcer.

Antacids. Although antacids are commonly used to treat peptic ulcer, they also present some risk. The most commonly used antacids are aluminum/magnesium compounds such as **Maalox, Mylanta,** and Digel. They may cause calcium and phosphorus depletion, aluminum toxicity, or the accumulation of aluminum in the brain. The sodium bicarbonate antacids—**Rolaids,** Alka-Seltzer, Bromo-Seltzer—can have an adverse effect upon heart and kidney function. The calcium carbonate antacids such as **Tums** can produce a rebound effect on gastric acid secretion, actually increasing acid after the beneficial effect wears off. They may also cause kidney stones.

Drugs blocking acid secretion or H2-receptor antagonists. Since histamine stimulates acid secretion in the stomach, these "anti-ulcer" drugs are technically antihistamines. However, they differ from the an-

tihistamines used to treat allergies (H1-receptor antagonists) because they act on a different histamine receptor. The most common examples of the anti-ulcer drugs are **Zantac, Tagamet,** Pepcid, and Axid. One could argue that peptic ulcer or hyperacidity has reached epidemic proportions in this country, given that Zantac has become the biggest-selling drug in pharmaceutical history. These anti-ulcer drugs are also highly expensive. Before **Pepcid-AC** became available over the counter (OTC) in 1995, it would often cost over $100 per month for a prescription. I expect that the OTC versions of this class of drug will soon be setting their own sales records. With a diagnosed ulcer, these drugs are usually prescribed for six weeks.

Like every other pharmaceutical drug, these H2 antihistamines also have significant side effects. In blocking the secretion of acid, a critical aspect of the digestive process, they can cause nausea, constipation, and diarrhea. Nutrient deficiencies may result because of impaired digestion. Other possible side effects include liver damage, allergic reactions, headaches, breast enlargement in men, hair loss, depression, insomnia, and impotence.

Antibiotics and bismuth subsalicylate. Both are used to kill HP, although bismuth is a naturally occurring mineral that can also act as an antacid. The most commonly used bismuth subsalicylate is Pepto-Bismol, which is relatively safe when taken in prescribed dosages.

Risk Factors and Causes

Physical Factors

- **NSAIDs (nonsteroidal anti-inflammatory drugs), steroids, and alcohol** can cause a breakdown in the protection of the mucosal lining of the stomach and duodenum.

- Discovered in 1982 by Australian physician Barry Marshall, **Helicobacter pylori (HP)** is a bacteria found between the stomach lining and the mucous membrane. HP is present in 70 percent of gastric ulcers and 90 to 100 percent of duodenal ulcers. It has not yet been determined whether HP is a direct cause or merely a contributor to ulcer formation.

- Increased incidence, diminished response to ulcer therapy, and increased mortality due to peptic ulcer are all related to **smoking.** This may occur because smoking decreases pancreatic bicarbonates, increases reflux of bile salts into the stomach, and accelerates gastric emptying into the duodenum.

- **Food allergies**. Milk is highest on the list of potential food allergens. Studies have shown that populations of higher milk drinkers have a greater incidence of ulcers. Milk also significantly increases hydrochloric acid secretion.

- **Fiber** is necessary for the proper maintenance of healthy bacteria in the intestine. Too little fiber aggravates pathogenic bacterial overgrowth, irritating the gut lining, making it vulnerable to inflammation and infection. Fiber also helps promote mucin, a protective layer in the stomach and intestine, and it acts as a buffering agent. Eating a diet rich in plant fibers is beneficial both preventively as well as therapeutically.

Mental and Emotional Factors

Just as with IBS, the mental and emotional issues related to the **third chakra** are associated with peptic ulcer. In her book *You Can Heal Your Life*, Louise Hay describes the probable emotional cause of ulcers as: "Fear. A strong belief that you are not good enough. What is eating away at you?" And for stomach problems: "Dread. Fear of the new. Inability to assimilate the new."

The mental and emotional issues that contribute to peptic ulcers directly address the greatest sources of stress impacting men today. The energy of the solar plexus chakra relates to **fear, trust, care of oneself,** and **self-confidence.** As I've mentioned throughout Part I, men are doers and our greatest concern is our **performance.** The fire burning holes in the bellies of millions of men with hyperacidity and peptic ulcer dis-ease is fueled by the **fear of not being good enough, of making mistakes, and of not having enough time to perform well enough.** As a result of this self-imposed pressure, we have **neglected ourselves** to the point where our digestive juices are eating away at our tissues.

Holistic Medical Treatment and Prevention

Physical Health Recommendations

The objective of both treatment and prevention is to restore and **maintain the integrity of the gut lining** by reducing irritants, maximizing mucosal recoverability, and reducing bacterial invasion and infection. Just as with the mucous membrane lining the respiratory tract, infection can only occur when the membrane is weak.

Diet. Follow a low-allergy, low-saturated-fat, and low-to-medium-fiber diet (beans, raw fruits, and vegetables), with **deliberate chewing** and relaxing before and during eating. Fatty foods delay the emptying of the stomach, which also delays the healing of an ulcer. If you do eat red meat, it should be as rare as possible to enhance the function of its digestive enzymes. **Avoid nicotine, caffeine, alcohol, refined sugars, white flour,** and **processed food. Eliminate milk** and **eggs** for three to six weeks. Increase daily fiber gradually to two to five grams per day. Drink at least your daily minimum requirement of **water,** but avoid drinking a lot with meals.

Vitamins, minerals, and nutritional supplements. **Deglycyrrhizinated licorice (DGL):** This licorice extract is a highly effective anti-ulcer "drug." Some studies have shown it to be more effective than Tagamet and Zantac. Commonly used in the United Kingdom, it works by stimulating the normal defense mechanisms of the mucosal lining that prevent ulcer formation. Although ordinary licorice or licorice root (*Glycyrrhiza glabra*) might cause potassium loss or increase blood pressure, DGL is extremely safe. The recommended dosage is two to four 380-mg chewable tablets either between or twenty minutes before meals. Dosage should be continued for eight to sixteen weeks, depending on the response. DGL is available at most health food stores.

L-glutamine. The most abundant amino acid in the body, L-glutamine is the most popular treatment for peptic ulcers throughout Asia. Glutamine is used by the intestinal lining as a primary fuel source for the mucosa to restore and maintain itself. It can be taken at the onset of treatment in a dose of two to eight grams per day in divided doses three times a day for four weeks, then reduced to a maintenance dose of 500 to 1,500 mg before meals.

Zinc picolinate. Essential for intestinal-lining repair, the dosage is 30–60 mg/day. Along with the zinc it is helpful to take *copper sebacate,* 4 mg/day.

Vitamins A, E, and C. Vitamin A contributes to healing the mucosal lining and should be taken in a dosage of 25,000–50,000 IU/day. This dose should be reduced within three to six months. When taking this high a dose of vitamin A, it is important to also take vitamin E at 800 IU/day. At least 1 gram 3x/day of vitamin C is also recommended.

Essential fatty acids (EFAs). EFAs, especially in the form of evening primrose oil (EPO) and flaxseed oil, help manage inflammation, buffer excess acid, and maintain the health of the mucosal lining. One capsule of EPO 3x/day and 2–5 tsp of organic, cold-pressed, fresh flaxseed oil daily supply the proper balance of EFAs.

Juicing. Raw cabbage juice has been used since the 1950s for peptic ulcers following the research of Dr. Garnett Cheney at Stanford University School of Medicine. Green cabbage juice appears to be best and can be mixed with celery and carrot juice daily. The juice is best diluted by one-third with water. Cheney and his colleagues showed that in many cases ulcers could be healed in seven days with this regimen.

For acid reflux or heartburn symptoms. Take two to three slippery elm bark capsules before meals. Slippery elm is a demulcent herb that is soothing and absorbs excess acid. A liquid calcium/magnesium preparation can be useful in acute situations, especially for nighttime reflux. Calcium carbonate–based antacids should not be used long term as they mask ulcer symptoms and will eventually interfere with protein and mineral digestion and assimilation. Be sure the preparation does not contain aluminum.

Mental and Emotional Health Recommendations

To effectively treat peptic ulcer dis-ease, **learn to let go of "what's eating you . . . or gnawing at you!"** The source of this pain is most often the fear of not performing well enough within a limited time. You may choose to work with a therapist, but whatever emotional therapy you commit to, your primary goal is to learn to **honestly express the deeply held feelings of fear stored deep in your gut.** Assertive expression of these feelings will help to restore self-confidence and facilitate greater acceptance of your limitations and imperfections. Louise Hay's **affirmation** for ulcers is "I love and approve of myself. I am at peace. I am calm. All is well." Many **visualizations** can be used to heal the ulcer crater, reduce acidity, and strengthen the protective layer of tissue lining the stomach and intestine. You may want to review these techniques in chapter 2.

These healing images can be incorporated into a meditative practice that is quite healing for the suffering gut. There are a number of variations on this so-called **soft-belly meditation.** This practice is based on the fact that most men with GI disease, out of fear and lack of trust, harden their bellies to guard against any violations or breaking of our boundaries. This usually occurs throughout the day, and as you learn to be a more sensitive observer of yourself or a regular practitioner of the body scan, you'll begin to notice when it happens and the circumstances that precipitate it. The soft-belly meditation allows for the easing of the hard-belly shield protecting us from emotional injury. (It may be protective, but it is also confining and prevents our gut from digesting and assimilating the world we live in.)

One variation of the soft-belly meditation is taught by James Gordon, M.D., a holistic physician and psychiatrist on the faculty of Georgetown University School of Medicine. He suggests you begin by breathing in through your nose and saying the word *soft* to yourself as you relax and soften your belly to expand your inhalation. As you exhale through your nose, you silently say the word *belly*. This should be performed slowly and mindfully—with your full attention, for two to ten minutes. You may choose to do this meditation several times a day, whenever you became aware of the hard belly. This abdominal breathing exercise is similar to the Quiet Five, except that instead of silently counting numbers, you're saying the words *soft* and *belly* and the exhale is through the nose.

It is also helpful to ask yourself: "What is my suffering?" "What am I sick and tired of?" "What do I yearn for; or what does my heart really desire?" "What possible solutions do I see to alleviate my present circumstance?" "Can I take care of myself?" Many men with ulcers seem to forget they actually have a body requiring regular care. Your stomach's pain is a cry for help, alerting you to redirect your attention to nurturing yourself.

Refer to the "Mental and Emotional Health Recommendations" for IBS. They can also be used for treating peptic ulcer.

The primary contributors to this chapter are John Mizenko, D.O., a holistic gastroenterologist practicing in Warrensville Heights, Ohio, and Todd Nelson, N.D., a naturopathic physician providing wellness education and clinical natural-health services with a focus on gastrointestinal disorders in Denver and Boulder, Colorado.

The Specialty of Holistic Medicine

The American Holistic Medical Association (AHMA) was founded in 1978. Its active members are licensed M.D.'s and D.O.'s representing nearly every medical specialty. Associate members of the AHMA must be licensed or certified in the state in which they practice. Among these holistic practitioners are naturopathic physicians (N.D.'s), chiropractors (D.C.'s), doctors of Chinese medicine (O.M.D.'s), homeopathic physicians, nurses, dentists, podiatrists, psychologists, social workers and physical therapists, dietitians, pharmacists, optometrists, and physician assistants.

All members adhere to the following principles:

PRINCIPLES OF HOLISTIC MEDICAL PRACTICE

Adopted by the American Holistic Medical Association, March 9, 1993

1. Holistic physicians embrace a variety of safe, effective options in diagnosis and treatment, including:
   (a) education for lifestyle changes and self-care;
   (b) complementary approaches; and
   (c) conventional drugs and surgery.
2. Searching for the underlying causes of disease is preferable to treating symptoms alone.
3. Holistic physicians expend as much effort in establishing what kind of patient has a disease as they do in establishing what kind of disease a patient has.
4. It is preferable to diagnose and treat patients as unique individuals rather than as members of a disease category.
5. When possible, lifestyle modifications are preferable to drugs and surgery as initial therapeutic options.
6. Prevention is preferable to treatment and is usually more cost-effective. The most cost-effective approach evokes the patient's own innate healing capabilities.
7. Illness is viewed as a manifestation of a dysfunction of the whole person, not as an isolated event.
8. In most situations encouragement of patient autonomy is preferable to decisions imposed by physicians.
9. The ideal physician-patient relationship considers the needs, desires, awareness,

and insight of the patient as well as those of the physician.

10. The quality of the relationship established between physician and patient is a major determinant of healing outcomes.

11. Physicians significantly influence patients by their example.

12. Illness, pain, and the dying process can be learning opportunities for patients and physicians.

13. Holistic physicians encourage patients to evoke the healing power of love, hope, humor, and enthusiasm and to release the toxic consequences of hostility, shame, greed, depression, and prolonged fear, anger, and grief.

14. Unconditional love is life's most powerful medicine. Physicians strive to adopt an attitude of unconditional love for patients, themselves, and other practitioners.

15. Optimal health is much more than the absence of sickness. It is the conscious pursuit of the highest qualities of the spiritual, mental, emotional, physical, environmental, and social aspects of the human experience.

In 1996, the American Board of Holistic Medicine (ABHM) was created. This exciting development reflects the rapid evolution of conventional medicine. I believe it is the first step toward the approval of holistic medicine by the American Board of Medical Specialties, establishing it as medicine's newest specialty. The ABHM will certify physicians (M.D.'s and D.O.'s) in holistic medicine. Certification will be determined by the applicant's commitment to holistic health and a written examination. The body of knowledge to be tested encompasses the following topics:

CORE CURRICULUM

Body (Physical and Environmental Health)
1. Nutritional medicine
2. Physical activity/exercise
3. Environmental medicine

Mind (Mental and Emotional Health)
4. Behavioral medicine

Spirit (Spiritual and Social Health)
5. Spiritual attunement
6. Energy medicine
7. Social health

Specialized Areas
1. Botanical medicine
2. Ethnomedicine—traditional Chinese medicine, Ayurvedic medicine, Native American medicine
3. Manual medicine
4. Homeopathay
5. Biomolecular diagnosis and therapy

The core topics will require a much higher degree of proficiency than the specialized areas, which will be more superficially tested. You can see from the scope of the specialty of holistic medicine that *it encompasses alternative medicine*, since almost every one of the more common alternative therapies is included within one of the core or specialized topics of holistic medicine (see the following table). "Alternative medicine" is a popular but ambiguous term that has been loosely used to refer to anything that isn't taught in medical schools.* In keeping with the medical school orientation, alternative medicine, like conventional medicine, is primarily focused on treating disease. However, instead of drugs and surgery as the chief therapeutic options, herbs, acupuncture, or a number of other therapies provide additional choices as alternatives or as a complement to the conventional treatment. If you're not in need of medical treatment, many of the alternative "therapies" can still be used as part of an optimal health program. Nutritional medicine, biofeedback, and regular massages can easily enhance one's health whether or not one has a disease.

A physician practicing alternative medicine is not necessarily considered a holistic physician merely because he or she is treating patients with a therapy beyond the scope of conventional medicine. Unless the practitioner alone, or as part of a therapeutic team, is treating the whole person—body, mind, and spirit—he or she is not truly practicing holistic medicine. A strong emphasis on optimal health also distinguishes the holistic physician from his alternative and conventional brethren. The fact that every board-certified holistic physician will be a licensed

M.D. or D.O. will ensure that conventional medical therapies, such as drugs and surgery, are possible options. Holistic medicine could be best described as "complementary medicine." Many insurance companies and large employers are now interested in covering alternative medical services but are concerned about the lack of standards and the variable quality and competence of the practitioners. The creation of the specialty and board certification for holistic physicians will provide the standardization and the well-trained physicians that most of the public and insurers are seeking. It should also help to establish a leadership position for holistic medicine as it becomes a standard-bearer for twenty-first-century health care.

ALTERNATIVE/COMPLEMENTARY MEDICINE = HEALING ARTS AND DISCIPLINES NOT TRADITIONALLY TAUGHT IN ALLOPATHIC (M.D.) MEDICAL SCHOOLS

Osteopathic medicine
    Holistic philosophy
    Osteopathic manipulative therapy
    (OMT), including
    craniosacral therapy
Naturopathic medicine
Nutritional medicine
Environmental medicine
Movement therapies
    Aerobic exercise
    Strength conditioning
    Yoga
    Tai chi
    Feldenkrais

*Until the early to mid 1990s, none of the alternative therapies was being taught in allopathic medical schools. Today, approximately forty-five medical schools are teaching one or more of these healing arts.

Behavioral medicine
    Biofeedback
    Guided imagery/visualization
    Neurolinguistic programming
       (NLP)
    Breath therapy
    Journaling
Energy medicine
    Healing touch
    Therapeutic touch
    Reiki
    Jin shin jyutsu
    Light, color, and sound healing
       techniques
    Qi (chi) gong
    Magnetic therapy
    Kinesiology
    Aromatherapy
Spiritual counseling—focuses on the
       practice and awareness of
    Prayer
    Meditation
    Using intuition

    Spiritual laws
    Experiencing unconditional love
Relationship counseling
Botanical or herbal medicine
Homeopathic medicine
Biomolecular therapies
    Bio-oxidative therapies (ozone,
       hydrogen peroxide)
    Chelation therapy
    Hormonal therapies
    The unconventional use of
       conventional drugs
Ethnomedicine
    Traditional Chinese medicine
       including acupuncture,
       acupressure, and Chinese herbs
    Ayurveda
    Native American medicine
Manual medicine
    Massage therapy
    Rolfing
    Reflexology
    Chiropractic

Some of the Alternative/ Complementary Health Care Therapies Practiced by Holistic Physicians

Allopathic or Western medicine (practiced by M.D.'s) is the primary system practiced in this country. The cause of disease is believed to be physical and ultimately visible; treatment is generally restricted to surgery and pharmaceutical medications. The technology developed within allopathic medicine makes it well-suited for trauma and acute, life-threatening problems.

Ayurveda, a branch of traditional Indian medicine, is one of the most ancient and complete of all systems. Only the yogic exercises and meditation practices are well known in the United States. Disease is seen as an imbalance in the life force (prana) or may be karmically preordained. Health is an enlightened integration of the elements of the body and mind.

Behavioral medicine is an emerging therapeutic system based on the idea that behavior, including attitude and feelings, is a fundamental source of health and disease. Much of the research on behavioral medicine comes from the science of psychoneuro-immunology. Emotional stress is considered

Courtesy of the American Holistic Medicine Association.

to be a major cause of disease and behavioral therapists employ a variety of stress-reduction techniques to treat people with intractable pain, heart disease, cancer, stroke, and other chronic or "terminal" conditions.

Chinese medicine (practiced by O.M.D.'s) is believed to be one of the oldest medical systems in existence, dating back almost 5,000 years. Disease is viewed as an imbalance between the body's nutritive substances, called yin, and the functional activity of the body, called yang. This imbalance causes a disruption of the flow of vital energy (chi) that circulates through pathways in the body known as meridians. The practice of acupuncture rebalances the body's energy through stimulation of specific points along the meridians. Chinese medicine also includes Chinese herbology, moxabustion, massage, diet, exercise, and meditation.

Chiropractic (practiced by D.C.'s) aims to normalize the nervous system through manipulation of the bones and joints. The theory of chiropractic holds that spinal misalignment is the cause of a multitude of diseases, including arthritis, hormonal imbalances, and gastrointestinal disorders.

Energy medicine utilizes both subtle

bioenergy and conventional microcurrent and magnetic energies. Examples include hands-on healing techniques such as Reiki, therapeutic touch, and jin shin jyutsu; remote techniques such as distance healing, prayer and meditation; light, color, and sound techniques; movement therapies such as qi (chi) gong and tai chi; magnetic therapy; and microcurrent therapies (Voll, Acusope, cranial electrical stimulation devices).

Environmental medicine deals with environmental hazards including chemicals, ionizing radiation, air pollution, sensitizing substances, social and work settings, and communicable disease. It addresses the preservation and enhancement of the quality of the human environment and the prevention of harmful effects of environmental toxins. It includes occupational, climatological, and social environmental concerns. In addition to addressing individual aspects of these experiences, the group, community, and societal aspects fall within the purview of this specialty. The vehicle for improvement of health is the improvement of the environment in which individuals and society exist.

Homeopathy, a major force in American medicine until the turn of the century, is based on the doctrine that "like cures like." Homeopaths identify substances that cause symptoms of a particular disease when taken in large doses by healthy people. The patient with that disease is then administered an extremely dilute solution of that substance to assist the natural healing capacity. The cardinal doctrine of homeopathy is that there is vital force in the body that strives for health.

Disease or disruption of this force cannot be classified but is unique to each person.

Native American medicine differs according to tribal custom with some elements in common. Disease is caused by some disharmony in the cosmic order, as well as by hexing, breaking a taboo, fright, or soul loss. Healing materials and techniques include chants, songs, drumming, sweat lodges, crystals, herbalism, and rituals.

Naturopathic medicine (practiced by N.D.'s) as a distinct American health care profession is almost 100 years old. The basic principles of naturopathy are based on the concept that the body is a self-healing organism. Naturopathic physicians enhance the body's own natural healing responses through noninvasive measures and health promotion. They treat both acute and chronic diseases using nutrition, herbal or botanical medicine, homeopathy, traditional Chinese medicine, physical medicine, exercise therapy, counseling, and hydrotherapy. Naturopathy is making its greatest contributions to the healing arts in the fields of immunology, clinical nutrition, and botanical medicine.

Nutritional medicine addresses the preventive and therapeutic application of dietary intervention and nutritional supplementation (both in physiological and pharmacological doses). Basic aspects of nutritional medicine include uses of whole, unprocessed foods, identification of food allergies, and appropriate supplementation with vitamins, minerals, amino acids, fatty acids, accessory food factors, metabolic intermediates, and identical-to-natural hormones.

Osteopathic medicine (practiced by D.O.'s) was founded by an M.D., Andrew Taylor Still, in 1874. He believed that physicians should study prevention as well as cure, and treat "patients," not "symptoms." The predecessor of holistic medicine, osteopathic medicine is based on a body, mind, spirit approach to evaluating and treating patients. The hands-on approach to diagnosis and treatment, called Osteopathic Manipulative Treatment (OMT), is based on the interrelationship of structure and function. In addition to its holistic philosophy, use of OMT is the other major characteristic distinguishing it from conventional medicine. In most other aspects of osteopathic training and practice it differs very little from conventional medicine.

Bibliography

Allard, Norman, and Glenn Barnett. "The Power of Breath: Part I." *Massage and Bodywork Quarterly,* Spring 1993.

Anand, Margo. *The Art of Sexual Ecstasy.* Los Angeles: J. P. Tarcher, 1989.

Anderson, Robert A. *Wellness Medicine.* New Canaan, Conn.: Keats, 1990.

Bandler, Richard. *Using Your Brain for a Change.* Moab, Utah: Real People Press, 1985.

Bauer, Cathryn. *Acupressure for Everybody.* New York: Henry Holt, 1991.

Benedict, Martha S. "Holistic Approaches to Colds and Flu." *Body Mind Spirit,* February/March 1995.

Borysenko, Joan. *Minding the Body, Mending the Mind.* New York: Bantam Books, 1987.

Burns, David D. *The Feeling Good Handbook: Using the New Mood Therapy in Everyday Life.* New York: Penguin Books, 1989.

Byrd, Randolph C. "Positive Therapeutic Effects of Intercessory Prayer in a Coronary Care Unit Population." *Southern Medical Journal,* July 1988.

Carey, Benedict. "A Jog in the Smog." *Hippocrates,* May/June 1989.

Carpenter, Betsy. "Is Your Water Safe?" *U.S. News & World Report,* July 29, 1991.

Challem, Jack. "Defend Yourself Against Supergerms." *Natural Health,* March/April 1995.

Chopra, Deepak. *Ageless Body, Timeless Mind.* New York: Harmony Books, 1993.

———. *Quantum Healing.* New York: Bantam Books, 1989.

———. *The Seven Spiritual Laws.* San Rafael, Calif.: New World Library, 1994.

Cooper, Robert K. *Health and Fitness Excellence.* New York: Houghton Mifflin, 1989.

Cousens, Garbriel. *Conscious Eating.* Santa Rosa, Calif.: Vision Books International, 1992.

Crerand, Joanne. "Home Remedy: Insomnia." *Natural Health,* March/April 1992.

Dockery, Douglas W., C. Arden Pope III, Xiphing Xu, John D. Spengler, James H. Ware, Martha E. Fay, Benjamin G. Ferris, Jr., and Frank E. Speizer. "An Association Between Air Pollution and Mortality in Six U.S. Cities." *The New England Journal of Medicine*, December 9, 1993.

Dossey, Larry. *Healing Words*. San Francisco: HarperSanFrancisco, 1993.

Douillard, John. *Body, Mind, and Sport*. New York: Harmony Books, 1994.

Dreher, Henry. "Why Did the People of Roseto Live So Long?" *Natural Health*, September/October 1993.

Epstein, Gerald. *Healing Visualizations— Creating Health Through Imagery*. New York: Bantam Books, 1989.

Gaby, Alan R. "Human Canaries and Silent Spring." *Holistic Medicine: Magazine of the American Holistic Medical Association*, Fall/Winter 1992.

Gantz, Nelson M., Donald Kaye, and C. Wayne Weart, "Antibiotics '95: Back to Basics." *Patient Care*, January 15, 1995.

Gawain, Shakti, *Creative Visualization*. San Rafael, Calif.: Whatever Publishing, Inc., 1978.

Goleman, Daniel. *Emotional Intelligence*. New York: Bantam Books, 1995.

Growald, Eileen Rockefeller, and Allan Luks. "The Healing Power of Doing Good." *American Health*, March 1988.

Gurian, Michael. *The Wonder of Boys*. New York: Tarcher-Putnam, 1996.

Guyton, Arthur C. *Textbook of Medical Physiology*, Philadelphia: W. B. Saunders Company, 1968.

Hassell, Randall. *The Karate Experience: A Way of Life*. Rutland, Vt.: Charles E. Tuttle Company, 1980.

———. *Zen, Pen and Sword*. St. Louis: Focus Publications, 1993.

Hay, Louise L. *You Can Heal Your Life*. Santa Monica, Calif.: Hay House, 1984.

Hendrix, Harville. *Getting the Love You Want: A Guide for Couples*. New York: Harper & Row, 1988.

Henning, Arthur. "Four Ways to Be a Better Father." *Men's Confidential*, June 1994.

Ivker, Robert S. *Sinus Survival: The Holistic Medical Treatment for Allergies, Asthma, Bronchitis, Colds, and Sinusitis*. New York: Tarcher-Putnam, 1995.

Jampolsky, Gerald. *Love Is Letting Go of Fear*. New York: Bantam Books, 1979.

Johnson, Don Hanlon. *Body: Recovering Our Sensual Wisdom*, Berkeley, Calif.: North Atlantic Books, 1983.

Johnson, Robert A. *HE: Understanding Masculine Psychology*. New York: Harper & Row, 1974.

Joy, Brugh. *Joy's Way*. New York: Tarcher-Putnam, 1979.

Kaptchuk, Ted. *The Web That Has No Weaver*. Chicago: Congdon & Weed, 1983.

Langs, Robert. "Understanding Your Dreams." *New Age Journal*, July/August 1988.

LaPerriere, Arthur, Gail Ironson, Michael H. Antoni, Neil Schneiderman, Nancy Klimas, and Mary Ann Fletcher. "Exercise and Psychoneuroimmunology." *American College of Sports Medicine,* 1994.

Laskow, Leonard. *Healing with Love.* San Francisco: HarperSanFrancisco, 1992.

Lau, D.C. Lao Tzu, *Tao Te Ching,* London: Penguin Books, 1963.

Lazear, Jonathan. *Meditations for Men Who Do Too Much.* New York: Simon & Schuster, 1992.

Levine, Stephen. *Healing into Life and Death.* New York: Anchor Press/Doubleday, 1987.

Lukeman, Alex. *What Your Dreams Can Teach You.* St. Paul, Minn.: Llewellyn Publications, 1990.

Maharishi Ayur-Veda Newsletter. "Sleep Like a Baby: The Ayurvedic Approach to Insomnia," September 1992.

Masters, William H., and Virginia E. Johnson. *Human Sexual Response.* Boston: Little, Brown, 1966.

McCarthy, Barry. *Male Sexual Awareness.* New York: Carroll and Graf, 1988.

Miller, Alice. *The Drama of the Gifted Child.* New York: Basic Books, 1981.

Millman, Dan. *Way of the Peaceful Warrior.* Tiburon, Calif.: H. J. Kramer, 1980.

Moody, R. *The Light Beyond.* New York: Bantam Books, 1988.

Murphy, Michael, and Rhea A. White. *The Psychic Side of Sports.* Reading, Mass.: Addison-Wesley, 1978.

Myss, Carolyn. *Anatomy of the Spirit.* Harmony Books: New York, 1996.

Ornstein, Robert, and David Sobel. *Healthy Pleasures.* New York: Addison-Wesley, 1989.

Parker, Sharon. "Drugs versus the Bug." *Utne Reader,* March/April 1995.

Patent, Arnold. *You Can Have It All.* Great Neck, N.Y.: Money Mastery, 1984.

Peck, M. Scott. *The Road Less Traveled.* New York, Simon & Schuster, 1978.

Perry, Leroy R. "What You Don't Know About Water Could Save Your Life." *Parade Magazine,* October 22, 1989.

Pipher, Mary. *The Shelter of Each Other.* New York: Grosset/Putnam, 1996.

Powell, Joanna. *Things I Should Have Said to My Father.* New York: Avon Books, 1994.

Rapp, Doris. *Allergies and Your Family.* Buffalo, N.Y.: Practical Allergy, 1990.

Reid Clyde. *Celebrate the Temporary.* New York: Harper & Row, 1972.

Reid, Daniel. *The Complete Book of Chinese Health and Healing.* Boston, Mass.: Shambhala Publications, Inc., 1994.

Rossman, Martin L. *Healing Yourself.* New York: Pocket Books, 1987.

Scarf, Maggie. *Intimate Partners.* New York: Random House, 1987.

Sears, Barry. *The Zone.* New York: HarperCollins, 1995.

Shih, Tsu Kuo. *The Chinese Art of Healing with Energy: Qi Gong Therapy.* Barrytown, N.Y.: Station Hill Press, 1994.

Siegel, Bernie S. *Love, Medicine, and Miracles.* New York: Harper & Row, 1986.

Spangler, Tina. "The Solution for Indoor Pollution." *Natural Health,* January/February 1996.

Vital and Health Statistics, from the Centers for Disease Control and Prevention/National Center for Health Statistics. "Current Estimates from the National Health Interview Survey," U.S. Department of Health and Human Services, 1992.

Warga, Claire. "You Are What You Think." *Psychology Today,* September 1988.

Weil, Andrew. *Natural Health, Natural Medicine.* Boston: Houghton-Mifflin, 1990.

Wilbur, Ken. *A Brief History of Everything.* Boston and London: Shambhala, 1996.

Zilbergeld, Bernie. *Male Sexuality.* New York: Bantam Books, 1978.

PERMISSIONS

Index

If you are interested in sharing or in receiving additional information on men's health, or in *Thriving: A Men's Health Newsletter,* please send your name and address to:

Thriving
P.O. Box 620236
Littleton, CO 80162-0236